国际经典内科学教科书

第10版

Cecil Essentials of Medicine

希氏内科学精要

中英双语版

原　著　**Edward J. Wing, MD, FACP, FIDSA**
Former Dean of Medicine and Biological Sciences
Professor of Medicine
Warren Alpert Medical School of Brown University, Providence, Rhode Island

Fred J. Schiffman, MD, MACP
Sigal Family Professor of Humanistic Medicine
Vice Chair, Department of Medicine
Warren Alpert Medical School of Brown University, Providence, Rhode Island

中英双语版　编辑委员会　主任委员　王　辰

第 6 分册

肿瘤疾病

主　译　王　洁　巴　一

北京大学医学出版社

XISHI NEIKEXUE JINGYAO（DI 10 BAN） DI 6 FENCE ZHONGLIU JIBING（ZHONGYING SHUANGYU BAN）

图书在版编目（CIP）数据

希氏内科学精要：第10版.第6分册，肿瘤疾病：汉、英／（美）爱德华·温（Edward J. Wing），（美）弗雷德·谢夫曼（Fred J. Schiffman）原著；王洁，巴一主译. -- 北京：北京大学医学出版社，2024. 11. -- ISBN 978-7-5659-3247-2

Ⅰ. R5

中国国家版本馆CIP数据核字第2024TW6304号

北京市版权局著作权合同登记号：图字：01-2024-4518

Elsevier (Singapore) Pte Ltd.
3 Killiney Road, #08-01 Winsland House I, Singapore 239519
Tel: (65) 6349-0200; Fax: (65) 6733-1817

Cecil Essentials of Medicine, Tenth Edition
Copyright © 2022 by Elsevier, Inc. All rights are reserved, including those for text and data mining, AI training, and similar technologies.
Publisher's note: Elsevier takes a neutral position with respect to territorial disputes or jurisdictional claims in its published content, including in maps and institutional affiliations.
Previous editions copyrighted 2016, 2010, 2007, 2004, 2001, 1997, 1993, 1990, and 1986.
ISBN-13: 978-0-323-72271-1

This translation of Cecil Essentials of Medicine, Tenth Edition by Edward J. Wing and Fred J. Schiffman was undertaken by Peking University Medical Press and is published by arrangement with Elsevier (Singapore) Pte Ltd.
Cecil Essentials of Medicine, Tenth Edition by Edward J. Wing and Fred J. Schiffman 由北京大学医学出版社进行翻译，并根据北京大学医学出版社与爱思唯尔（新加坡）私人有限公司的协议约定出版。
《希氏内科学精要（第10版）第6分册 肿瘤疾病（中英双语版）》（王洁 巴一 主译）
ISBN: 978-7-5659-3247-2
Copyright © 2024 by Elsevier (Singapore) Pte Ltd. and Peking University Medical Press.
All rights reserved. No part of this publication may be reproduced or transmitted in any form or by any means, electronic or mechanical, including photocopying, recording, or any information storage and retrieval system, without permission in writing from Elsevier (Singapore) Pte Ltd. and Peking University Medical Press.

注 意

本译本由北京大学医学出版社独立完成。相关从业及研究人员必须凭借其自身经验和知识对文中描述的信息数据、方法策略、搭配组合、实验操作进行评估和使用。由于医学科学发展迅速，临床诊断和给药剂量尤其需要经过独立验证。在法律允许的最大范围内，爱思唯尔、译文的原文作者、原文编辑及原文内容提供者均不对译文或因产品责任、疏忽或其他操作造成的人身及（或）财产伤害及（或）损失承担责任，亦不对由于使用文中提到的方法、产品、说明或思想而导致的人身及（或）财产伤害及（或）损失承担责任。

Published in China by Peking University Medical Press under special arrangement with Elsevier (Singapore) Pte Ltd. This edition is authorized for sale in the People's Republic of China only, excluding Hong Kong SAR, Macau SAR and Taiwan. Unauthorized export of this edition is a violation of the contract.

希氏内科学精要（第10版） 第6分册 肿瘤疾病（中英双语版）

主　　译：王　洁　巴　一
出版发行：北京大学医学出版社
地　　址：（100191）北京市海淀区学院路38号　北京大学医学部院内
电　　话：发行部 010-82802230；图书邮购 010-82802495
网　　址：http://www.pumpress.com.cn
E-mail：booksale@bjmu.edu.cn
印　　刷：北京信彩瑞禾印刷厂
经　　销：新华书店
策划编辑：高　瑾
责任编辑：高　瑾　　责任校对：靳新强　　责任印制：李　啸
开　　本：889 mm×1194 mm　1/16　印张：10.25　字数：376千字
版　　次：2024年11月第1版　2024年11月第1次印刷
书　　号：ISBN 978-7-5659-3247-2
定　　价：80.00元
版权所有，违者必究

（凡属质量问题请与本社发行部联系退换）

中英双语版　编辑委员会

主任委员

王　辰

委　　员（按姓氏笔画排序）

王　洁	王伊龙	王建祥	巴　一	代华平	宁　光	宁晓红	朱　兰
任景怡	刘海鹰	李小鹰	李梦涛	李雪梅	杨爱明	张福杰	郑金刚
房静远	赵　晶	赵明辉	郝　伟	姜　辉	栗占国	贾继东	夏维波
黄　慧	黄晓军	曹　彬	彭　斌	潘　慧			

第 1 分册　　内科学概论·呼吸与危重症医学·术前和术后照护
　　　　　　主译　王　辰　代华平　赵　晶　黄　慧

第 2 分册　　心血管疾病
　　　　　　主译　郑金刚　任景怡

第 3 分册　　肾脏疾病
　　　　　　主译　李雪梅　赵明辉

第 4 分册　　胃肠疾病·肝脏与胆道系统疾病
　　　　　　主译　房静远　杨爱明　贾继东

第 5 分册　　血液疾病
　　　　　　主译　黄晓军　王建祥

第 6 分册　　肿瘤疾病
　　　　　　主译　王　洁　巴　一

第 7 分册　　内分泌疾病与代谢疾病·女性健康·男性健康·骨与骨矿物质代谢疾病
　　　　　　主译　宁　光　朱　兰　姜　辉　夏维波　潘　慧

第 8 分册　　肌肉骨骼与结缔组织疾病
　　　　　　主译　栗占国　李梦涛

第 9 分册　　感染性疾病
　　　　　　主译　刘海鹰　张福杰　曹　彬

第 10 分册　神经疾病·老年医学·缓和医疗·酒精和物质使用
　　　　　　主译　彭　斌　王伊龙　李小鹰　宁晓红　郝　伟

医学名词审定指导

任慧玲　李晓瑛　冀玉静　张燕舞　李军莲

中英双语版 序言

让我国医学生与国际医学生站在同一起跑线上的首要之事，是为其提供具有世界先进水平的标准教材。我们应争取使每一位医学生都能接触到内容经典、充分代表现代医学水平的国际权威原文教材并力求准确翻译，提供原文与中文双语对照版本，使医学生和医生在学习中形成双语医学词语、概念、概念间逻辑及由此构成的医学知识体系。在这样的思想驱动下，国际经典内科学教科书《希氏内科学精要（第10版）》中英双语版应运而生。

《希氏内科学》原著以其论述严谨准确、系统全面，被誉为"标准的内科学参考书"。自1927年首次出版以来，在内科学领域渐享世界级声誉，成为全球众多优秀医学院校，包括哈佛医学院、斯坦福大学医学院、约翰斯·霍普金斯大学医学院、牛津大学医学部、剑桥大学医学院、墨尔本大学医学院、新加坡国立大学医学院及多伦多大学医学院等普遍采用的内科学参考书。首版《希氏内科学精要》则诞生于1986年，旨在凝炼其全本的精华和要点，以最为简洁明确的方式向以医学生为主体的医学界精辟传达《希氏内科学》的核心信息，包括书中所体现出的人文精神。此后，每版精要本都力求凝炼地反映当时最新医学成果和医疗实践指南，愈来愈成为各国医学生、住院医师、专培医师及教师学习和传授内科学的主要教本，在世界医学教材体系中居引领地位。《希氏内科学》和《希氏内科学精要》两个版本不仅在英语国家被广泛使用，更被翻译为葡萄牙语、西班牙语、希腊语、意大利语、日语、简体中文版，为全球医学界广泛采用。

中国的医学生、住院医师、专培医师需要培养国际专业信息获取能力。将精要本原文引进并准确翻译，以中英文对照的形式呈现，便于读者进行双语对照阅读和学习，使之在学习理解国际标准医学内容的同时，学习好中英文医学词语，为国际医学交流打好基础。相信此举对于提高我国的医学教育水平，培养国际型医学人才至为有益。

《希氏内科学精要》精练地涵盖了内科学的所有主要领域，包括心血管疾病、呼吸疾病与危重症、消化疾病、肾脏疾病、内分泌和代谢疾病、风湿疾病、血液疾病、肿瘤、感染性疾病、神经与老年疾病等，构建了较为系统的知识体系。在翻译引进过程中，我们遵循将相关内容集中的原则，将原书按系统器官拆分为十个分册，使其更具有专科阅读的对应性，以更加灵活轻便的形式为读者提供多样化的阅读选择。

为确保译文质量，我们在译者遴选上采取了严谨的标准。从《希氏内科学（第26版）》翻译团队中择优选取责任心强、译文优质的译者，同时吸纳了临床医学专业"101"计划核心教材的编者团队。每个分册均由主译专家带领各自译者团队完成翻译、审校、交叉互审、通审四级审校工作。这些译者具备扎实的英语与专业能力，他们在翻译过程中，深入理解原文，准确阐述作者思想，并多角度审视译文的准确性、流畅性与风格一致性，确保译文的忠实性、规范性与可读性，在不同的语言和文化间架起坚实的桥梁。尤其值得称赞的是，对原著中疏漏或不够完善之处，译文中以"译者注"的形式加以适当解释和说明，使译文内容在忠实于原著的基础上更为准确。

本书读者定位于具有一定学习能力和基础的高等医学院校医学专业8年制、5年制学生以及相关医学专业人员，可作为医务人员的内科学参考书、住院医师规范化培训和专科医师规范化培训辅导教材、研究生入学考试辅导教材、内科学教师参考书、内科学各专科医师复习回顾其他专科知识的重要读本。

呼吸与危重症医学教授
中国医学科学院院长
北京协和医学院校长
2024年11月

对学习者教科书重要。

对学医者内科学重要。

世界上的内科学教科书，

首推《希氏内科学精要》。

中文是中国医生主要执业用语。

英文是国际医学交流的主要文字。

学习医学，当以双语对应阅读为好。

如此，可获纵横国际之效。

本书力求有助于此。

In Memoriam

Thomas E. Andreoli, MD

Dr. Thomas Andreoli, along with Drs. Lloyd Hollingsworth (Holly) Smith, Jr., Fred Plum, and Charles C.J. Carpenter, was one of the four founding editors of *Cecil Essentials of Medicine*. He served as editor for editions one through eight before he passed away on April 14, 2009. Dr. Andreoli was born in the Bronx, New York, in 1935, attended Catholic primary and high schools, and graduated from St. Vincent College and the Georgetown School of Medicine. He trained as a resident at Duke University under legendary Chair of Medicine Dr. Eugene Stead, who recognized him as a brilliant physician and scientist and encouraged his research career. Dr. Andreoli received his research training at the NIH and then in the laboratory of Dr. Tosteson at Duke. His research focused on the biochemical and biophysical properties of renal tubular cell membranes and their role in water and electrolyte transport. He made fundamental discoveries on the normal renal physiology, illuminating the way to subsequent work by many others on renal health and disease. His research was recognized with numerous awards and election to honorific societies both in the United States and in Europe. Dr. Andreoli also served as editor of *The American Journal of Physiology: Renal Physiology* and Editor in Chief of *Kidney International*.

Tom's national prominence and leadership qualities were recognized early in his career when he became head of Nephrology at the University of Alabama in Birmingham. There he helped faculty and trainees develop outstanding research, organized clinical services, and created a hemodialysis program to build one of the outstanding Divisions of Nephrology in the country. In 1979, Dr. Andreoli was appointed Chair of the Department of Internal Medicine at the University of Texas, Houston, where he assembled an outstanding faculty focused on research, clinical care, and teaching. In 1988, he accepted the position as Chairman of Internal Medicine at the University of Arkansas School of Medicine, a position he held until his death. There he again assembled a distinguished faculty who were outstanding researchers but also dedicated to outstanding clinical care and teaching. Morning report and clinical rounds with Dr. Andreoli were rigorous and riveting, focusing on the individual patient, not only their diagnoses and treatment but also on each patient's personal concerns and well-being. Dr. Andreoli was revered by medical students, his house staff, faculty, and colleagues, and I (EJW) personally can attest to what he regarded as his most cherished role—the mentorship and education of the next generation of physicians.

One of Dr. Andreoli's great interests was *Cecil Essentials of Medicine*, for which he was the editor/chief editor for eight of its ten editions, an interest that reflected his commitment to the education of students, house staff, and other physicians in the "essentials" of Internal Medicine.

Dr. Andreoli was devoted to his family. He was married to Elizabeth Berglund Andreoli from 1987 until his death. He was previously married to Dr. Kathleen Gainor Andreoli, mother of his three children and their ten grandchildren. Being of Italian ancestry and from Bronx, New York, it is not surprising that Dr. Andreoli was a passionate fan of the New York Yankees, Italian opera, which he could sing in Italian, and Frank Sinatra.

Dr. Andreoli's legacy lives on in his numerous previous students, house staff, colleagues, and in this book.

缅 怀

托马斯·安德里奥利博士

托马斯·安德里奥利（Thomas E. Andreoli）博士携手李奥德·霍灵斯沃斯·史密斯［Lloyd Hollingsworth（Holly）Smith］博士、弗雷德·普拉姆（Fred Plum）博士和查尔斯·卡彭特（Charles C.J. Carpenter）博士同为《希氏内科学精要》的创始编者。他在2009年4月14日去世前，曾担任该书第1至第8版的编者。安德里奥利博士于1935年出生于美国纽约布朗克斯区，就读于天主教小学和中学，后毕业于圣文森特学院和乔治城大学医学院。他在杜克大学医学院接受住院医师培训期间师从著名内科主任尤金·斯特德（Eugene Stead）博士，后者将其视为杰出的医生和科学家，并鼓励他投身科研事业。安德里奥利博士在美国国立卫生研究院接受科研训练后，前往杜克大学托斯特森（Tosteson）博士的实验室继续深造。他重点研究肾小管细胞膜的生化和生物物理特性及其在水和电解质转运中所发挥的作用。他在正常肾脏生理学方面的重要发现为后续关于肾脏健康和疾病的研究铺平了道路。安德里奥利博士的研究工作荣获多个学术奖项，并入选美国和欧洲的多个荣誉学会。他还担任《美国生理学杂志：肾脏生理学篇》（The American Journal of Physiology: Renal Physiology）的编辑以及《国际肾脏杂志》（Kidney International）的主编。

安德里奥利博士担任阿拉巴马大学伯明翰分校肾脏病学系主任后不久，即因其杰出领导力而赢得全美业内声誉。他帮助本校师生们取得科研突破，负责临床业务的组织实施，并因开创血液透析业务而使该科跻身全美顶级肾脏内科之列。1979年，安德里奥利博士被任命为得克萨斯大学休斯敦分校内科学系主任，他在该系组建了一支科研、临床诊疗和教学并重的优秀教职团队。自1988年起，他担任阿肯色大学医学院内科学系主任，直至辞世。在这里他再次组建了一支卓越的教职团队，他们不仅科研工作出色，临床诊疗和教学工作也出类拔萃。安德里奥利博士带领的晨会报告和查房非常严谨而引人入胜，不仅尽心竭力于每位患者的诊断和治疗，还关注到他们每个人的个体情况和福祉。安德里奥利博士深受医学生、住院医师、教职人员和同事的崇敬，我（EJW）可以证明，他最珍视的角色当属培养和教育下一代医生。

安德里奥利博士对《希氏内科学精要》倾注了满腔热忱，先后担任了该书10版中8版的编者/主编，践行他为医学生、住院医师和其他各科医生们传授内科学"精要"的承诺。

安德里奥利博士高度重视家庭。他与第二任妻子伊丽莎白·伯格兰德·安德里奥利（Elizabeth Berglund Andreoli）的婚姻从1987年延续到辞世。他与第一任妻子凯瑟琳·盖娜·安德里奥利（Kathleen Gainor Andreoli）博士育有三个子女和十个孙辈。作为意大利裔和纽约布朗克斯人，安德里奥利博士是纽约洋基队、意大利歌剧（他能用意大利语演唱）和美国著名歌手、演员、主持人弗兰克·辛纳屈（Frank Sinatra）的忠实拥趸。安德里奥利博士将永远被他的众多学生、住院医师和同事怀念，并因本书而流芳百世。

In Memoriam

Charles C.J. Carpenter, MD

Dr. Charles C.J. Carpenter joined Drs. Thomas Andreoli, Lloyd Hollingsworth Smith, Jr., and Fred Plum as a founder of *Cecil Essentials of Medicine.* He served as editor for seven editions and was followed in that role by Dr. Ivor Benjamin and then Dr. Edward Wing. Sadly, Chuck passed away on March 19, 2020, surrounded by his wife and children. He was Professor Emeritus of Medicine at The Warren Alpert Medical School of Brown University and Physician-in-Chief Emeritus at The Miriam Hospital.

Chuck was born in Savannah, Georgia, on January 5, 1931. He attended college at Princeton and medical school at Johns Hopkins where he also did his house staff training, including chief residency, and then joined the Johns Hopkins faculty. With his young family, he travelled to Calcutta, India, where he carried out landmark studies for the treatment of cholera.

Before coming to Brown in 1986, he was Chair of Medicine at Baltimore City Hospital and Case Western Reserve University.

His contributions to medical science and clinical care were many. While in Calcutta, using basic scientific evidence coupled with practical approaches, Dr. Carpenter developed "oral rehydration therapy" to address the cholera epidemic there. This treatment has saved millions of lives. While at Case, one of his innovations was to develop the nation's first Division of Geographic Medicine because of his strong belief that all physicians should be medical citizens of the world. In 1987, as he became deeply involved in the clinical management of persons living with HIV, he initiated a unique program in which Brown University faculty and trainees assumed responsibility for all HIV care in the Rhode Island State prison system.

Dr. Carpenter served as Chairman of the American Board of Internal Medicine and President of the Association of American Physicians. He has been a member of the NIH AIDS Executive Committee, the National Advisory Allergy and Infectious Diseases Council, and the USPHS AIDS Task Force. He was Chair of the Antiretroviral Treatment Panel of the International AIDS Society-USA and authored their recommendations on antiretroviral treatment. He also served as Chair of the Treatment Committee to evaluate the President's Emergency Plan for HIV/AIDS Relief. He became the director of the Brown University International Health Institute and the director of the Lifespan/Brown Center for AIDS Research with several Boston hospitals.

Throughout his career, Dr. Carpenter was the recipient of many international, national, and regional awards, accepting each with characteristic humility. With both small and large groups of learners, Chuck made certain that every member of his team was well educated, and each felt that they contributed to the well-being of their patients. His ability to sit calmly at the bedside, hold the patient's hand, comfort them, and listen in a genuinely focused way, influenced so many physicians. He was truly grateful for the opportunity to care for those less fortunate than he, and the feeling of being privileged to do so was clearly transmitted to all. Dr. Carpenter was a wonderful blend of profound compassion combined with the adherence to scholarship and teaching. Sir William Osler wrote that physicians should "Do the kind thing and do it first." Chuck lived by this precept. Vigor and insight characterized his approach to clinical and ethical challenges, always with younger colleagues at his side. In a recent tribute to him, many emphasized that Dr. Carpenter dedicated his life to his patients, many of whom were the most vulnerable members of society. We hope that we will have some of his strength and use his example as our compass as we are challenged to reduce suffering and improve the health of all for whom we are responsible.

He is survived by his wife of 61 years, Sally; three sons, Charles, Murray, and Andrew; and seven grandchildren.

缅 怀

查尔斯·卡彭特博士

查尔斯·卡彭特（Charles C.J. Carpenter）博士与 托马斯·安德里奥利（Thomas E. Andreoli）博士、李奥德·霍灵斯沃斯·史密斯（Lloyd Hollingsworth Smith）博士和弗雷德·普拉姆（Fred Plum）博士共同开创了《希氏内科学精要》。他共担任了 7 版的编者，嗣后由艾弗·本杰明（Ivor Benjamin）博士和爱德华·温（Edward Wing）博士接任。查尔斯·卡彭特博士于 2020 年 3 月 19 日在妻子和子女们的陪伴下辞世。他曾担任布朗大学沃伦·阿尔珀特医学院的内科学系名誉教授和米里亚姆医院的名誉主任医师。

查尔斯·卡彭特博士于 1931 年 1 月 5 日出生于美国佐治亚州萨凡纳市。他在普林斯顿大学获得学士学位后进入约翰斯·霍普金斯大学医学院，并完成了包括住院总医师在内的住院医师培训，随后加入了约翰斯·霍普金斯大学的教职团队。他曾携妻子和年幼的孩子前往印度加尔各答，在当地对霍乱的治疗进行了具有里程碑意义的研究工作。

在 1986 年入职布朗大学之前，他曾担任巴尔的摩市医院和凯斯西储大学医学院的内科学主任。

他在医学科学研究和临床诊疗领域建树颇多。在加尔各答期间，基于基础科学证据及临床实践，查尔斯·卡彭特博士开创了"口服补液疗法"以遏制当地的霍乱疫情。这一疗法拯救了数百万人的生命。秉承医生无国界的世界公民理念，他在凯斯西储大学做了一项开创性工作，建立了美国首个地缘医学部（研究地理环境因素对人体健康和疾病影响的学科）。1987 年，他深度参与人类免疫缺陷病毒（HIV）携带者的临床管理，并发起了一个独特的项目——由布朗大学教职团队和医学生们承担罗德岛州监狱系统内所有艾滋病相关诊疗工作。

查尔斯·卡彭特博士曾担任美国内科医师委员会主席和美国医师协会主席。他曾是美国国立卫生研究院艾滋病行政委员会、美国国家过敏与传染病咨询委员会以及公共卫生服务部艾滋病工作组的成员。他还曾担任国际艾滋病学会-美国分会抗逆转录病毒治疗组主席，并撰写了抗逆转录病毒治疗建议。他还担任过艾滋病治疗委员会主席，该委员会负责评估美国总统防治艾滋病紧急救援计划；曾担任布朗大学国际健康研究所所长，以及大学与多家波士顿当地医院合办的生命周期/布朗大学艾滋病研究中心主任。

查尔斯·卡彭特博士在职业生涯中获得过诸多国际性、全美和地区性奖项，同时展现其谦逊品格。无论学员人数多寡，查尔斯·卡彭特博士都会确保人人都能受到良好教育，并让他们感到自己也对患者的健康做出了贡献。他能够安静地坐在病床边，握住患者的手，安慰他们，并全神贯注地听取患者倾诉，这一举动深深地感染了许多医生。他十分珍视诊治不幸染病者的机会，并且能够将这种殊荣感传递给所有人。查尔斯·卡彭特博士完美地融汇了对患者的宅心仁厚与对学术和教学的坚守。威廉·奥斯勒（William Osler）爵士曾写道，医生应该"行善事，为人先"，而这正是查尔斯·卡彭特博士一生奉行的信条。他在面对临床和伦理挑战时充满活力和洞察力，始终重视提携年轻同事。许多人的悼词中都重点指出，查尔斯·卡彭特博士将毕生致力于患者福祉，其中许多人属于社会上最弱势群体。我们希望，在我们面临减少患者痛苦及改善其健康状况的挑战时，能够拥有他的力量，并以他为榜样获得指引。

查尔斯·卡彭特博士与妻子萨丽（Sally）共度了 61 年的婚姻时光，育有查尔斯（Charles）、穆雷（Murray）和安德鲁（Andrew）三子以及七个孙辈。

ABOUT THE EDITORS

Dr. Edward J. Wing was an editor of *Cecil Essentials of Medicine,* editions 8 and 9, and is the lead editor of edition 10. He graduated from Williams College in 1967 and from the Harvard Medical School in 1971. He was a resident in Internal Medicine at the Peter Bent Brigham and completed an Infectious Diseases Fellowship at Stanford University. Joining the faculty at the University of Pittsburgh in 1975, he focused his NIH-funded research on mechanisms of cell-mediated immunity as well as various clinical aspects of Infectious Diseases. From 1990 to 1998, the University and UPMC appointed him as Physician-in-Chief at Montefiore Hospital, then Chief of Infectious Diseases, and finally Interim Chair of Medicine.

In 1998, Dr. Wing became Chair of Medicine at Brown University (1998–2008) where he consolidated the department across hospitals, practice plans, and training programs. As Dean of Medicine and Biological Sciences at Brown University (2008–2013) he strengthened ties with affiliated hospitals (Lifespan and Care New England), increased research, and oversaw the construction of a new medical school building. International exchange programs with medical schools in Kenya, the Dominican Republic, and Haiti were established during his years as chairman and dean. Dr. Wing has cared for patients with HIV since the beginning of the epidemic in outpatient clinics. He continues to be active in research, clinical care, and teaching.

Dr. Fred J. Schiffman, who along with Dr. Edward Wing is editor of *Cecil Essentials of Medicine,* 10th edition, attended Wagner College and then the New York University School of Medicine, from which he graduated in 1973. He performed his early house staff training at Yale-New Haven Hospital and then spent two years at the National Cancer Institute. He returned to Yale as Chief Medical Resident followed by a hematology fellowship. He became Medical Director of Yale's Primary Care Center before coming to Brown University in 1983, where he has been a leader in the medical residency program as well as Associate Physician-in-Chief at The Miriam Hospital.

Dr. Schiffman holds The Sigal Family Professorship in Humanistic Medicine at The Warren Alpert Medical School of Brown University. His scholarly interests include the structure and function of the human spleen and the intersection of the arts and medical care. He has directed or championed many projects and programs, including those that encourage and reinforce wellness and resilience in patients, families, and caregivers. He began a novel program that places medical students and physicians with other nonmedical professionals as they share in the viewing of works of art in the Museum of the Rhode Island School of Design. Dr. Schiffman recently led a Brown University edX course entitled, "Artful Medicine: Art's Power to Enrich Patient Care," with worldwide participation. Dr. Schiffman has also edited texts on hematologic pathophysiology, consultative hematology, and the anemias.

原著主编

爱德华·温（Edward J. Wing）博士是《希氏内科学精要》第8版和第9版的编者，以及第10版的主编。他先后于1967年和1971年毕业于威廉姆斯学院和哈佛医学院。他曾在彼得·本特·布里格姆医院任内科住院医师，后在斯坦福大学完成了传染病学的专科医师（Fellowship）课程。自1975年加入匹兹堡大学医学院以来，他通过美国国立卫生研究院资助的研究项目，探索细胞介导免疫的机制以及传染病学各领域的临床诊疗工作。1990—1998年期间，他先后被匹兹堡大学及其医学中心任命为蒙特菲奥里医院的主任医师、传染病科主任，后担任内科临聘主任。

1998年起，温博士担任布朗大学医学院的内科主任（1998—2008年）。在此期间，他在不同医院、实践计划和培训项目间对内科进行整合。在担任布朗大学医学与生物科学院院长（2008—2013年）期间，他加强了与各附属医院（Lifespan医院和Care New England医院）间的联系，提升了科研工作的水准，并为医学院建成了一座新楼。在担任主任和院长期间，他还建立了与肯尼亚、多米尼加共和国和海地的医学院的国际交流项目。温博士自艾滋病流行初期便在门诊诊治艾滋病患者，并始终工作在科研、临床和教学一线。

弗雷德·谢夫曼（Fred J. Schiffman）博士与爱德华·温（Edward Wing）博士共同担任《希氏内科学精要》第10版的主编。他就读于瓦格纳学院，随后进入纽约大学医学院，并于1973年毕业。他在耶鲁大学附属纽黑文医院接受早期住院医师培训，随后在美国国家癌症研究所工作了两年。回到耶鲁大学后，他担任住院总医师，然后完成了血液学专科医师课程，随后成为耶鲁初级保健中心医学主任。他于1983年入职布朗大学，领导医学住院医师项目并担任米里亚姆医院的副主任医师。

谢夫曼博士担任布朗大学沃伦·阿尔珀特医学院人文医学系的西格尔家庭医学教授。他的学术兴趣涵盖人体脾脏的结构和功能，以及艺术与医疗的交叉融合。他主持或参与了许多项目和计划，其中包括许多旨在鼓励和加强患者、家人和医护人员的福祉与康复能力的项目。他所创办的一个新项目可以让医学生和医生与其他非医学专业人士一起，共同欣赏罗德岛设计学院博物馆的艺术作品。谢夫曼博士近期还主持了布朗大学名为"艺术与医学：艺术赋能患者照护"的edX课程，此课程的参与者来自全球多个国家。谢夫曼博士还出版了有关血液病理生理学、血液科会诊和贫血的著作。

原著者名单

Jinnette Dawn Abbott, MD
Rajiv Agarwal, MD
Marwa Al-Badri, MD
Hyeon-Ju Ryoo Ali, MD
Jason M. Aliotta, MD
Khaldoun Almhanna, MD, MPH
Mohanad T. Al-Qaisi, MD
Zuhal Arzomand, MD
Akwi W. Asombang, MD, MPH
Su N. Aung, MD, MPH
Christopher G. Azzoli, MD
Christina Bandera, MD
Debasree Banerjee, MD
Mashal Batheja, MD
Jeffrey J. Bazarian, MD, MPH
Selim R. Benbadis, MD
Ivor J. Benjamin, MD, FAHA, FACC
Eric Benoit, MD
Marcie G. Berger, MD
Clemens Bergwitz, MD
Nancy Berliner, MD
Jeffrey S. Berns, MD
Pooja Bhadbhade, DO
Ratna Bhavaraju-Sanka, MD
Tanmayee Bichile, MD
Ariel E. Birnbaum, MD
Charles M. Bliss, Jr., MD
Andrew S. Blum, MD, PhD
Bryan J. Bonder, MD
Russell Bratman, MD
Glenn D. Braunstein, MD
Alma M. Guerrero Bready, MD
Richard Bungiro, PhD
Anna Marie Burgner, MD, MEHP
Jonathan Cahill, MD
Andrew Canakis, DO
Benedito A. Carneiro, MD, MS
Brian Casserly, MD
Abdullah Chahin, MD, MA, MSc
Philip A. Chan, MD
Kimberle Chapin, MD
William P. Cheshire, Jr., MD
Waihong Chung, MD, PhD
Emma Ciafaloni, MD

Joaquin E. Cigarroa, MD
Michael P. Cinquegrani, MD
Andreea Coca, MD, MPH
Harvey Jay Cohen, MD
Scott Cohen, MD, MPH
Beatrice P. Concepcion, MD, MS
Nathan T. Connell, MD, MPH
Maria Constantinou, MD
Roberto Cortez, MD
Timothy J. Counihan, MD, FRCPI
Anne Haney Cross, MD
Cheston B. Cunha, MD, FACP
Joanne S. Cunha, MD
Susan Cu-Uvin, MD
Noura M. Dabbouseh, MD
Kwame Dapaah-Afriyie, MD, MBA
Erin M. Denney-Koelsch, MD
Andre De Souza, MD
An S. De Vriese, MD, PhD
Neal D. Dharmadhikari, MD
Leah Dickstein, MD
Don Dizon, MD, FACP, FASCO
Robyn T. Domsic, MD, MPH
Kim A. Eagle, MD
Michael G. Earing, MD
Pamela Egan, MD
Wafik S. El-Deiry, MD, PhD, FACP
Mitchell S. V. Elkind, MD, MS
Tarra B. Evans, MD
Michael B. Fallon, MD
Dimitrios Farmakiotis, MD
Francis A. Farraye, MD
Ronan Farrell, MD
Panayotis Fasseas, MD, FACC
Mary Anne Fenton, MD
Fernando C. Fervenza, MD, PhD
Sean Fine, MD
Arkadiy Finn, MD
Timothy Flanigan, MD
Brisas M. Flores, MD
Andrew E. Foderaro, MD
Theodore C. Friedman, MD, PhD
Joseph Metmowlee Garland, MD, AAHIVM

Eric J. Gartman, MD
Abdallah Geara, MD
Raul Macias Gil, MD
Timothy Gilligan, MD, FASCO
Michael Raymond Goggins, MB BCh BAO, MRCPI
Geetha Gopalakrishnan, MD
Vidya Gopinath, MD
Susan L. Greenspan, MD, FACP
Osama Hamdy, MD, PhD
Johanna Hamel, MD
Sajeev Handa, MD, SFHM
Mitchell T. Heflin, MD, MHS
Robert G. Holloway, MD, MPH
Christopher S. Huang, MD
Zilla Hussain, MD
T. Alp Ikizler, MD
Iris Isufi, MD
Carlayne E. Jackson, MD
Paul G. Jacob, MD, MPH
Matthew D. Jankowich, MD
Niels V. Johnsen, MD, MPH
Jessica E. Johnson, MD
Rayford R. June, MD
Tareq Kheirbek, MD, ScM, FACS
Alok A. Khorana, MD, FACP, FASCO
Sena Kilic, MD
David Kim, MD
James Kleczka, MD
James R. Klinger, MD
Patrick Koo, MD, ScM
Pooja Koolwal, MD
Mary P. Kotlarczyk, PhD
Nicole M. Kuderer, MD
Awewura Kwara, MD
Jennifer M. Kwon, MD, MPH
Richard A. Lange, MD, MBA
Jerome Larkin, MD
Alfred I. Lee, MD, PhD
Daniel J. Levine, MD
David E. Lewandowski, MD
Kelly V. Liang, MD, MS
Kimberly P. Liang, MD, MS
David R. Lichtenstein, MD

扫描二维码了解更多信息

Douglas W. Lienesch, MD
Geoffrey S.F. Ling, MD, PhD
Ester Little, MD, FACP
Yi Liu, MD
Nicole L. Lohr, MD, PhD
John R. Lonks, MD, FACP, FIDSA, FSHEA
Gary H. Lyman, MD, MPH
Jeffrey M. Lyness, MD
Shane Lyons, MD, MRCPI, MRCP(UK)
Diana Maas, MD
Talha A. Malik, MD, MSPH
Sonia Manocha, MD
Susan Manzi, MD, MPH
Frederick J. Marshall, MD
F. Dennis McCool, MD
Russell J. McCulloh, MD
Kelly McGarry, MD, FACP
Eavan Mc Govern, MD, PhD
Robin L. McKinney, MD
Anthony Mega, MD
Shivang Mehta, MD
Douglas F. Milam, MD
Maria D. Mileno, MD
Abhinav Kumar Misra, MBBS, MD
Orson W. Moe, MD
Niveditha Mohan, MBBS
Larry W. Moreland, MD
Alan R. Morrison, MD, PhD
Steven F. Moss, MD
Christopher J. Mullin, MD, MHS
Sinéad M. Murphy, MB, BCh, MD, FRCPI
Sagarika Nallu, MD, FAAP, FAAN, FAASM
Javier A. Neyra, MD, MSCS
Ghaith Noaiseh, MD

Thomas A. Ollila, MD
Steven M. Opal, MD
Biff F. Palmer, MD
Jen Jung Pan, MD, PhD
Anna Papazoglou, MD
Aric Parnes, MD
Nayan M. Patel, DO, MPH
Ari Pelcovits, MD
Mark A. Perazella, MD
Michael F. Picco, MD, PhD
Kate E. Powers, DO
Laura A. Previll, MD, MPH
Nilum Rajora, MD
Adolfo Ramirez-Zamora, MD
John Reagan, MD
Rebecca Reece, MD
Harlan Rich, MD, AGAF, FACP
Jennifer H. Richman, MD
Lisa R. Rogers, DO
Ralph Rogers, MD
Michal G. Rose, MD
James A. Roth, MD
Sharon Rounds, MD
Jason C. Rubenstein, MD
Abbas Rupawala, MD
Jenna Sarvaideo, DO
Ramesh Saxena, MD, PhD
Fred J. Schiffman, MD, MACP
Ruth B. Schneider, MD
Kristin A. Seaborg, MD
Anil Seetharam, MD
Stuart Seropian, MD
Jigme Michael Sethi, MD
Sanjeev Sethi, MD, PhD
Elizabeth Shane, MD
Esseim Sharma, MD

Shani Shastri, MD, MPH
Barry S. Shea, MD
Lauren Shevell, MD, MPH
Joseph A. Smith, Jr., MD
Robert J. Smith, MD
Davendra P.S. Sohal, MD, MPH
Christopher Song, MD, FACC
Thomas Sperry, MD
Jeffrey M. Statland, MD
Emily M. Stein, MD
Jennifer L. Strande, MD, PhD
Rochelle Strenger, MD
Thomas R. Talbot, MD, MPH
Christopher G. Tarolli, MD, MSEd
Yael Tarshish, MD
Pushpak Taunk, MD
Philip Tsoukas, MD
Allan R. Tunkel, MD, PhD
Jeffrey M. Turner, MD
Zoe G.S. Vazquez, MD
Stacie A. F. Vela, MD
Paul M. Vespa, MD, FCCM, FAAN, FANA, FNCS
Wanpen Vongpatanasin, MD
Marcella D. Walker, MD
Eunice S. Wang, MD
Sharmeel K. Wasan, MD
Thomas J. Weber, MD
Brandon J. Wilcoxson, MD
Edward J. Wing, MD, FACP, FIDSA
Ellice Wong, MD
John J. Wysolmerski, MD
Rayan Yousefzai, MD
Thomas R. Ziegler, MD
Rebecca Zon, MD

ACKNOWLEDGMENTS

Dr. Schiffman and I wish to thank first of all, the authors of the 128 chapters that make up the tenth edition of *Cecil Essentials of Medicine*. They have worked diligently to compose the material for each chapter and apply their mastery as they added the newest information, in clear language, to the text. Their efforts are apparent in the excellence of the book, and we are immensely grateful for their work. We wish to also thank Marybeth Thiel, Jennifer Ehlers, and Dan Fitzgerald from Elsevier who guided and supported our work as editors and whose expertise has made this volume possible. Finally, we are always thankful to our wives, Dr. Rena Wing and Ms. Gerri Schiffman, without whose love, support, and especially humor, this book would not have happened.

致 谢

谢夫曼博士和我首先要致谢《希氏内科学精要》第10版全书128章的各位作者。感谢他们精益求精地撰写每一章节，并运用其专业知识，以简明的语言将前沿资讯呈现在书中。正是他们的辛勤努力确保了本书的卓越地位，对他们唯有由衷的感激。我们还要感谢爱思唯尔出版集团的玛丽贝丝·蒂尔（Marybeth Thiel）、詹妮弗·埃勒斯（Jennifer Ehlers）和丹·菲茨杰拉德（Dan Fitzgerald），他们对本书的编辑工作给予了指导和支持，其专业水准保障了本书的完稿。最后，要特别感谢我们的妻子——蕾娜·温（Rena Wing）博士和盖瑞·谢夫曼（Gerri Schiffman）女士，对她们的爱和支持，特别是积极乐观的心态始终心存感激，她们为本书的圆满完成发挥了不可或缺的作用。

总目录

第 1 分册

- 第 1 篇　内科学概论　Introduction to Medicine
- 第 2 篇　呼吸与危重症医学　Pulmonary and Critical Care Medicine
- 第 3 篇　术前和术后照护　Preoperative and Postoperative Care

第 2 分册

心血管疾病　Cardiovascular Disease

第 3 分册

肾脏疾病　Renal Disease

第 4 分册

- 第 1 篇　胃肠疾病　Gastrointestinal Disease
- 第 2 篇　肝脏与胆道系统疾病　Diseases of the Liver and Biliary System

第 5 分册

血液疾病　Hematologic Disease

第 6 分册

肿瘤疾病　Oncologic Disease

第 7 分册

- 第 1 篇　内分泌疾病与代谢疾病　Endocrine Disease and Metabolic Disease
- 第 2 篇　女性健康　Women's Health
- 第 3 篇　男性健康　Men's Health
- 第 4 篇　骨与骨矿物质代谢疾病　Diseases of Bone and Bone Mineral Metabolism

第 8 分册

肌肉骨骼与结缔组织疾病　Musculoskeletal and Connective Tissue Disease

第 9 分册

感染性疾病　Infectious Disease

第 10 分册

第 1 篇　神经疾病　Neurologic Disease
第 2 篇　老年医学　Geriatrics
第 3 篇　缓和医疗　Palliative Care
第 4 篇　酒精和物质使用　Alcohol and Substance Use

第6分册

肿瘤疾病

第 6 分册译者名单

主　译

王　洁　巴　一

译　者（按姓氏笔画排序）

万　蕊　中国医学科学院肿瘤医院	何　焱　浙江省肿瘤医院
王　洁　中国医学科学院肿瘤医院	应红艳　中国医学科学院北京协和医院
王　湘　中国医学科学院北京协和医院	张智旸　中国医学科学院北京协和医院
王志杰　中国医学科学院肿瘤医院	张锦松　中国医学科学院肿瘤医院
王晰程　中国医学科学院北京协和医院	邵亚娟　中国医学科学院北京协和医院
公小蕾　中国医学科学院北京协和医院	周　娜　中国医学科学院北京协和医院
巴　一　中国医学科学院北京协和医院	周光飚　中国医学科学院肿瘤医院
朱以香　四川省肿瘤医院	周建凤　中国医学科学院北京协和医院
仲　佳　中国医学科学院肿瘤医院	赵　林　中国医学科学院北京协和医院
庄　威　中国医学科学院肿瘤医院	段建春　中国医学科学院肿瘤医院
刘　媛　中国医学科学院北京协和医院	郭玉峰　中山大学肿瘤防治中心
李宁宁　中国医学科学院北京协和医院	葛郁平　中国医学科学院北京协和医院
李孝远　中国医学科学院北京协和医院	程月鹃　中国医学科学院北京协和医院
邱　维　中国医学科学院北京协和医院	

第 6 分册目录

肿瘤疾病　Oncologic Disease

1. Cancer Biology, 4
   肿瘤生物学，5

2. Cancer Epidemiology, 20
   癌症流行病学，21

3. Principles of Cancer Therapy, 32
   癌症治疗原则，33

4. Lung Cancer, 44
   肺癌，45

5. Gastrointestinal Cancers, 56
   胃肠道癌症，57

6. Genitourinary Cancers, 68
   泌尿生殖系统肿瘤，69

7. Breast Cancer, 80
   乳腺癌，81

8. Gynecological Cancer, 92
   妇科癌症，93

9. Other Solid Tumors (Head and Neck, Sarcomas, Melanoma, Unknown Primary), 108
   其他实体瘤（头颈癌、肉瘤、黑色素瘤、原发部位不明的癌症），109

10. Complications of Cancer and Cancer Treatment, 118
    肿瘤并发症及其治疗，119

索引 Index，128

CECIL ESSENTIALS OF MEDICINE

Oncologic Disease

Oncologic Disease

1   Cancer Biology, 4

2   Cancer Epidemiology, 20

3   Principles of Cancer Therapy, 32

4   Lung Cancer, 44

5   Gastrointestinal Cancers, 56

6   Genitourinary Cancers, 68

7   Breast Cancer, 80

8   Gynecological Cancer, 92

9   Other Solid Tumors (Head and Neck, Sarcomas, Melanoma, Unknown Primary), 108

10   Complications of Cancer and Cancer Treatment, 118

肿瘤疾病

1 肿瘤生物学，5

2 癌症流行病学，21

3 癌症治疗原则，33

4 肺癌，45

5 胃肠道癌症，57

6 泌尿生殖系统肿瘤，69

7 乳腺癌，81

8 妇科癌症，93

9 其他实体瘤（头颈癌、肉瘤、黑色素瘤、原发部位不明的癌症），109

10 肿瘤并发症及其治疗，119

1

Cancer Biology

Andre De Souza, Wafik S. El-Deiry

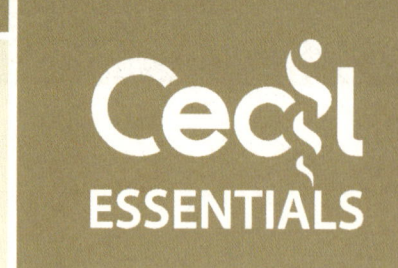

INTRODUCTION

Cancer is a complex genetic disease that is defined by the transition of a normal cell, governed by processes that control its replication, into a cancer cell that is typified by unrestrained proliferation and dissemination. The underlying landscape of cancer genetics is now fully defined for many cancers, aided by the evolving technologies in gene sequencing. Many therapeutic advances of the last decade have successfully focused on targets identified by the study of genetic mutations. This chapter reviews the essential elements of cancer biology and key underlying genetic alterations driving this biology.

THE GENETICS OF CANCER

Cancer is a genetic disease. Carcinogens are chemical mutagens or physical insults that result in DNA alterations. Each of these insults produce different alterations with distinct outcomes for a cancer cell. These alterations can also be derived from random mutations enabled by failure of DNA repair mechanisms.

The most common gene alterations in cancer are nonsynonymous point mutations. A synonymous point mutation is a single nucleotide exchange (also called single nucleotide polymorphism [SNP] or single nucleotide variant [SNV]) that does not affect the final resultant amino acid and therefore does not affect the function of a protein. By contrast, a nonsynonymous mutation will result in an amino acid change that may be beneficial for the survival of a cancer cell. Dr. Bert Volgelstein described the stepwise acquisition of mutations as drivers of cancer progression. Using the progressive histopathological stages of colorectal cancer as a model, he depicted carcinogenesis as a sequence of alterations in genes such as APC, KRAS, TP53, and SMAD4 (small mothers against decapentaplegic 4). In recognizing TP53 as a tumor suppressor gene and determining its central role in the transformation of a preneoplastic adenoma to colorectal cancer, Dr. Volgelstein linked the most common tumor suppressor gene to one of the most prevalent human malignancies. He further unraveled the role of mutations as "drivers" and "passengers" in the pathogenesis of cancer and its heterogeneity. The genetic changes associated with cancer paved the way for screening tests that could be used for early detection and prevention of cancer development.

Copy number variation or gene amplification denotes the loss or gain of a whole copy of a gene. When a cell has extra copies of genes, it can produce twice or more the amount of proteins. On the other hand, when just parts of a gene are lost (deletions) or anomalous sequences are inserted amid the full gene sequence (insertions), these events are called indels (insertions and deletions). Indels have a knack for activating the immune system. Why? When proteins transcribed from genes with indels are presented in the regular health cellular checkup we call antigen presentation, they look more foreign to immune cells than point mutations. Lastly, mitosis malfunction may be conducive to fusion of distinct segments of chromosomes. Natural selection can then favor gene fusions from translocational events that stimulate cell survival. Much progress has been made in the past several decades to unravel oncogenic fusions in various leukemias and solid tumors (Fig. 1.1). The classical Philadelphia chromosome in chronic myelogenous leukemia creates a fusion of the *BCR-ABL* genes. Tyrosine kinase inhibitors such as Imatinib block the transforming ability of *BCR-ABL* and have led to prolonged patient survival. The *BCL-2* gene translocated in follicular lymphoma can be therapeutically inhibited by venetoclax, while various NRTK fusions driving cancer can be treated with larotrectinib or entrectinib. Other common translocations in Burkitt's lymphoma, Ewing's sarcoma, or prostate cancer are well-known but not yet therapeutically targeted.

THE TUMOR MICROENVIROMENT

Tissues are made of a myriad of cells, each contributing to a state of homeostasis that controls unchecked growth of individual cells. Our understanding of cancer is evolving from a cellular disease to an infirmity of tissues.

There is a growing body of evidence that bone marrow–derived and stromal–derived cells contribute to the evolution of cancer. Myeloid-derived suppressor cells (MDSCs) have been shown to suppress NK and cytotoxic T cells (CD8$^+$) in the tumor microenvironment, whereas cancer-associated fibroblasts (CAFs) synthesize the thick extracellular matrix (desmoplasia) that serves as a scaffold and a shield for drugs targeting stroma-rich tumors such as pancreatic cancer (Fig. 1.2). The tumor microenvironment (TME) is complex and includes multiple immune, stromal, endothelial cells, altered extracellular matrix, proinflammatory, immunosuppressive, and chemoattracting cytokines, and physical changes such as hypoxia, altered tumor metabolism leading to low pH, a dysregulated metabolome. The TME promotes cancer progression and resistance to therapy.

HALLMARKS OF CANCER

The hallmarks of cancer were established by Hanahan and Weinberg and updated in 2011. These hallmarks are products of driver mutations that incapacitate selective pressures restricting tumor growth. The hallmarks include acquisition of immortality, genomic instability, hyperactive proliferative signaling pathways, growth checkpoint disruption, angiogenesis, metabolism reprogramming, invasion and metastasis, and immune escape.

Immortality: Apoptosis Suppression, and Telomerase Activation

Apoptosis or programmed cell death occurs in adult cells when DNA damage or other forms of cellular stress elicit a suicidal program to

肿瘤生物学

郭玉峰 译 周光飚 王志杰 审校 王洁 通审

引言

肿瘤是一类错综复杂的基因疾病，源自正常细胞在一系列调控其增殖机制的因素作用下，异常转变为增殖不受控制的癌细胞，具备潜在的播散与转移能力。在基因测序技术进步的推动下，多种肿瘤的遗传学特征图谱已逐渐被清晰描绘。近10年来，治疗领域的显著进展尤为体现在精准医疗上，即通过深入研究基因突变，成功锁定了多个治疗靶点。本章回顾了肿瘤生物学的基础架构及其中关键的驱动性基因改变。

肿瘤遗传学

肿瘤作为一种基因疾病，于化学诱变剂或物理损伤等致癌因素作用下引起DNA发生改变而发生。这些不同的损伤因素能够引起肿瘤细胞内特定的DNA改变，并产生不同的生物学效应。而DNA修复机制异常亦能引发随机突变导致DNA改变。

非同义点突变是肿瘤最为常见的基因变异类型之一。该类突变通过改变氨基酸序列，可能为肿瘤细胞提供生存优势。与之相对，同义点突变，即单核苷酸的替换［也称为单核苷酸多态性（SNP）或单核苷酸变异（SNV）］，由于不会影响氨基酸的最终生成，故不会影响蛋白质功能。Bert Vogelstein博士提出肿瘤进展由基因突变逐渐累积所驱动。利用结直肠癌组织病理学多阶段演进模型，他提出肿瘤发生是通过APC、KRAS、TP53和SMAD4（small mothers against decapentaplegic 4）等基因发生一系列改变而引起的。Vogelstein博士鉴定出TP53是一种抑癌基因，证实其在癌前腺瘤至结直肠癌转化中发挥核心作用，从而将最常见的抑癌基因与一种最普遍的人类恶性肿瘤联系起来。此外，他还进一步揭示"驱动"和"乘客"突变在肿瘤发病机制及其异质性中的作用。肿瘤相关基因改变为早期检测和预防肿瘤进展的筛查奠定了基础。

拷贝数变异或基因扩增是指整个基因拷贝的丧失或增加。当拥有额外的基因拷贝时，细胞可产生两倍或更多量的蛋白质；此外，仅一部分基因丧失（缺失）或异常序列插入完整基因序列（插入）则称为插入/缺失。插入/缺失可激活免疫系统，原因在于其产生的蛋白质在免疫系统中具有更强的外源性特征，更易被免疫系统识别，从而可能激活免疫应答；最后，细胞分裂异常可能导致染色体不同片段的融合，而自然选择会倾向于保留那些促进细胞生存的基因融合事件。在过去的几十年中，有关揭示多种白血病和实体肿瘤致癌性基因融合的研究取得诸多进展（图1.1）。如慢性髓细胞性白血病中经典的费城染色体形成*BCR-ABL*基因融合，而酪氨酸激酶抑制剂如伊马替尼可阻断*BCR-ABL*转化能力从而延长患者生存期；维奈托克可有效抑制在滤泡性淋巴瘤中发生易位的*BCL-2*基因；拉罗替尼或恩曲替尼可治疗多种NRTK融合驱动型肿瘤。然而，对于伯基特淋巴瘤、尤因肉瘤或前列腺癌中的其他常见易位尽管早已被发现，但仍缺乏有效的靶向治疗方法。

肿瘤微环境

人体组织由大量细胞组成，每个细胞均参与维持环境稳态，以遏制异常的细胞增殖。人们对肿瘤的认识正在发生深刻转变，从单一的细胞疾病演变为一种组织学层面的疾病。越来越多的证据表明，骨髓来源细胞和间质来源细胞参与肿瘤进化。髓系来源的抑制性细胞（MDSC）已被证实在肿瘤微环境中抑制NK细胞和细胞毒性T细胞（$CD8^+$），而肿瘤相关成纤维细胞（CAF）能合成致密的细胞外基质（硬化症），在靶向富含间质型肿瘤（如胰腺癌）药物治疗时，起到支架和保护屏障作用（图1.2）。肿瘤微环境（TME）成分复杂，不仅包括多种免疫细胞、间质细胞、内皮细胞、异常的细胞外基质，以及促炎性、免疫抑制性和趋化性细胞因子，还存在低氧、肿瘤代谢改变引起的低pH值和代谢组异常等物理变化。TME促进肿瘤进展以及治疗耐药。

肿瘤的特征

肿瘤的特征由Hanahan和Weinberg确立并于2011年拓展更新。这些特征源于驱动基因突变，以突破限制肿瘤生长的选择性压力，包括永生能力获得、基因组不稳定、增殖信号通路过度激活、生长检查点破坏、血管生成、代谢重编程、侵袭和转移，以及免疫逃逸。

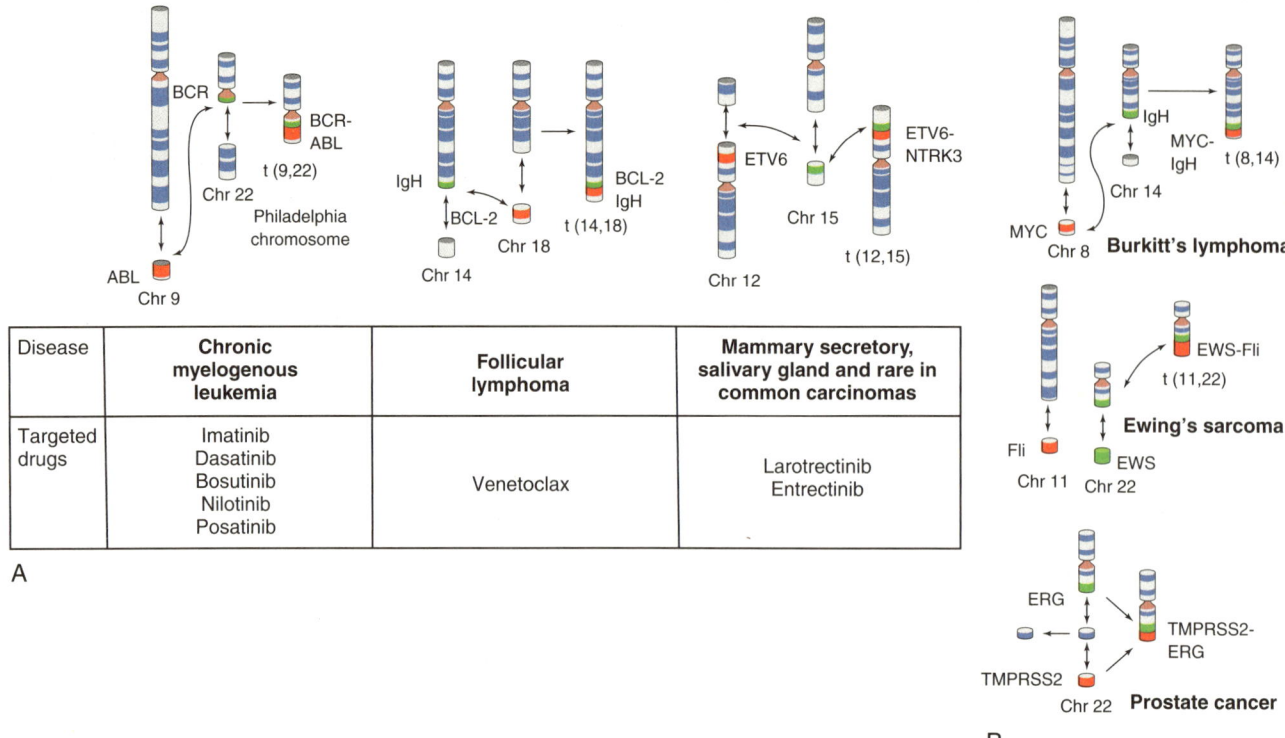

Fig. 1.1 Chromosomal translocations and oncogene activation in human cancer. (A) Depicted are several classical translocations associated with different types of cancer and the FDA-approved drugs used to treat them. These include chronic myelogenous leukemia t(9,22)(BCR-ABL), follicular lymphoma t(14,18) *(IgH/BCL2)*, and *NTRK* gene fusions that occur in various solid tumors (e.g., *ETV-6/NTRK3*). (B) Major chromosomal translocations associated with Burkitt's lymphoma t(8,14) *(MYC/IgH)*, Ewing's and other sarcomas *(EWS/FLI)*, and prostate cancer *(TMPRSS2/ERG)*. Other translocations are being recognized as they contribute to therapy resistance including *ESR1* whose translocation (not shown) confers resistance to hormonal therapy in breast cancer. Not shown are common translocations in mantle cell lymphoma t(11,14) (Cyclin D, IgH) or other *NTRK* genes such as *NTRK1* and *NTRK2*.

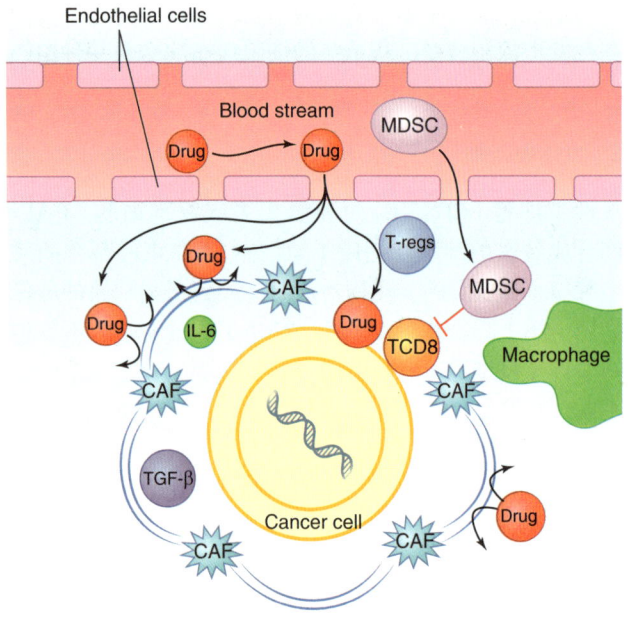

Fig. 1.2 The tumor microenvironment promotes cancer progression and impedes cancer therapy. The tumor microenvironment (TME) is composed of different cell types in addition to cancer cells. The TME of a growing tumor typically has hypoxic regions, low pH due to altered metabolism, and low levels of nutrients. Cancer associated fibroblasts (CAF) create a thick connective tissue mesh which acts as a mechanical barrier to drug delivery to cancer cells. This connective tissue shell is also known as desmoplasia, here stylized as *blue concentric curves*. A small molecule or biologic drug is represented as *red circles* crossing through the endothelial lining of a blood vessel. Although some drug does make it to the tumor cell, some bounces off the desmoplastic shell. Once cancer evolves, the body tries to fight it off with an adaptative immune response, which ultimately delivers cytotoxic T cells (TCD8) to kill cancer cells, enabled by chemical mediators such as Interleukin-6 (IL-6) and attenuated by immunosuppressive factors such as transforming growth factor β (TGF-β). Immunosuppressive cells include macrophages and T regulatory cells (T-regs). The cytotoxic T cells are characterized by specific transmembrane receptors, the cluster of differentiation (CD) 8 proteins, and are regulated in part by myeloid-derived suppressor cells (MDSCs), which dampen an overstimulated immune response that otherwise would result in autoimmune disease. MDSCs are generated in the bone marrow and also cross endothelial cell gaps to render TCD8 cells anergic. MDSCs are hijacked by tumors to serve as one of the mechanisms of immune evasion. Some of these concepts have been recently summarized in a review of the physical hallmarks of cancer (Nia HT, Munn LL, Jain RK: *Science* October 2020; 370[546]: 1–11).

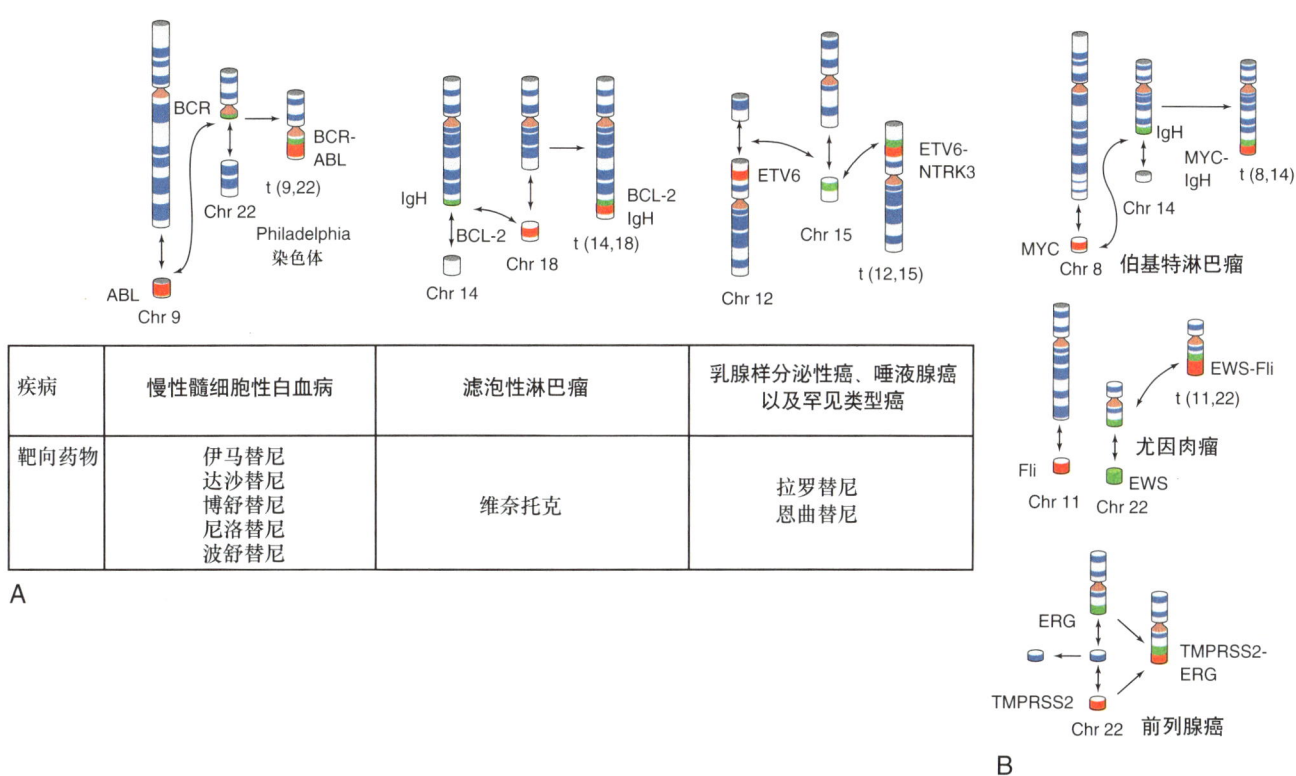

图1.1 人类肿瘤中染色体易位和癌基因激活。（**A**）与不同类型肿瘤相关的几种经典易位以及FDA批准的靶向药物，包括慢性髓细胞性白血病 t（9,22）（*BCR-ABL*）、滤泡性淋巴瘤 t（14,18）（*IgH/BCL2*）和发生于多种实体肿瘤中的 *NTRK* 基因融合（如 *ETV-6/NTRK3*）。（**B**）与伯基特淋巴瘤 t（8,14）（*MYC/IgH*）、尤因和其他肉瘤（*EWS/FLI*）以及前列腺癌（*TMPRSS2/ERG*）相关的主要染色体易位；其他与治疗耐药相关的易位正在被鉴定，例如 *ESR1* 易位（未显示）促进乳腺癌对内分泌治疗耐药；未显示的常见易位还包括套细胞淋巴瘤 t（11,14）（Cyclin D, IgH）和其他 *NTRK* 基因如 *NTRK1* 和 *NTRK2*

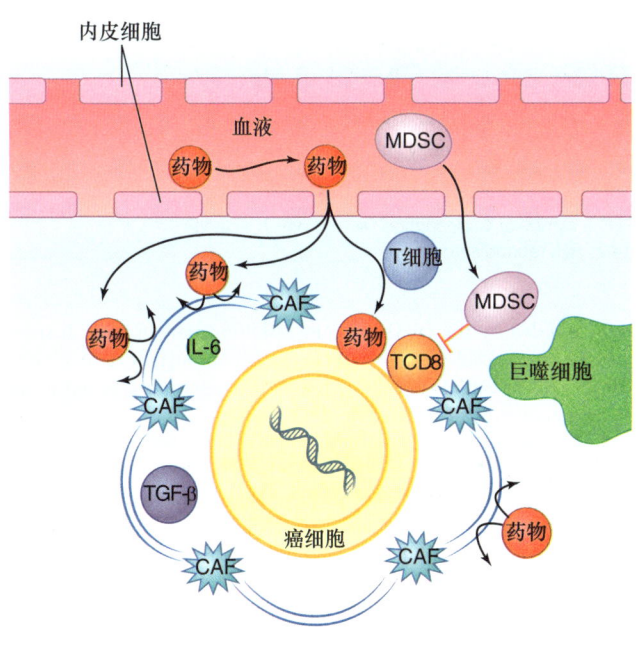

图1.2 肿瘤微环境促进肿瘤进展并阻碍肿瘤治疗。肿瘤微环境（TME）由癌细胞和其他不同的细胞类型组成。处于生长期的肿瘤，其TME通常具有缺氧区域、代谢改变导致的低pH值环境以及营养物质缺乏。肿瘤相关成纤维细胞（CAF）构建致密结缔组织网，作为一种机械屏障以阻止药物递送至肿瘤细胞。此种结缔组织外壳也被称为硬化症，在图中以蓝色同心曲线表示。小分子或生物药物穿过血管内皮，以红色圆圈表示。尽管部分药物可到达肿瘤细胞，仍有些药物被阻挡在硬化外壳之外。当肿瘤进展时，机体试图通过激活适应性免疫应答并最终输送细胞毒性T细胞（TCD8）以杀伤癌细胞。此种适应性免疫应答通过白细胞介素-6（IL-6）等化学介质所介导，也可被免疫抑制性因子如转化生长因子β（TGF-β）所抑制。免疫抑制性细胞包括巨噬细胞和调节性T细胞（T-regs）。细胞毒性T细胞的特征是具有特定跨膜受体，即分化簇（CD）8蛋白，其活性在一定程度上可由髓系来源抑制细胞（MDSC）调控。MDSC能抑制过度刺激的免疫反应以避免自身免疫性疾病的发生，主要产生于骨髓，可穿过内皮细胞间隙而诱导 CD8$^+$ T细胞失能。MDSC被肿瘤劫持操纵是免疫逃逸的重要机制之一。近来的一篇关于肿瘤物理特征的综述对其中一些概念进行了总结［Nia HT, Munn LL, Jain RK: Science October 2020；370（546）：1-11］

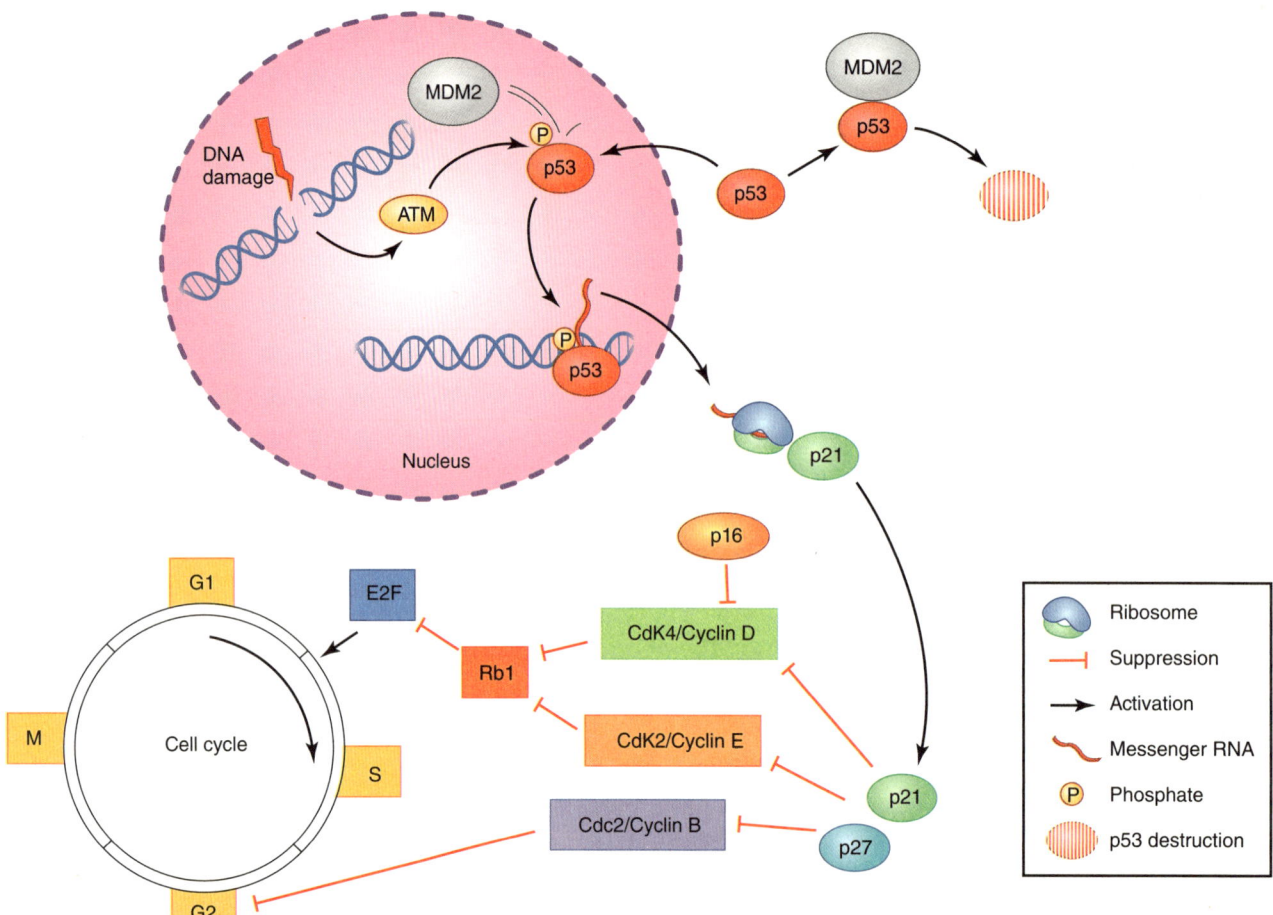

Fig. 1.3 DNA damage stalls the cell cycle. DNA damage, for example after exposure to ionizing radiation, triggers ATM phosphorylation of the p53 protein. Other kinases induced by DNA damage include ATR, Chk1, and Chk2 (not shown). The p53 protein is constitutively tagged to proteasomal destruction by the E3 ligase MDM2; p53 phosphorylation stabilizes the protein by blocking its binding to MDM2. The p53 protein transcriptionally activates the expression of the p21 gene *(CDKN1A, WAF1)*. The p21 protein is the cell checkpoint of all three CDK and cyclin complexes (CDK4/Cyclin D, CDK2/Cyclin E, CDC2/Cyclin B). Therefore, p53, through p21, arrests the cell cycle to allow repair after DNA damage and thereby prevent cancer. *TP53* is the most commonly mutated gene in human cancer. The p27 protein is another universal inhibitor of CDK complexes. By contrast, the p16 protein, encoded by the *CDKN2A* gene, inhibits CDK4/Cyclin D. Inhibition of CDK4 and CDK2 complexes allows unphosphorylated RB to bind E2F proteins and inhibit entry of cells into S-phase where the DNA is replicated. CDK4 and 6 inhibitors are approved for therapy of estrogen receptor positive breast cancer. MDM2, ATR, ATM, Chk1, and Chk2 inhibitors are currently in clinical trials for cancer therapy. The "*p*" denotes protein, followed by molecular weight in Kilodaltons, as in p21 and p53. *Arrows* indicate activation processes in a pathway. *Red "T"* symbols indicate suppression of a pathway. *ATM,* Ataxia telangiectasia mutated; *CDK,* cyclin-dependent kinase; *E2F,* a family of transcription factors which activate genes required for S-phase; *MDM2,* mouse double minute 2; *RB,* retinoblastoma.

save the organism as a whole. This program is actioned by extracellular ligands (extrinsic pathway) or intracellular mediators (intrinsic pathway). The extracellular ligand FASL or TRAIL (in immune cells) or soluble ligands (in the extracellular space) bind to FAS and TRAIL receptors in the cell that undergoes apoptosis. The intrinsic pathway culminates in release of cytochrome c to the cytosol. Caspase activation in response to either the extrinsic or intrinsic cell death pathways results in proteolytic cleavage of thousands of cellular proteins that result in cell detachment, shrinkage, nuclear fragmentation and engulfment by macrophages. Several pro- and anti-apoptotic regulator proteins, such as Bcl-2, are deregulated in cancer (Figs. 1.3 – 1.5). Telomere shortening is the prime cellular timekeeper process only avoided by the enzyme telomerase, dormant in most tissues. Telomerase reactivation induces cancer cell immortality and is a key early event in carcinogenesis. However, the telomerase target is yet to be meaningfully exploited in cancer therapy.

Genomic Instability: Impairing DNA Repair Genes

Alterations in DNA repair genes increase tumor mutation burden. It was also observed that some cancer cells had frail chromosomes, prone to breakage. While some tumor cells have chromosomal instability, others have microsatellite instability characterized by mutations including frequently at repetitive DNA sequences. This microsatellite instability (MSI) is a result of mutations in DNA repair

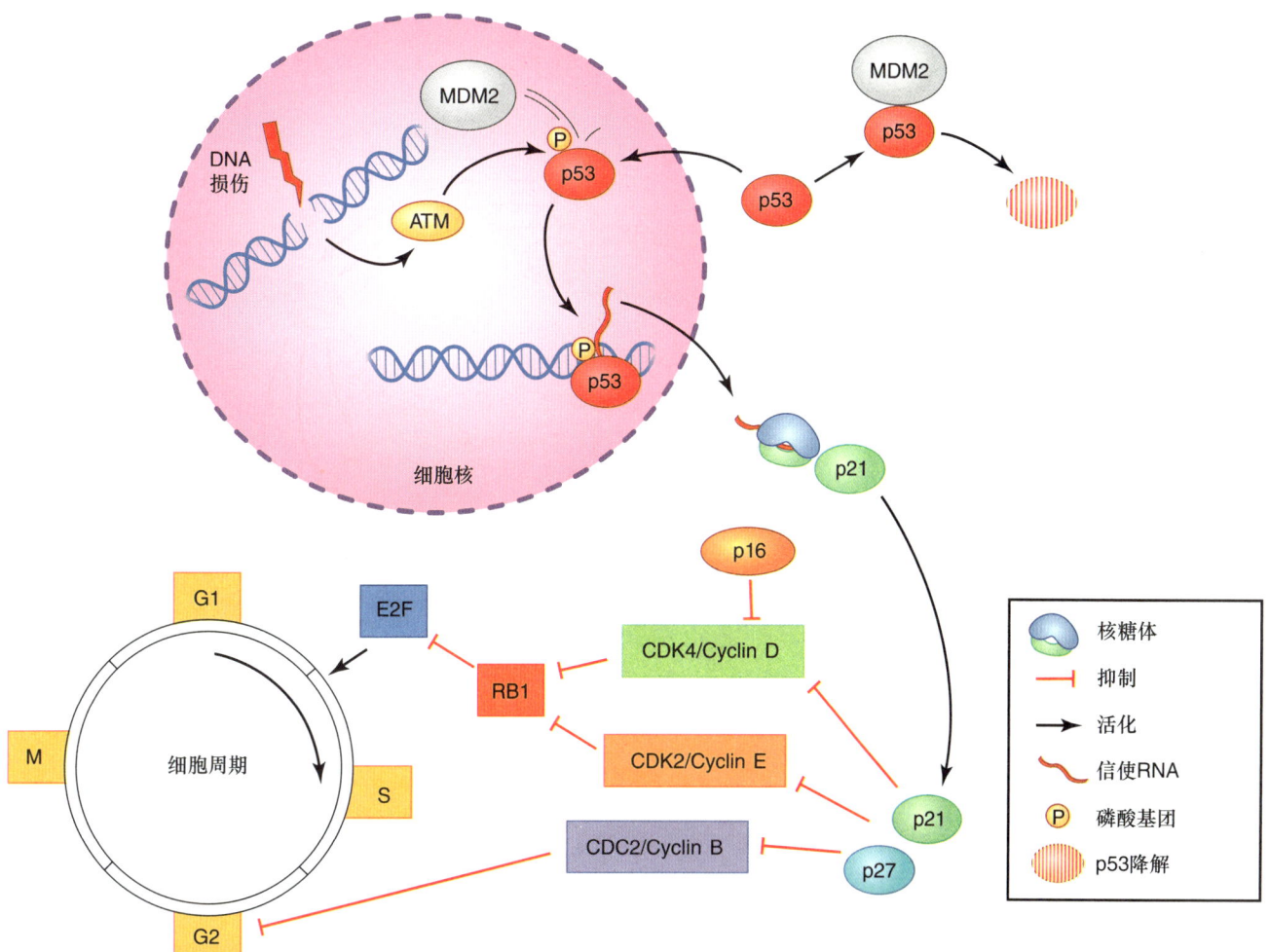

图1.3 DNA 损伤诱导细胞周期停滞。DNA 损伤，例如暴露于电离辐射后，能引发 ATM 对 p53 蛋白的磷酸化。由 DNA 损伤诱导的其他激酶包括 ATR、Chk1 和 Chk2（未显示）。p53 蛋白由 E3 连接酶 MDM2 进行组成性标记后被蛋白酶体降解；p53 磷酸化阻止其与 MDM2 结合从而增加蛋白稳定性。p53 蛋白转录激活 p21 基因（CDKN1A，WAF1）表达，后者是三个 CDK 和细胞周期蛋白复合物 [CDK4/细胞周期蛋白（Cyclin）D、CDK2/细胞周期蛋白 E 和 CDC2/细胞周期蛋白 B] 的细胞检查点。因此，p53 通过 p21 诱导细胞周期停滞以允许 DNA 损伤后修复，从而阻碍肿瘤的发生。TP53 是人类肿瘤中最常见的突变基因。p27 蛋白则是另一个广谱 CDK 复合物抑制剂；相比之下，由 CDKN2A 基因编码的 p16 蛋白可抑制 CDK4/细胞周期蛋白 D。抑制 CDK4 和 CDK2 复合物使非磷酸化 RB 结合 E2F 蛋白，从而阻止细胞进入 DNA 复制的 S 期。CDK4 和 6 抑制剂已被批准用于治疗雌激素受体阳性乳腺癌；MDM2、ATR、ATM、Chk1 和 Chk2 抑制剂目前正在进行药物临床试验（译者注：MDM2 抑制剂的作用机制主要是阻止 MDM2 介导 p53 降解；而 ATR、ATM、Chk1 和 Chk2 抑制剂的作用机制则表现在：当肿瘤细胞 DNA 损伤时，抑制 ATM/ChK2 和 ATR/ChK1 通路能够阻碍肿瘤细胞的自我修复，从而达到增强杀伤肿瘤细胞的作用）。"p"表示蛋白质，后面跟随以千道尔顿为单位的分子量，如 p21 和 p53，箭头表示通路中的活化进程，红色"T"符号表示通路抑制作用。ATM，共济失调毛细血管扩张突变；CDK，细胞周期依赖性激酶；E2F，一类激活 S 期所需基因的转录因子家族；MDM2，鼠双微体 2；RB，视网膜母细胞瘤

永生能力：凋亡抑制和端粒酶激活

凋亡或程序性细胞死亡是指成体细胞经历 DNA 损伤或其他形式的细胞应激时，通过引发凋亡程序，以维持生物体内的稳态。凋亡程序由细胞外配体（外在途径）或细胞内介质（内在途径）所介导。细胞外配体 FASL、TRAIL（免疫细胞）或可溶性配体（细胞外空间）与正在发生凋亡细胞的 FAS 和 TRAIL 受体结合；内在途径最终导致细胞色素 c 释放至细胞质。外在或内在细胞死亡途径激活 caspase 通路，引起数千种蛋白质裂解，导致细胞分离、皱缩、核碎裂以及被巨噬细胞吞噬。多种促凋亡和抗凋亡的调节蛋白（如 Bcl-2）在肿瘤中失调

（图 1.3 至图 1.5）。端粒作为细胞寿命的"有丝分裂钟"，其不可逆的缩减趋势仅能被端粒酶所抑制。然而，端粒酶在机体大多数组织中通常处于休眠状态。端粒酶的重新激活诱导肿瘤细胞永生化是癌变早期的关键事件，然而靶向端粒酶的治疗手段尚未得到实质性应用。

基因组不稳定性：DNA 损伤修复基因

DNA 错配修复基因改变增加了肿瘤突变负荷，而某些肿瘤细胞也被观察到具有易断裂的染色体。某些肿瘤细胞具有染色体不稳定性，而某些肿瘤细胞具有微卫星不稳定性（MSI），其特征是在 DNA 重复序列中频繁出现突变，是 DNA 修复基因突变的结果。错配

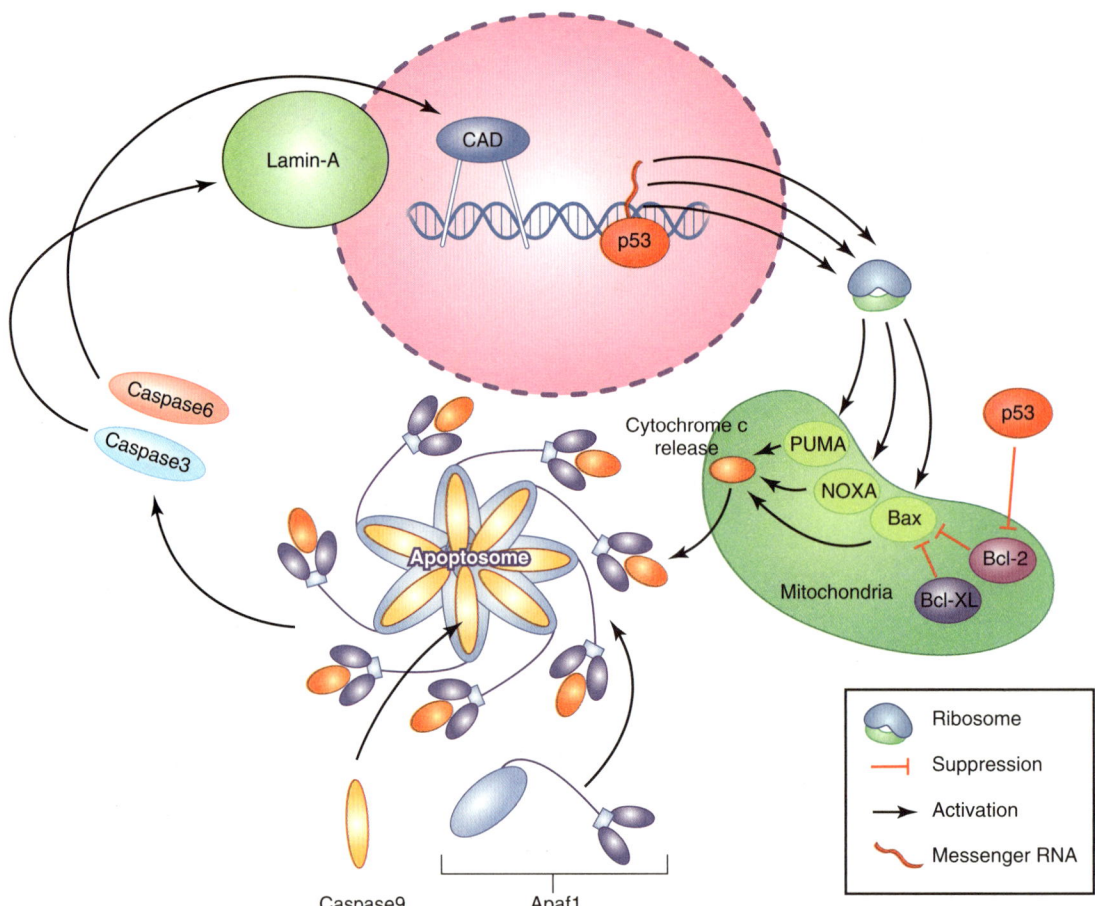

Fig. 1.4 DNA damaging chemotherapy activates p53 leading to tumor cell death through the intrinsic apoptosis pathway. This figure shows the central role of the p53 protein in the intrinsic apoptosis pathway, which culminates in apoptosome activation. Oncogene activation or cytotoxic DNA damaging chemotherapies stabilize and activate the p53 protein. If the damage is repaired, cells survive and do not become transformed. If there is too much damage, cells undergo p53-dependent cell death. When p53 is mutated in cancer, its tumor suppressor function is lost. As part of its normal function after DNA damage, the p53 protein modulates the intrinsic apoptosis pathway by regulating the balance of the proapoptotic proteins PUMA, NOXA, and BAX and the antiapoptotic proteins BCL-XL and BCL-2, resulting in the release of cytochrome c from the mitochondria. When cytochrome c binds to the apoptosome, a multimer of caspase 9 and APAF1, it activates caspases 3 and 6, which promote nuclear membrane destruction by Lamin-A and DNA fragmentation by CAD. The *"p"* denotes protein, followed by molecular weight in Kilodaltons, as in p53. *Arrows* indicate activation processes in a pathway. *Red "T" symbols* indicate suppression of a pathway. *APAF1,* Apoptosis protease activating factor 1; *BAX,* BCL-associated X; *BCL-2,* B-cell lymphoma 2; *BCL-XL,* BCL-extra-large; *CAD,* caspase-activated deoxyribonuclease; *NOXA,* Latin for damage; *PUMA,* p53 upregulated mediator of apoptosis. For a more detailed review of the apoptosis pathway and its exploitation in cancer therapy, see Carneiro BA, El-Deiry WS, *Nat. Rev. Clin. Oncol.* 2020 Jul;17(7):395–417.

genes. When the repair system is defective, the number of mutations increases. The total number of mutations in a cancer cell is called tumor mutation burden. MSI correlates with tumor mutation burden. The processing of the mutant proteins from MSI-high tumor cells in the endoplasmic reticulum and their presentation by the main histocompatibility complex-I (MHC-I) as neo-antigens predicts response to immunotherapy. Furthermore, mutations in components of the FANC complex (including BRCA genes) affect DNA double-strand break repair, resulting in homologous recombination deficiency (HRD) observed in subsets of ovarian, breast, prostate, and pancreatic cancer patients. Some of these cancers use a rescue DNA repair system, the poly-ADP ribose polymerase (PARP) system, which can be targeted with inhibitors, a concept often named synthetic lethality (specifically in the BRCA-mutated cells). PARP inhibitors are oral medications available in the oncology clinic for patients with HRD. Both MSI and HRD may be acquired through germline (inherited from parents) or somatic (originated in the tumor) mutations.

Oncogenes Unleash Proliferation

Oncogene mutations convert a normal cell into a cancerous cell (Fig 1.6). Oncogenes often activate pathways that are important for cancer. For example, chronic myelogenous leukemia (CML) occurs when the proto-oncogene ABL from chromosome 9 translocates to

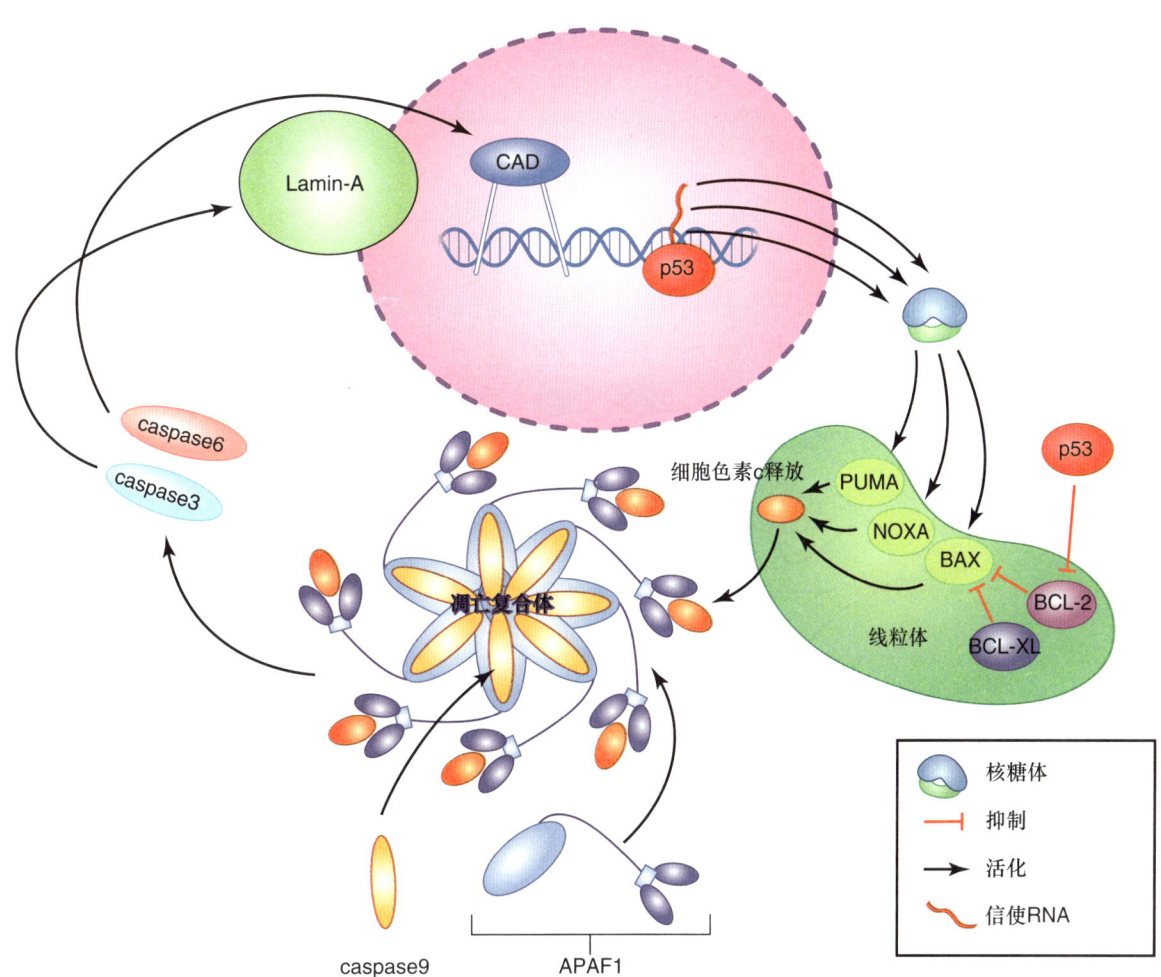

图 1.4 在化疗诱导的 DNA 损伤下，p53 蛋白作为核心调控因子，通过内源性的凋亡通路激活，触发肿瘤细胞的程序性死亡机制。本图展示 p53 蛋白在内在凋亡途径中的中心作用并最终激活凋亡复合体。癌基因激活或细胞毒性 DNA 损伤化疗药物可稳定并激活 p53 蛋白。若损伤被修复，细胞得以存活且不会发生恶性转化；反之，若损伤程度超出正常范围，细胞则经历 p53 介导的细胞死亡。在肿瘤发展的进程中，p53 基因的突变往往导致其抑癌功能的丧失。在正常生理条件下，p53 蛋白在 DNA 损伤后通过调控促凋亡蛋白 PUMA、NOXA 和 BAX 以及抗凋亡蛋白 BCL-XL 和 BCL-2 的平衡而调节内在凋亡途径，导致线粒体释放细胞色素 c。当细胞色素 c 结合至凋亡复合体（由 caspase 9 和 APAF1 组成的多聚体），可激活 caspase 3 和 6，进而分别通过 Lamin-A 和 CAD 促进核膜破坏和 DNA 碎片化。"p"表示蛋白质，后面跟随以千道尔顿为单位的分子量，如 p53。箭头表示通路中的活化进程，红色"T"符号表示通路抑制作用。APAF1，凋亡蛋白酶激活因子 1；BAX，BCL 相关 X；BCL-2，B 细胞淋巴瘤 2；BCL-XL，B 细胞淋巴瘤 XL；CAD，caspase 激活脱氧核糖核酸酶；NOXA，拉丁文，意为损伤；PUMA，p53 上调凋亡介质。有关凋亡途径及其在肿瘤治疗中应用的更详细综述，请参见 Carneiro BA, El-Deiry WS, Nat. Rev. Clin. Oncol. 2020 Jul；17（7）：395-417.

修复系统缺陷会增加突变基因的数量，肿瘤细胞突变基因总数则称为肿瘤突变负荷。MSI 与肿瘤突变负荷相关，高 MSI（MSI-H）肿瘤细胞在内质网中合成突变蛋白，并通过主要组织相容性复合体 -Ⅰ（MHC-Ⅰ）呈递这些突变蛋白为新抗原。这一过程已成为预测免疫治疗反应性的重要生物标志物。此外，部分卵巢癌、乳腺癌、前列腺癌和胰腺癌患者存在 FANC 复合体成分（包括 *BRCA* 基因）突变，影响 DNA 双链断裂修复进而产生同源重组修复缺陷（HRD）。MSI 和 HRD 可由胚系（从父母遗传）突变或体细胞（来源于肿瘤）突变获得。其中某些肿瘤存在替代性 DNA 修复系统，即聚腺苷二磷酸核糖聚合酶（PRAP）系统，这为利用 PARP 抑制剂通过合成致死机制治疗肿瘤（特别是在 BRCA 突变细胞中）提供了可能。PARP 抑制剂作为口服用药可用于同源重组修复缺陷的肿瘤患者。

癌基因促发增殖

癌基因的突变是肿瘤发生发展过程中的关键驱动力之一，其通过激活对细胞增殖至关重要的信号通路，将原本正常的细胞转变为不受控制的肿瘤细胞（图 1.6），例如，慢性髓细胞性白血病（CML）发生于 9 号染色体原癌基因 *ABL* 转位至 22 号染色体 *BCR* 基因，形成 *BCR-*

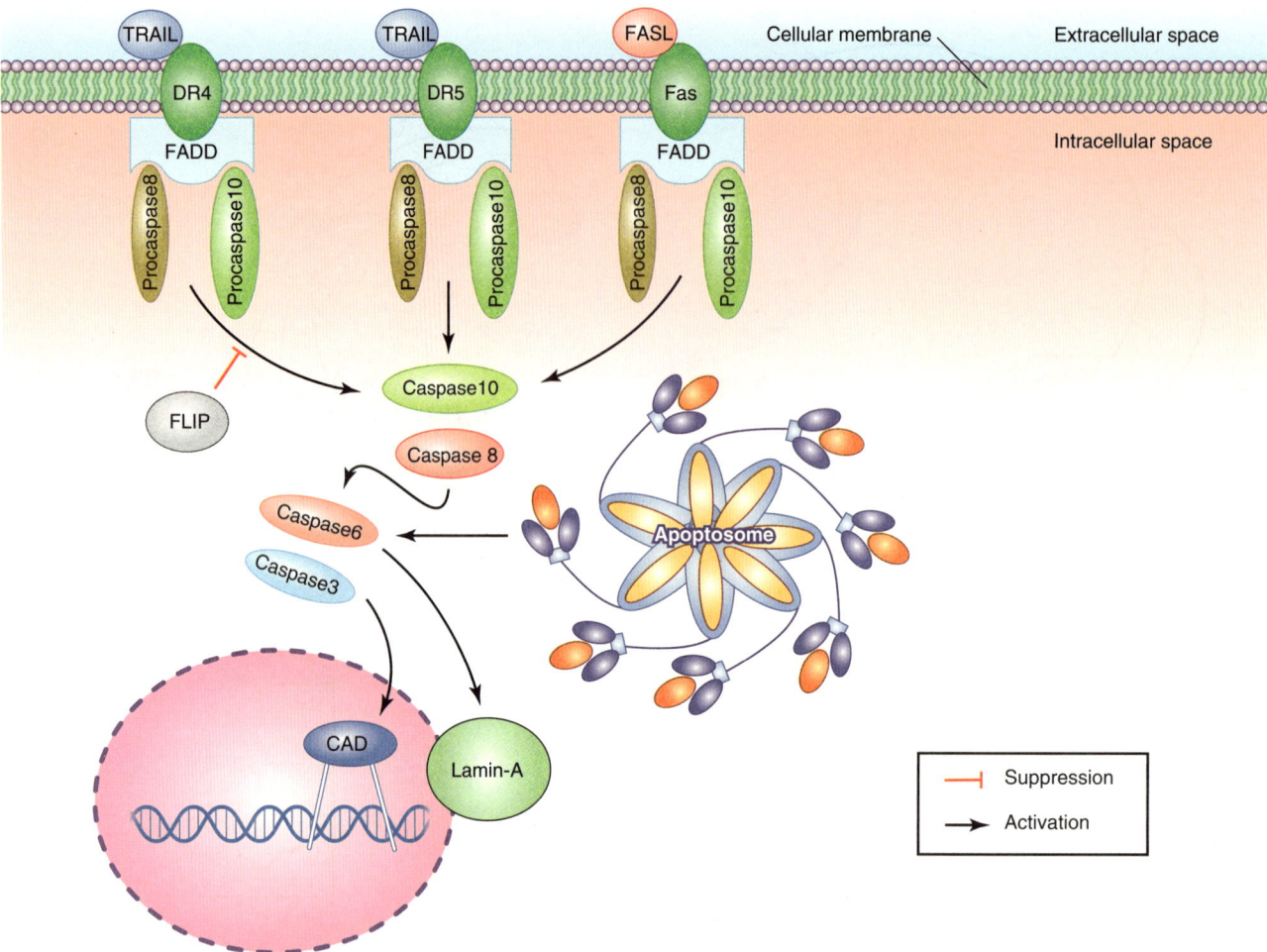

Fig. 1.5 The innate immune system, through the extrinsic apoptosis pathway, eliminates transformed cells. Extracellular molecules (TRAIL and FASL) bind to transmembrane receptors (DR4, DR5, and FAS), anchoring the intracellular adaptor protein FADD to the cellular membrane. Then, FADD recruits initiators Pro-caspase 8 and Pro-caspase 10, which are then cleaved to their active forms, caspase 8 and caspase 10. This activation reaction is tightly regulated by c-FLIP. The apoptosome, a multimer of caspase 9 and APAF1, leads to activation of executioner caspases 3 and 6, promoting nuclear membrane destruction by Lamin-A and DNA fragmentation by CAD, respectively. The *TRAIL, DR5,* and *FAS* genes are regulated by p53. The *"p"* denotes protein, followed by molecular weight in Kilodaltons, as in p53. *Arrows* indicate activation processes in the pathway. *"T" symbols* indicate suppression of a pathway. *DR,* Death receptor; *FADD,* FAS-associated protein with death domain; *FAS,* FS-7 (a cell line)-associated surface antigen; *FASL,* FAS ligand; *FLIP,* FADD-like interleukin 1 beta-converting enzyme inhibitory protein; *TRAIL,* tumor necrosis factor-related apoptosis inducing ligand. For a more detailed review of the apoptosis pathway and its exploitation in cancer therapy, see Carneiro BA, El-Deiry WS, *Nat. Rev. Clin. Oncol.* 2020 Jul;17(7):395–417.

the *BCR* gene on chromosome 22. The new protein formed by expression of the combined gene *BCR-ABL* sends unchecked growth-promoting signals to the nucleus. An activating mutation in one allele of an oncogene is usually sufficient to promote tumorigenesis (e.g., *KRAS*).

Because oncogenes activate pathways that drive cancer growth, their discovery has led to specifically designed drugs that target the products of these genes and the pathways they control. For example, among patients with breast cancer, HER2 amplification serves as a biomarker that identifies those who will benefit from treatment with the anti-HER2 monoclonal antibody trastuzumab. Similarly, activating mutations in EGFR serve to identify patients with non–small cell lung cancer who will improve with the use of drugs (erlotinib, gefitinib, afatinib, dacomitinib, osimertinib) that specifically inhibit the mutated form of EGFR. Another example is BRAF mutations in melanoma, which are inhibited by the FDA-approved drugs dabrafenib, vemurafenib, and encorafenib. This paradigm—identify a mutated oncogene, find a specific drug that inhibits the activated mutant protein, and treat patients who have the specific mutation with a drug that affects the mutated protein—has

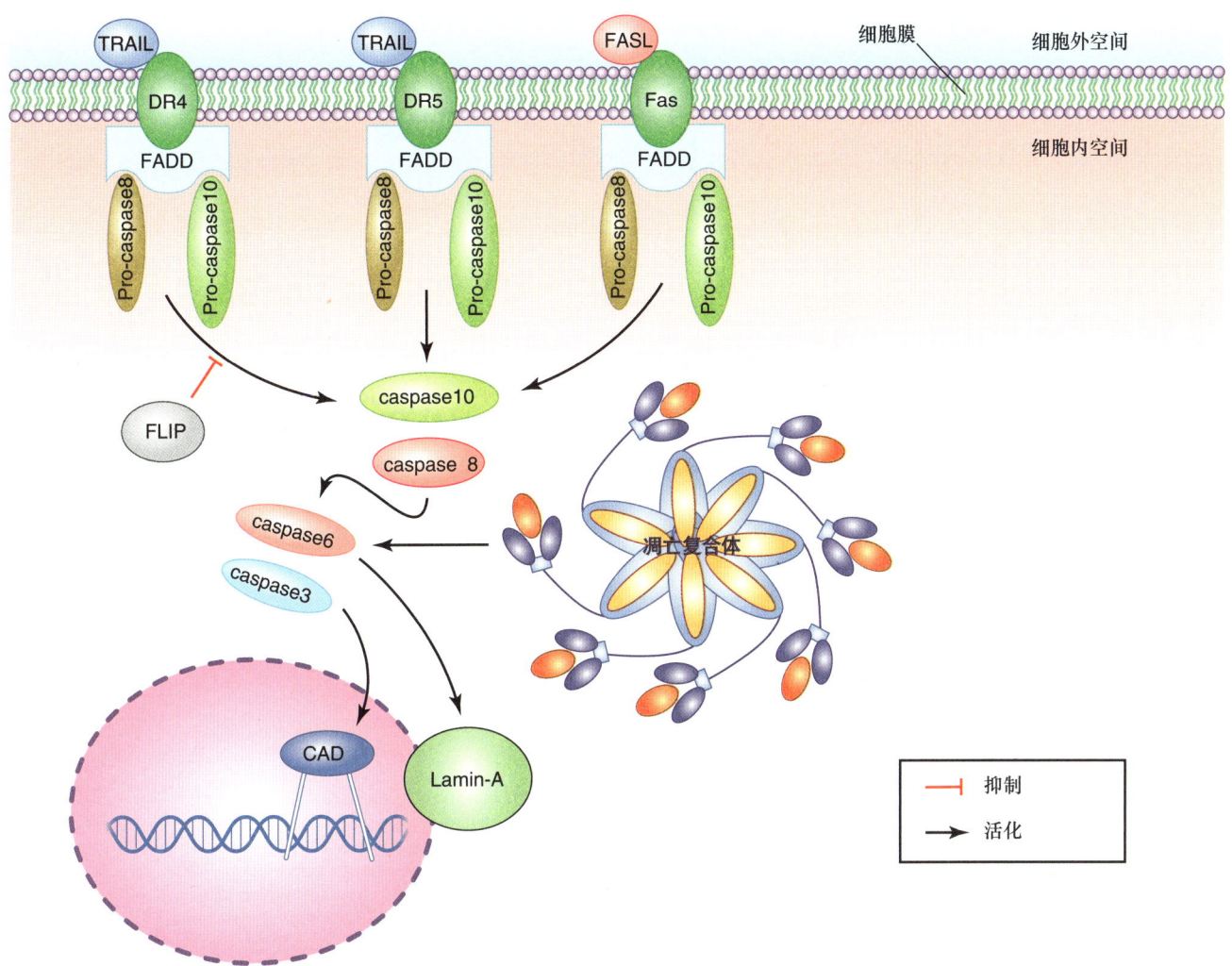

图 1.5 先天免疫系统经外在凋亡途径清除转化细胞。细胞外分子（TRAIL 和 FASL）与跨膜受体（DR4、DR5 和 FAS）结合，将细胞内接头蛋白 FADD 锚定至细胞膜。FADD 募集启动型 Pro-caspase 8 和 Pro-caspase 10，后两者随后被切割为活性形式，即 caspase 8 和 caspase 10。上述激活反应由 c-FLIP 严密调控。由 caspase 9 和 APAF1 组成的凋亡复合体激活执行蛋白 caspase 3 和 6，分别通过 Lamin-A 和 CAD 促进核膜破坏和 DNA 碎片化。*TRAIL*、*DR5* 和 *FAS* 基因由 p53 调节。"p"表示蛋白质，后面跟随以千道尔顿为单位的分子量，如 p53。箭头表示通路中的活化进程，红色"T"符号表示通路抑制作用。DR，死亡受体；FADD，FAS 相关蛋白，具有死亡结构域；Fas，FS-7（一种细胞系）相关表面抗原；FASL，FAS 配体；FLIP，FADD 样白介素 1β 转化酶抑制蛋白；TRAIL，肿瘤坏死因子相关凋亡诱导配体。有关凋亡途径及其在肿瘤治疗中应用的更详细综述，请参见 Carneiro BA，El-Deiry WS，Nat. Rev. Clin. Oncol. 2020 Jul；17（7）：395-417。

ABL 融合基因并表达全新蛋白质，而这种蛋白质能向细胞核发送不受控制的促生长信号。癌基因中一个等位基因的激活突变通常足以促进肿瘤发生（例如 *KRAS*）。

鉴于癌基因激活肿瘤生长相关通路，研究人员设计出特异性药物以靶向癌基因产物及其调控的相关通路。例如，HER2 扩增作为一种生物标志物可鉴定出对抗 HER2 单克隆抗体曲妥珠单抗治疗获益的乳腺癌患者；类似地，EGFR 突变可用于筛选对特异性抑制 EGFR 突变类药物（厄洛替尼、吉非替尼、阿法替尼、达克替尼、奥希替尼）治疗获益的非小细胞肺癌患者；此外，FDA 批准药物达拉非尼、维莫非尼和恩科拉非尼可抑制黑色素瘤 BRAF 突变。通过鉴定突变癌基因并找到抑制活化突变蛋白的特异性药物，这一治疗模式已被广泛验证为针对携带特定癌基因突变的肿瘤患

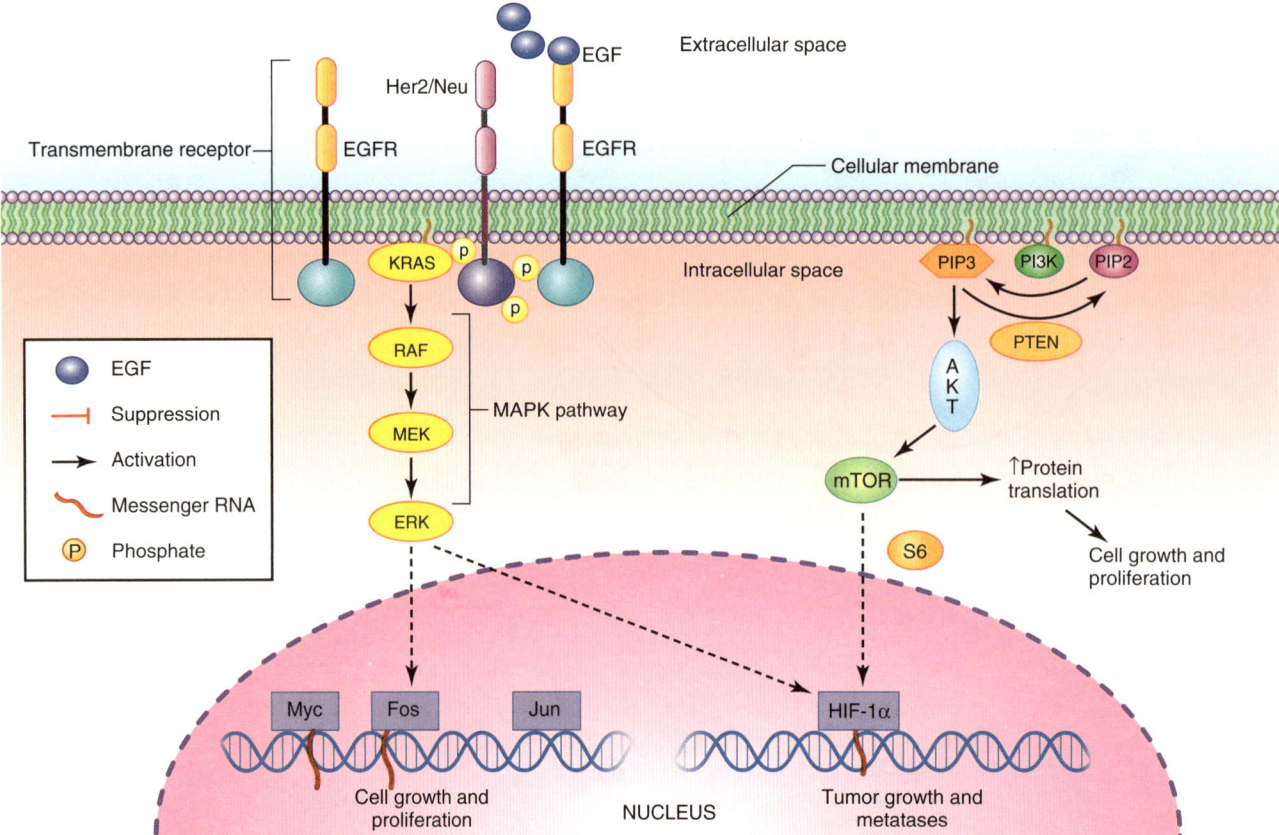

Fig. 1.6 Principles of intracellular cancer signaling and targeted therapeutics. Ligands are extracellular molecules such as the epidermal growth factor (EGF) which binds to a transmembrane receptor known as the EGF receptor (EGFR), to activate intracellular cancer pathways. Illustrated here are the MAPK (mitogen-activated protein kinase) and the phosphatidyl inositol-3 kinase/mammalian target of rapamycin (PI3K/mTOR) pathways. These pathways converge into proliferative genetic programs mediated by transcription factors including myelocytomatosis (Myc), Fos, Jun, hypoxia-inducing factor-1α (HIF-1α), and others. These transcription factors turn on genes that promote cell growth and proliferation as well as tumor growth and metastases. The major effect of mTOR signaling is to stimulate protein translation that is required for cell growth and proliferation. Modern cancer therapy has evolved to include therapeutic agents targeting most of these tumor promoting proteins. Examples include trastuzumab (Her2/neu), cetuximab (EGFR), dabrafenib (RAF), trametinib (MEK), copanlisib (PI3K), mTOR (everolimus), and many others. *Yellow "p"* denotes phosphate. *Arrows* indicate activation processes in the pathway. *Red "T" symbols* indicate suppression of a pathway. Activation of Myc, Fos, and Jun by the MAPK pathway and HIF-1α by mTOR and S6 kinase is indirect. *AKT*, AK mouse strain transforming retrovirus (AKT is also known as PKB [protein kinase B]); *ERK*, extracellular signal regulated kinase; *Her2/neu*, human EGF receptor 2/neural; *KRAS*, Kirsten rat sarcoma; *MEK*, MAP (mitogen-activated protein)/ERK kinase; *PIP3*, phosphatidylinositol (3,4,5)-trisphosphate; *PTEN*, phosphatase and tensin homolog; *RAF*, rapidly accelerating fibrosarcoma.

repeatedly been proven to be a successful approach. Recently, targeting of a specific KRAS G12C driver mutation has been achieved through a small molecule that covalently attaches to the cysteine, and this appears efficacious in some patients with non-small cell lung cancer and colon cancer. Other significant advances involved the development and FDA-approval of Ret inhibitors selpercatinib and pralsetinib for multiple tumor types including non-small cell lung cancer. Capmatinib inhibits Met exon-skipping mutant non-small cell lung cancers and sonic hedgehog pathway inhibitors vismodegib and sonidegib are used for the treatment of advanced basal cell carcinoma. Ongoing research aims to target additional oncogenic cancer pathways such as the Wnt/Beta-catenin and Notch pathways (Fig. 1.7).

Tumor Suppressor Genes Disrupt Growth Checkpoints

The inactivation of both alleles of a tumor suppressor gene (e.g., retinoblastoma, *RB1*) results in cancer, most commonly by an inherited mutation in an allele followed by loss of heterozygosity due to epigenetic events or aneuploidy (loss or gain of part of chromosomes). The tumor suppressor gene *TP53* is the most commonly mutated gene in human cancer. The p53 protein is a transcription factor that activates various genes such as p21 (WAF1) and multiple genes that induce cell death (Figs. 1.3–1.5). Mutation of this *TP53* gene can be inherited (Li-Fraumeni syndrome) in families that have higher rates of a variety of leukemia, sarcoma, breast, and brain tumors, or most commonly is acquired during cancer growth. Loss of two copies of a tumor suppressor gene leading

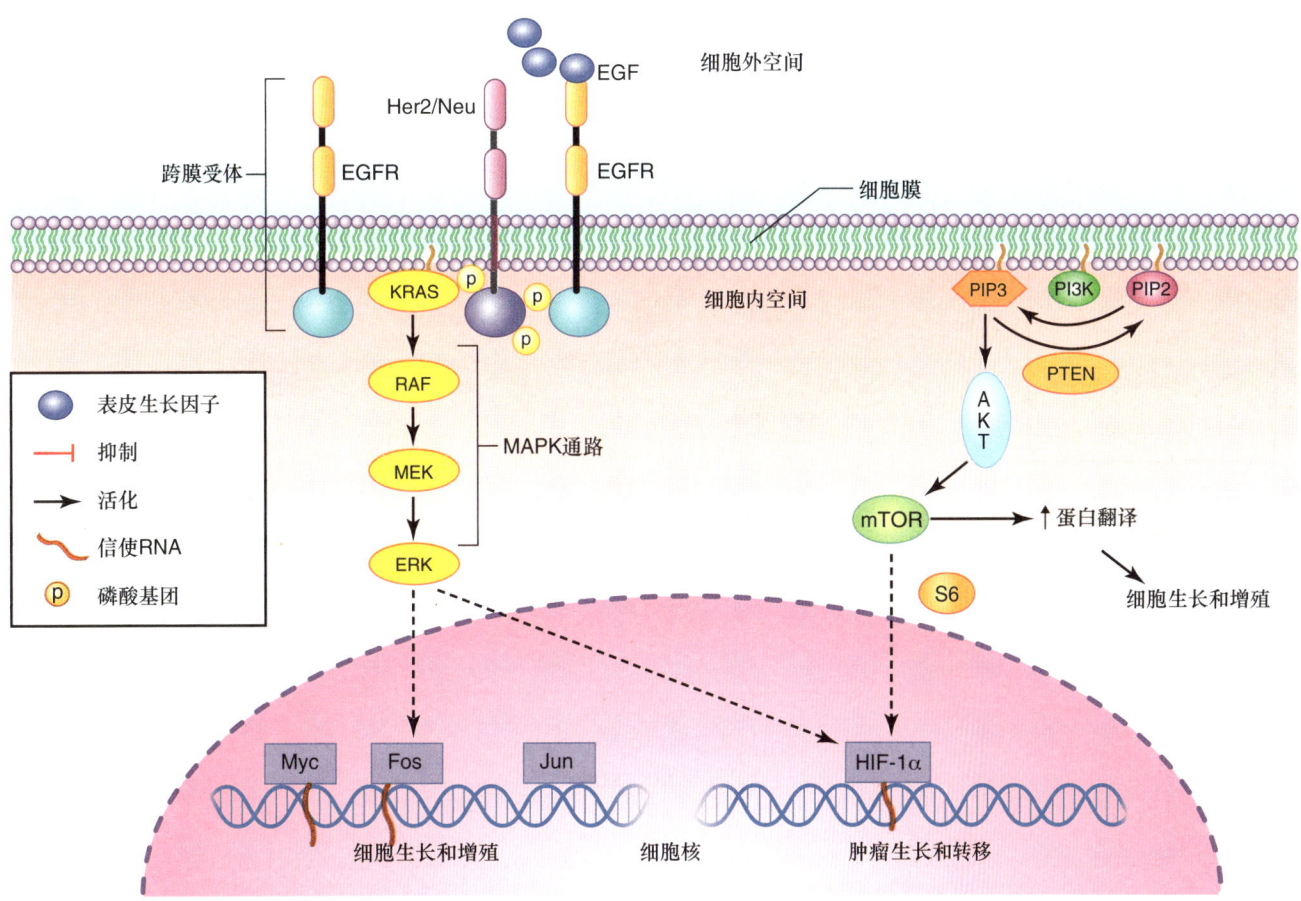

图 1.6 胞内肿瘤信号传导及靶向治疗的原理。细胞外分子作为配体，如表皮生长因子（EGF），与跨膜受体如 EGF 受体（EGFR）结合，以激活胞内促肿瘤通路。此处展示的是 MAPK（丝裂原活化蛋白激酶）和磷脂酰肌醇-3 激酶 / 哺乳动物雷帕霉素靶蛋白（PI3K/mTOR）通路。这些通路汇聚至由髓细胞组织增生蛋白（Myc）、Fos、Jun、缺氧诱导因子-1α（HIF-1α）等转录因子介导的增殖基因程序。这些转录因子可启动促进细胞生长、增殖以及肿瘤生长和转移的基因表达。mTOR 信号传导的主要作用是增强细胞生长和增殖所需的蛋白质翻译。现代肿瘤学治疗已囊括了大多数可靶向上述促肿瘤蛋白的药物，例如曲妥珠单抗（Her2/Neu）、西妥昔单抗（EGFR）、达拉非尼（RAF）、曲美替尼（MEK）、考比利斯（PI3K）、mTOR 抑制剂依维莫司和其他药物。黄色"p"表示磷酸基团，箭头表示通路中的活化进程，红色"T"符号表示通路抑制作用。MAPK 通路对 Myc、Fos 和 Jun 的激活作用以及 mTOR 和 S6 激酶对 HIF-1α 的激活作用均是间接的。AKT，AK 小鼠品系转化逆转录病毒［AKT 也称为 PKB（蛋白激酶 B）］；ERK，细胞外信号调节激酶；Her2/Neu，人 EGF 受体 2/ 神经；KRAS，克里斯顿大鼠肉瘤；MEK，MAP（丝裂原活化蛋白）/ERK 激酶；PIP3，磷脂酰肌醇（3,4,5）- 三磷酸；PTEN，磷酸酶和张力蛋白同源物；RAF，快速加速纤维肉瘤

者的高效策略。近年来，通过共价结合半胱氨酸的小分子以特异性靶向 KRAS G12C 驱动突变，已在某些非小细胞肺癌和结肠癌患者中显示出疗效。其他重要进展包括：获 FDA 批准的 RET 抑制剂塞尔帕替尼和普拉替尼，可用于包括非小细胞肺癌在内的多种肿瘤类型；MET 外显子跳跃突变抑制剂卡马替尼治疗非小细胞肺癌；音猬因子通路抑制剂维斯莫德吉和索尼德吉用于治疗晚期基底细胞癌；正在进行的研究旨在探索靶向 Wnt/β - 连环蛋白和 Notch 通路等其他的致癌基因通路的潜在疗法（图 1.7）。

抑癌基因干扰生长检查点

抑癌基因（例如视网膜母细胞瘤基因 *RB1*）的双等位基因失活会导致肿瘤发生。最常见的情况是一个等位基因中存在遗传性突变，随后由于表观遗传事件或非整倍体（染色体部分减少或增加）引起的杂合性缺失而导致双等位基因失活。*TP53* 作为人类肿瘤中最常突变的基因之一，其编码的 p53 蛋白作为关键转录因子激活多种基因如 p21（WAF）和诱导细胞死亡基因（图 1.3 至图 1.5）。*TP53* 基因突变可通过遗传获得（Li-Fraumeni 综合征），携带有此突变的家系患白血病、肉瘤、乳腺癌和脑肿瘤等肿瘤的概率更高，而大多数情况下此突变在肿瘤生长的过程中获得。抑癌基因双拷

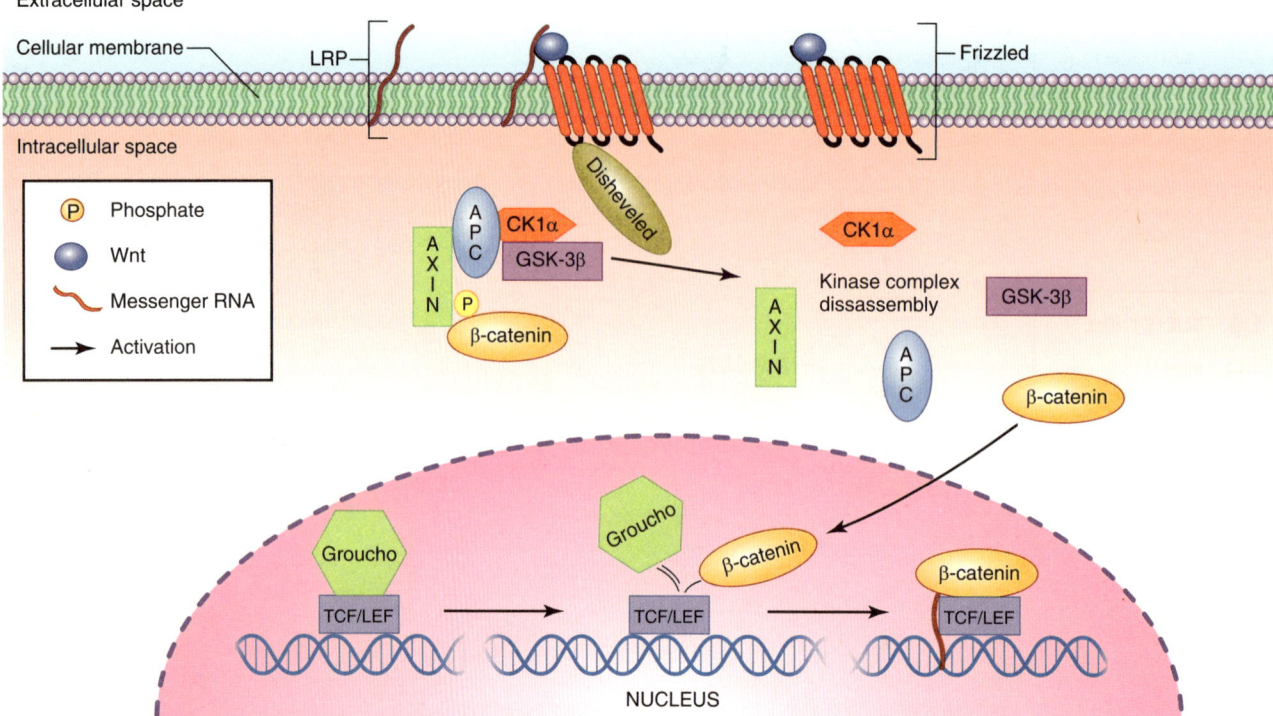

Fig. 1.7 The beta-catenin intracellular cancer signaling pathway is involved in cancer development. The extracellular molecule Wnt engages the transmembrane proteins LDL receptor related protein (LRP) and Frizzled, which activate the intracellular adaptor protein Disheveled. Then, Disheveled disassembles the kinase complex composed of the proteins Adenomatous Polyposis Coli (APC), Axin, Glycogen Synthase Kinase-3β (GSK-3β), and Casein Kinase-1α (CK-1α). This kinase complex usually breaks down beta-catenin by tagging it for destruction through phosphorylation. However, the activation of Disheveled by Frizzled bound to Wnt promotes kinase complex disassembly, stabilizing beta-catenin. Finally, beta-catenin crosses the nuclear membrane displacing the transcription repressor Groucho, which enables TCF/LEF transcriptional activity that activates target genes such as *MYC* and the Cyclin D gene (*CCND1*). This pathway is deregulated in most colon cancers through *APC* mutation (both sporadic and inherited forms of colon cancer such as Familial Adenomatous Polyposis). In other tumors, β-catenin mutations are more commonly observed. This pathway remains largely untapped for cancer therapeutic development. Inhibitors of GSK-3β, Wnt, and β-catenin are currently under development. *Arrows* indicate activation processes in a cellular pathway. *TCF/LEF*, T-cell factor/lymphoid enhancer-binding factor; *Wnt*, wingless/integrated.

to cancer was predicted by Knudson's two-hit hypothesis. Tumor suppressor genes can be inactivated by viral genes including Human Papilloma Virus (HPV) E6 and E7 that target p53 and Rb. HPV types 16 and 18 can cause cervical cancer and head and neck cancer, and there is a preventative vaccine.

Hypoxia, Angiogenesis, Invasion, and Metastases

Under hypoxic pressure from the tumor microenvironment, cancer cells shift their metabolism towards aerobic glycolysis. This so-called Warburg effect diverts Krebs cycle intermediate metabolites towards nucleic acid and amino acid production, favoring cell growth. Although mutations affecting enzymes from the Krebs cycle are uncommon in cancer (i.e., fumarate hydratase in certain kidney tumors and succinate dehydrogenase in pheochromocytomas), isocitrate dehydrogenase (IDH) 1 or 2 are commonly mutated in certain brain, bile duct, and acute myelogenous leukemia and are targeted by the FDA-approved drugs ivosidenib (mutant IDH1 inhibitor) and enasidenib (mutant IDH2 inhibitor). Also, the upregulation of a transcription factor known as hypoxia-inducing factor induces overexpression of the vascular endothelial growth factors (VEGF). VEGF then co-opts endothelial cells to form new aberrant vessels (angiogenesis), allowing the growing mass to survive hypoxia. These ill-walled vessels allow elopement of cancer cells to the bloodstream, priming distant organ colonization (metastasis). The angiogenesis inhibitors include the biologic agents bevacizumab, ramucirumab, and ziv-aflibercept and some small molecules such as sunitinib, sorafenib, regorafenib, lenvatinib, cabozantinib among others. Finally, hypoxia upregulates a series of transcription factors (Snail, Slug, TWIST, ZEB 1 and 2) that coordinate cell-to-cell adhesion dysregulation promoting phenotypic changes (epithelial-mesenchymal transition) that enable cell migration and metastasis. Such is the importance of the hypoxia

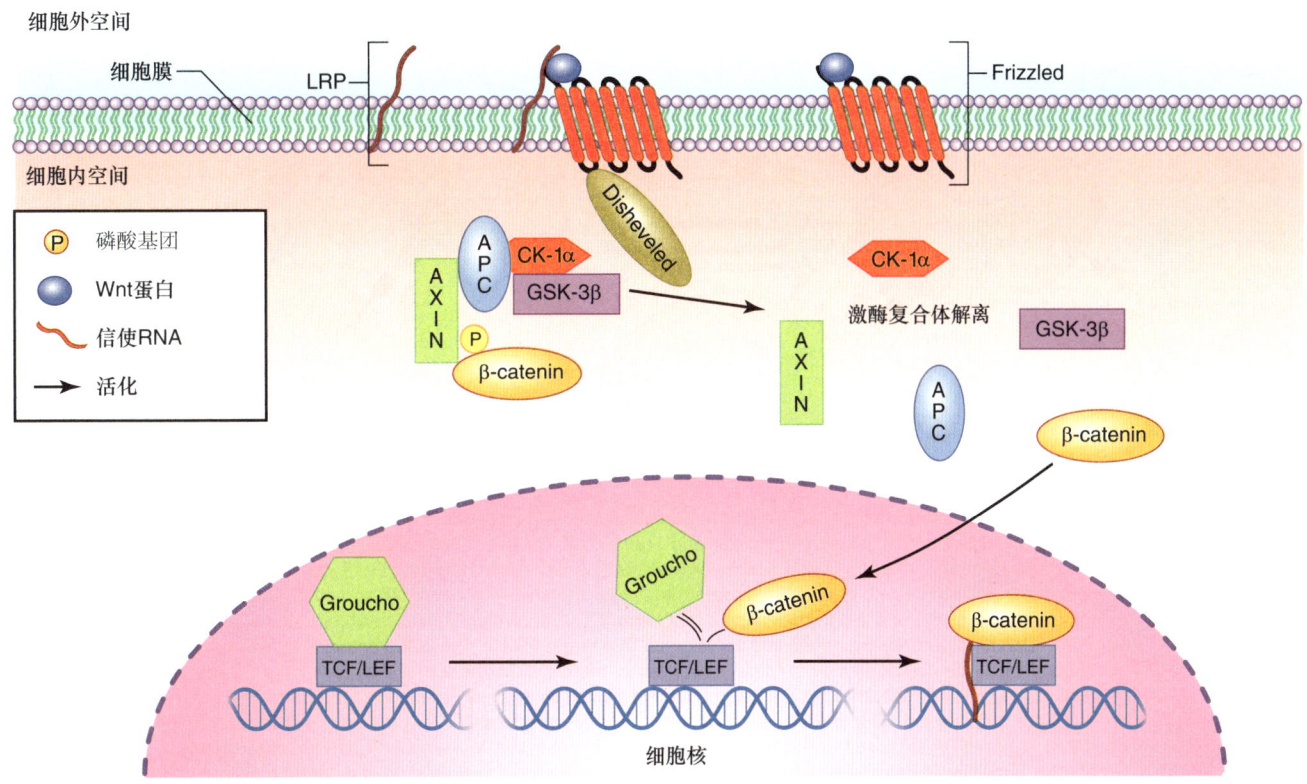

图 1.7 β-连环蛋白（catenin）胞内信号传导通路参与肿瘤发展。细胞外分子 Wnt 与跨膜蛋白 LDL 受体相关蛋白（LRP）和 Frizzled 结合，激活细胞内接头蛋白 Disheveled，后者可解离由腺瘤性息肉病蛋白（APC）、轴突蛋白（AXIN）、糖原合酶激酶 -3β（GSK-3β）和酪蛋白激酶 -1α（CK-1α）组成的激酶复合体。此激酶复合体通常利用 β-连环蛋白磷酸化对其标记并抑制其功能。然而，由 Frizzled 与 Wnt 结合激活的 Disheveled 促进激酶复合体解离，并稳定 β-连环蛋白。最后，β-连环蛋白穿过核膜，取代转录抑制因子 Groucho，从而启动 TCF/LEF 转录活性，激活 *MYC* 和细胞周期蛋白 D 基因（*CCND1*）等靶基因。在多数结肠癌（包括散发性和遗传性结肠癌，如家族性腺瘤性息肉病）中，*APC* 基因突变导致 Wnt/β-连环蛋白通路异常调控；而在其他肿瘤中，β-连环蛋白突变更为常见。此通路在肿瘤治疗方面的价值尚未被挖掘。针对 GSK-3β、Wnt 和 β-连环蛋白的抑制剂目前正在研发中。箭头表示细胞通路中的活化进程。TCF/LEF，T 细胞因子/淋巴增强子结合因子；Wnt，无翼（wingless）/整合（integrated）

贝缺失导致肿瘤发生被称为克努森二次打击假说。病毒基因如靶向 p53 和 Rb 的人乳头瘤病毒（HPV）E6 和 E7 等，可抑制抑癌基因活性。HPV 16 和 18 型能导致宫颈癌和头颈癌发生，目前已有针对 HPV 16 和 18 型的预防性疫苗。

缺氧、血管生成、侵袭和转移

Warburg 效应是指肿瘤细胞在微环境缺氧压力下将其代谢转向有氧糖酵解，将三羧酸循环中间代谢产物转向核酸和氨基酸生成，从而有利于肿瘤细胞生长。尽管在肿瘤中影响三羧酸循环酶的基因突变并不常见（例如某些肾脏肿瘤的富马酸水合酶和嗜铬细胞瘤的琥珀酸脱氢酶），但在某些脑肿瘤、胆道肿瘤和急性髓细胞性白血病中异柠檬酸脱氢酶（IDH）1 或 2 常常发生突变。这些 IDH 突变成为了治疗的新靶点，FDA 已批准艾伏尼布（针对 IDH1 突变）和恩西地平（针对 IDH2 突变）等抑制剂，为患者带来了新的治疗希望。此外，一种被称为缺氧诱导因子的转录因子上调会诱导血管内皮生长因子（VEGF）过表达。VEGF 随后诱导内皮细胞形成新的异常血管（血管生成），使不断生长的肿瘤得以在缺氧环境中生存，而这些薄壁血管可使肿瘤细胞进入血液，促发远隔器官定植（转移）。为应对这一挑战，目前已开发出血管生成抑制剂，包括生物制剂贝伐珠单抗、雷莫西尤单抗和阿柏西普以及小分子药物如舒尼替尼、索拉非尼、瑞格非尼、仑伐替尼、卡博替尼等。最后，缺氧会上调一系列转录因子如 Snail、Slug、TWIST、ZEB 1 和 ZEB2 等引起细胞间黏附失调，促进表型变化（上皮-间质转化），这有助于肿瘤细胞迁移和转移。上述表明缺氧通路在肿瘤发生发展中至关重要，因此 2019 年诺贝尔生理学或医

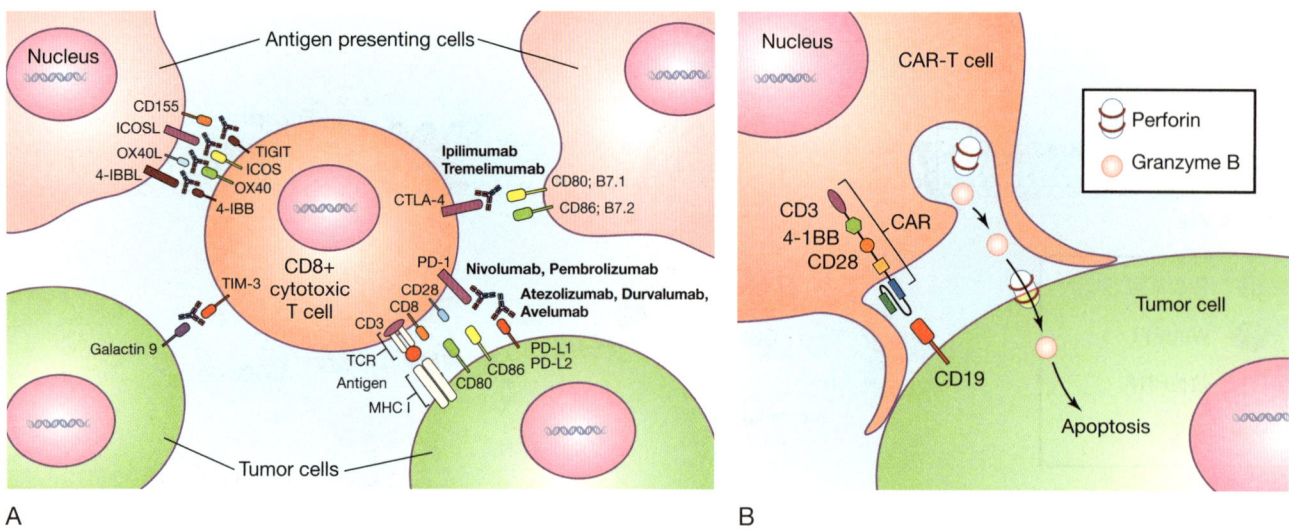

Fig. 1.8 Cancer immunotherapy. (A) Targets for cancer immune checkpoint therapy. Depicted here is a CD8+ cytotoxic T cell, an antigen presenting cell, and a tumor cell. These cell-cell interactions may take place within a primary tumor, draining lymph nodes, or metastatic sites. On the right of the T cell are immune checkpoints that have been successfully targeted in cancer therapy with now FDA-approved antibodies. Examples include ipilimumab and tremelimumab that target CTLA-4, nivolumab and pembrolizumab that target PD-1, and atezolizumab, avelumab, and durvalumab that target PD-L1. These therapeutics are currently being combined with chemotherapy or targeted therapy in the clinic. To the left of the T-cell are a number of checkpoints for which therapeutics are being tested in clinical trials. They include the T cell targets TIGIT, ICOS, OX40, TIM-3, and 4-1BB. (B) Cellular chimeric antigen receptor-T cell (CAR-T) therapy has been developed and is now FDA-approved in the treatment of acute lymphocytic leukemia and diffuse large B cell lymphoma. Shown is an engineered CAR-T cell with an immune synapse, with binding of different receptors, release of granzyme B and perforin, leading to apoptosis of a target tumor cell.

pathways in cancer that the Physiology or Medicine Nobel prize of 2019 was bestowed on William G. Kaelin, Gregg L. Semenza, and Peter J. Ratcliffe.

Immune Escape

The immune system is constantly killing cancer cells. Under pressure of this constant immune vigilance, cancer cells with random mutations that allow re-expression of useful genes that are usually dormant survive. Among the genes involved in this "immune escape," one of the best studied is *PD-L1* (programmed-death ligand 1). *PD-L1* usually is expressed in the placenta, preventing a mother's immune system from attacking her fetus, ultimately a foreign body. When tumors express *PD-L1* it binds its receptor PD-1 in cytotoxic T CD8+ cells, rendering them ineffective. One of the most revolutionary therapies in oncology is use of monoclonal antibodies to *PD-L1* and other so-called immune checkpoints (Fig. 1.8). They have been so successful that the scientists James Allison and Tasuku Honjo who were responsible to bring them to the clinic were awarded the Nobel Prize in Physiology or Medicine in 2018.

Dr. Steven Rosenberg observed that T cells fighting cancer could be removed from patients, cultured ex-vivo, and used as cancer therapies. This adoptive cell therapy acquired an iteration when Carl June selected patient-derived (autologous) cells through special magnetic beads, introduced genetically engineered antibodies linked to immune checkpoint receptors through viral vectors, and infused it back to the same patients who donated the cells. Chimeric antigenic receptor (CAR)-T cell therapy has been developed to target surface proteins in various tumors, such as CD19 in acute lymphocytic leukemia, which was approved by the FDA in 2017. The first patient treated in a clinical trial in 2012 is cancer free by 2020. Off-the-shelf CAR-T cells, extracted from allogeneic donors and engineered to avoid rejection by the recipient, are in development. Umbilical cord-derived CAR-natural killer (CAR-NK) cells are also under development.

SUGGESTED READINGS

Chae YK, Anker JF, Carneiro BA, et al: Genomic landscape of DNA repair genes in cancer, Oncotarget 7(17):23312–23321, 2016.

Classon M, Harlow E: The retinoblastoma tumour suppressor in development and cancer, Nat Rev Cancer 2(12):910–917, 2002.

El-Deiry WS: p21(WAF1) Mediates cell-cycle inhibition, relevant to cancer suppression and therapy, Cancer Res 76(18):5189–5191, 2016.

Hanahan D, Weinberg RA: Hallmarks of cancer: the next generation, Cell 144(5):646–674, 2011.

Kamps R, Brandão RD, Bosch BJ, et al: Next-Generation sequencing in oncology: genetic Diagnosis, Risk prediction and cancer classification, Int J Mol Sci (2)18, 2017.

Koike T, Kimura N, Miyazaki K, et al: Hypoxia induces adhesion molecules on cancer cells: a missing link between Warburg effect and induction of selectin-ligand carbohydrates, Proc Natl Acad Sci U S A 101(21):8132–8137, 2004.

Shay JW: Role of Telomeres and telomerase in Aging and cancer, Cancer Discov 6(6):584–593, 2016.

Vogelstein B, Lane D, Levine AJ: Surfing the p53 network, Nature 408(6810):307–310, 2000.

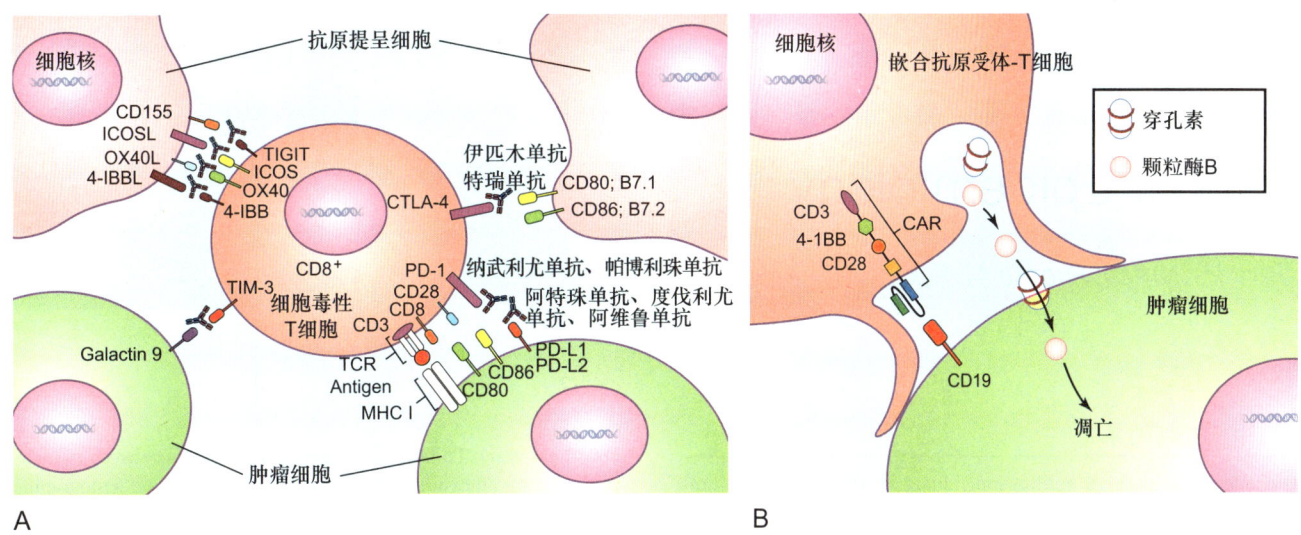

图 1.8 肿瘤免疫治疗。（**A**）肿瘤免疫检查点治疗靶点。此处展示的是一个 CD8⁺ 细胞毒性 T 细胞，一个抗原提呈细胞和一个肿瘤细胞。这些细胞间的相互作用可发生于原发肿瘤、引流淋巴结或转移部位。T 细胞右侧的免疫检查点，是可在抗肿瘤治疗中成功开发并已获 FDA 批准使用的抗体，例如靶向 CTLA-4 的伊匹木单抗和特瑞单抗，靶向 PD-1 的纳武利尤单抗和帕博利珠单抗，以及靶向 PD-L1 的阿特珠单抗、阿维鲁单抗和度伐利尤单抗。这些治疗方法目前在临床上与化疗或靶向治疗相联合；T 细胞的左侧多个检查点，对其治疗方式目前正在临床试验中进行检测，包括 T 细胞靶点 TIGIT、ICOS、OX40、TIM-3 和 4-1BB。（**B**）细胞嵌合抗原受体 -T 细胞（CAR-T）治疗已被开发并获得 FDA 批准用于治疗急性淋巴细胞白血病和弥漫大 B 细胞淋巴瘤。此处显示的是一个具有免疫突触的工程改造的 CAR-T 细胞，它与不同受体结合，释放颗粒酶 B 和穿孔素，导致靶点肿瘤细胞凋亡

学奖授予 William G. Kaelin、Gregg L. Semenza 和 Peter J. Ratcliffe。

免疫逃逸

免疫系统不断杀死肿瘤细胞，在此持续免疫监视压力下，部分肿瘤细胞因携带随机突变而重新表达通常处于休眠状态的重要基因，从而得以存活。在这些涉及免疫逃逸相关机制的基因中，*PD-L1*（程序性死亡配体 1）是最受瞩目的研究焦点之一。*PD-L1* 通常在胎盘中表达，以防止母体免疫系统攻击实际上以异物形式存在的胎儿。当肿瘤表达 *PD-L1* 时，可与细胞毒性 CD8⁺ T 细胞上 PD-1 受体结合，从而抑制其功能。应用针对 *PD-L1* 和其他免疫检查点的单克隆抗体（图 1.8），这一革命性的治疗方法在肿瘤学领域取得了巨大成功。因此 2018 年诺贝尔生理学或医学奖授予了作为免疫治疗先驱的科学家 James Allison 和 Tasuku Honjo。

Steven Rosenberg 博士提出杀伤肿瘤的 T 细胞能够从患者体内取出，进行离体培养后用于治疗肿瘤。Carl June 利用特殊磁珠分选患者来源（自体）细胞，通过病毒载体引入与免疫检查点受体相连接的基因工程抗体，随后将其回输至供体患者，是上述过继性细胞治疗的拓展。嵌合抗原受体（CAR）-T 细胞治疗已被开发用于靶向多种肿瘤的表面蛋白，如急性淋巴细胞白血病中的 CD19，并于 2017 年获 FDA 批准。最早在 2012 年一项临床试验中接受该治疗的患者，到 2020 年已实现无瘤生存。目前，从同种异体中提取并通过工程改造以避免受体排斥的"现货型"CAR-T 细胞，以及脐带来源的嵌合抗原受体-自然杀伤细胞（CAR-NK），均处于研发之中。

推荐阅读

Chae YK, Anker JF, Carneiro BA, et al: Genomic landscape of DNA repair genes in cancer, Oncotarget 7(17):23312–23321, 2016.

Classon M, Harlow E: The retinoblastoma tumour suppressor in development and cancer, Nat Rev Cancer 2(12):910–917, 2002.

El-Deiry WS: p21(WAF1) Mediates cell-cycle inhibition, relevant to cancer suppression and therapy, Cancer Res 76(18):5189–5191, 2016.

Hanahan D, Weinberg RA: Hallmarks of cancer: the next generation, Cell 144(5):646–674, 2011.

Kamps R, Brandão RD, Bosch BJ, et al: Next-Generation sequencing in oncology: genetic Diagnosis, Risk prediction and cancer classification, Int J Mol Sci (2)18, 2017.

Koike T, Kimura N, Miyazaki K, et al: Hypoxia induces adhesion molecules on cancer cells: a missing link between Warburg effect and induction of selectin-ligand carbohydrates, Proc Natl Acad Sci U S A 101(21):8132–8137, 2004.

Shay JW: Role of Telomeres and telomerase in Aging and cancer, Cancer Discov 6(6):584–593, 2016.

Vogelstein B, Lane D, Levine AJ: Surfing the p53 network, Nature 408(6810):307–310, 2000.

Cancer Epidemiology

Gary H. Lyman, Nicole M. Kuderer

INTRODUCTION

Globally, more than 18 million individuals are diagnosed with cancer and nearly 10 million die annually from the disease. At the same time, the number of cancer survivors worldwide is increasing dramatically each year. In the United States in 2020, it is estimated that more than 1.8 million individuals will be diagnosed with cancer, for an age-adjusted incidence rate of 448 per 100,000 population. At the same time, more than 600,000 individuals will die from cancer, for an age-adjusted death rate of 158 per 100,000. Cancer has become the leading cause of mortality among both women and men between the ages of 40 and 80 and the second leading cause of death for most other age groups, including children between 1 and 14 years of age.

The leading types of new invasive cancer cases and cancer-specific deaths are shown in Table 2.1. While breast cancer and prostate cancer are the most common noncutaneous forms of cancer in men and women, respectively, lung cancer is the leading cause of cancer-specific mortality accounting for nearly 30% of cancer deaths in both genders. While mortality rates for gastric and cervical cancers have decreased steadily for decades, overall cancer death rates have decreased some 20% since their height in the early 1990s, with the greatest declines for colorectal, prostate, and lung cancers in men and colorectal and breast cancer in women (Fig. 2.1). Disparities in cancer occurrence and mortality persist despite a reduction in the overall age-adjusted mortality from cancer. Cancer incidence remains highest in the United States among white individuals, likely due to their high rates of lung and female breast cancer. However, black men continue to have the highest gender-specific cancer incidence among men and the highest mortality rates despite considerable reductions in cancer mortality for all genders and races. While white women have the highest cancer incidence among women, black women have the highest gender-specific cancer mortality rate despite gradually falling rates for all races. Cancer mortality rates in developed countries are consistently higher among those from racial and ethnic minority groups, especially African Americans, and among those from lower socioeconomic strata. Greater mortality rates among racial and ethnic minorities are not fully explained by differences in the stage at diagnosis. Socioeconomic factors, access to appropriate treatment, and comorbidities represent additional determinants of greater cancer mortality.

CANCER EPIDEMIOLOGY METHODS

Epidemiologists study disease variation among populations and the factors that influence such variation. The proportion of individuals with disease in the population at a given point in time is the *prevalence* whereas *incidence and mortality rates* represent the number of events in a population over a defined period of time (e.g., cancers per 100,000 per year). To facilitate comparisons of rates between populations, rates are often adjusted for age, sex, race, or other demographic characteristics. The association between a characteristic or exposure with cancer risk is generally assessed in either cohort or case-control studies. *Cohort studies* are generally prospective and evaluate disease experience in exposed and unexposed individuals whereas *case-control studies* assess the exposure experience in individuals with and without disease. The *relative risk (RR)* is a measure of association between exposure and disease with estimates above 1.0 representing an increase in risk. In case-control studies, RR is estimated by the odds ratio because the sizes of the exposed and unexposed populations are often not known. The larger the study population, the more precise the estimate of association is between exposure and disease. However, proper interpretation of the results must explore whether any systematic error or bias has been introduced during the study design or analysis. Confounding factors may obscure or weaken a true association or create a false association because of an association between the factor and both the exposure and disease. Confounding can be evaluated and adjusted for in stratified or multivariate analysis if the potential confounder is recognized and has been properly measured in the data. It is generally not safe to assume that all possible confounding factors have been considered. Therefore, causal inference is seldom justified on the basis of a single study but evolves gradually with study repetition and consideration of other information including animal and other laboratory results, the strength of the association, and a careful consideration of likely confounding factors. Interventions for cancer prevention and screening are generally studied in randomized controlled trials requiring large numbers of participants, close monitoring for adherence in the intervention, long-term follow-up, and appropriate ascertainment of disease and disease-free status.

RISK FACTORS

Genetic

Risk factors for developing cancer can be grouped as either genetic (inherited) or acquired. While important for our understanding of carcinogenesis, only a small proportion of cancers are inherited in a mendelian fashion. Neoplasms inherited in an autosomal dominant manner include retinoblastomas, multiple endocrine neoplasia syndromes, and polyposis coli. Several additional pre-neoplastic conditions demonstrate mendelian inheritance with variable penetrance. Several common malignancies demonstrate familial risk patterns with low penetrance, including breast cancer and colorectal cancer. Genetic testing and potential preventative measures are available for several inherited cancer syndromes (Table 2.2). Although genetic testing is available for several identified cancer susceptibility genes, care must be

癌症流行病学

张锦松 译 仲佳 周光飚 审校 王洁 通审

引言

全球范围内，每年有超过1800万人确诊患有癌症，近1000万人死于癌症。与此同时，全球带癌生存人数正以惊人的速度增加。2020年美国有超过180万人被诊断出患有癌症，年龄调整后的发病率为每10万人448例。与此同时，有超过60万人死于癌症，年龄调整后的死亡率为每10万人158例。癌症已成为40～80岁女性和男性的首要死亡原因，也是其他大多数年龄组（包括1～14岁儿童）的第二大死亡原因。

表2.1显示了主要癌症类型的发病率和死亡率。虽然乳腺癌和前列腺癌分别是男性和女性最常见的非皮肤癌类型，但肺癌是导致癌症特异性死亡的最常见原因，在两性中占近30%的癌症死亡人数。在胃癌和宫颈癌的死亡率稳步下降的同时，几十年来，癌症总体死亡率自1990年代初达到峰值后下降了约20%（图2.1）。男性中，结直肠癌、前列腺癌和肺癌的下降幅度最大，女性中则是结直肠癌和乳腺癌。尽管癌症的年龄调整后总死亡率有所下降，但癌症发病率和死亡率的差异依然存在。在美国，白人的癌症发病率仍居最高，这可能与他们较高的肺癌和女性乳腺癌发病率有关。然而，尽管所有性别和种族的癌症死亡率都有显著下降，黑人男性的性别特定癌症发病率仍居男性最高，死亡率也最高。尽管所有种族的癌症死亡率都在逐渐下降，但白人女性的癌症发病率在女性中居最高，黑人女性的癌症死亡率在女性中仍居最高。在发达国家，来自少数族裔群体（尤其是非裔美国人）和低社会经济阶层的人的癌症死亡率始终更高。少数族裔群体具有的更高死亡率不能完全用诊断时的分期不同来解释。社会经济因素、获得适当治疗的机会以及合并症是导致更高癌症死亡率的其他决定性因素。

癌症流行病学研究方法

流行病学家研究人群中疾病的变异以及影响这种变异的因素。在特定时间点，人群中患有疾病的人数比例是患病率，而发病率和死亡率代表在定义的时间段内人群中发生的事件数量（例如，每年每百万人中的癌症数量）。为了便于比较不同人群的发病率，通常会根据年龄、性别、种族或其他人口统计特征对发病率进行调整。通常使用队列研究或病例对照研究来评估特征或暴露与癌症风险之间的关联。队列研究通常是前瞻性的，评估暴露和未暴露人群的疾病经历，而病例对照研究则评估有病和无病人群的暴露经历。相对风险（RR）是暴露与疾病之间关联程度的衡量指标，估计值大于1.0代表风险增加。在病例对照研究中，RR通过比值比来估计，因为暴露和未暴露人群的规模通常无法确定。研究人群越大，暴露与疾病之间的关联程度估计越精确。然而，为了保证结果解释正确性，应该考虑研究设计和分析过程中是否存在系统性误差或偏倚。混杂因素可能会掩盖或削弱真正的关联，或者由于因素与暴露和疾病之间的关联而产生虚假的关联。如果在数据中识别并正确测量了潜在的混杂因素，就可以在分层或多变量分析中进行评估和调整。通常不能假定所有可能的混杂因素都已被考虑，因此，基于单项研究的因果推断通常是不合理的，而是随着研究重复和考虑其他信息（包括动物和其他实验室结果、关联强度以及对可能的混杂因素的仔细考虑）而逐渐发展。癌症预防和筛查的干预措施通常在需要大量参与者的随机对照试验中进行研究，要求对干预措施进行密切监测以确保遵从，进行长期随访，并适当地确定疾病和无病状态。

风险因素

基因

癌症的发病风险因素可分为遗传性（遗传）或获得性两种。虽然有助于我们理解癌变过程，但只有一小部分癌症是以孟德尔方式遗传的。染色体显性遗传的肿瘤包括视网膜母细胞瘤、多内分泌腺瘤综合征和家族性息肉病。还有一些其他癌前病变具有可变外显率的孟德尔遗传方式。一些常见的恶性肿瘤表现出低外显率的家族遗传倾向，包括乳腺癌和结直肠癌。对于几种遗传性癌症综合征（表2.2），可以进行基因检测并采取相应的预防措施。尽管已经发现了一些已知的癌症易感基因，但进行基因检测时仍需谨慎。此类

TABLE 2.1 US 2020 Cancer Statistics

ESTIMATED NEW CANCER CASES[a]

Females (912,930)		Males (893,660)	
Breast	30%	Prostate	21%
Lung and bronchus	12%	Lung and bronchus	13%
Colon and rectum	8%	Colon and rectum	9%
Uterine corpus	7%	Urinary bladder	7%
Thyroid	4%	Melanoma of the skin	7%
Melanoma of the skin	4%	Kidney and renal pelvis	5%
Non-Hodgkin lymphoma	4%	Non-Hodgkin lymphoma	5%
Kidney and renal pelvis	3%	Oral cavity and pharynx	4%
Pancreas	3%	Leukemia	4%
Leukemia	3%	Pancreas	3%
All other sites	22%	All other sites	22%

ESTIMATED CANCER DEATHS

Females (285,360)		Males (321,160)	
Lung and bronchus	22%	Lung and bronchus	23%
Breast	15%	Prostate	10%
Colon and rectum	9%	Colon and rectum	9%
Pancreas	8%	Pancreas	8%
Ovary	5%	Liver and intrahepatic bile duct	6%
Uterine corpus	4%	Leukemia	4%
Liver and intrahepatic bile duct	4%	Esophagus	4%
Leukemia	3%	Urinary bladder	4%
Non-Hodgkin lymphoma	3%	Non-Hodgkin lymphoma	4%
Brain and other nervous system	3%	Brain and other nervous system	3%
All other sites	24%	All other sites	25%

Data from Siegel RL, Miller KD, Jemal A: Cancer statistics, 2020. CA: A Cancer Journal for Clinicians. (70)1:7-30, 2020.
[a]Excludes basal cell and squamous cell skin cancers and in situ carcinoma except urinary bladder.

utilized in selecting individuals for such testing. Such testing requires a reasonable understanding of cancer genetics as well as the target population along with relevant ethical, economic, and societal issues.

At the same time, acquired somatic mutations are universally identified in malignant cells with some clearly driving the development and progression of cancer. While random genetic mutations occur frequently, proto-oncogenes involved in cell growth and proliferation, tumor suppressor genes involved in regulation of cellular proliferation, and mismatch repair genes associated with chromosomal instability play critical roles in carcinogenesis, tumor growth, progression, invasion, and metastasis. Fortunately, the spontaneous mutation rate is relatively low, and more than one mutational event is usually necessary for complete carcinogenic transformation resulting in a malignancy.

Lifestyle

Acquired risk factors for cancer include lifestyle factors as well as occupational and other environmental exposure to carcinogenic substances. Major lifestyle risk factors include tobacco, alcohol and other dietary factors, as well as lack of physical activity (Table 2.3).

Tobacco

Tobacco products are, by far, the single greatest contributor to cancer incidence and mortality worldwide. Cigarette smokers have a 20-fold or greater risk for developing cancer compared with nonsmokers, with smoking being the single largest cause of lung cancer. Tobacco accounts for one third of all cancers in the United States, contributing to the more than 1 million people annually who are estimated to die from tobacco-induced cancers globally. The vast majority of lung cancers are attributable to cigarette smoking while exposure to secondhand smoke increases the risk for lung cancer in nonsmokers. Cigarette and cigar smoking and chewing tobacco are major risk factors for head, neck, mouth, and esophageal cancers and are associated with development of stomach, pancreas, kidney, bladder, and cervical cancer as well. While tobacco use has declined in the United States over the past two decades, it continues to be unacceptably high, especially among younger women, and continues to increase in many parts of the developing world.

Nutrition

Diet and body weight appear to play an important role in cancer causation. Excess alcohol use is clearly a significant risk factor for cancers of the liver, head and neck, esophagus, and breast. Obesity and dietary fat intake are associated with colon and breast cancers, but the exact nature of the relationship is still under investigation. Central or visceral adiposity in both men and women is associated with increased incidence and mortality from a number of cancers, including endometrium, breast in postmenopausal women, kidney, gallbladder, pancreas, esophagus, colon, and prostate.

Infection

Several chronic infections, including bacterial, viral, and parasitic, have been associated with an increased risk of different types of cancer. In certain parts of the developing world, infection with *Schistosoma haematobium* is a major cause of squamous cell carcinoma of the bladder.

表 2.1　美国 2020 癌症统计数据

预计新增癌症病例数 [a]			
女性（912 930）		**男性（893 660）**	
乳腺	30%	前列腺	21%
肺和支气管	12%	肺和支气管	13%
结肠和直肠	8%	结肠和直肠	9%
子宫体	7%	膀胱	7%
甲状腺	4%	皮肤黑色素瘤	7%
皮肤黑色素瘤	4%	肾脏和肾上腺	5%
非霍奇金淋巴瘤	4%	非霍奇金淋巴瘤	5%
肾脏和肾上腺	3%	口咽	4%
胰腺	3%	白血病	4%
白血病	3%	胰腺	3%
其他所有部位	22%	其他所有部位	22%
预计癌症死亡人数			
女性（285 360）		**男性（321 160）**	
肺和支气管	22%	肺和支气管	23%
乳腺	15%	前列腺	10%
结肠和直肠	9%	结肠和直肠	9%
胰腺	8%	胰腺	8%
卵巢	5%	肝和肝内胆管	6%
子宫体	4%	白血病	4%
肝和肝内胆管	4%	食管	4%
白血病	3%	膀胱	4%
非霍奇金淋巴瘤	3%	非霍奇金淋巴瘤	4%
脑和其他神经系统	3%	脑和其他神经系统	3%
其他所有部位	24%	其他所有部位	25%

引自 Siegel RL，Miller KD，Jemal A：Cancer statistics，2020. CA：A Cancer Journal for Clinicians.（70）1：7-30，2020.
[a]：不包括基底细胞癌和鳞状细胞皮肤癌以及尿道原位癌。

测试需要对癌症遗传学以及目标人群特性有合理的理解，并充分考虑相关的伦理、经济和社会问题。

与此同时，在恶性细胞中普遍发现了获得性体细胞突变，其中一些明显驱动了癌症的发生和进展。虽然随机的遗传突变经常发生，但参与细胞生长和增殖的原癌基因、参与细胞增殖调控的肿瘤抑制基因以及与染色体不稳定性相关的错配修复基因在癌症发生、肿瘤生长、进展、侵袭和转移中起着关键作用。幸运的是，自发突变率相对较低，并且通常需要多个突变事件才能导致完全的致癌转化并形成恶性肿瘤。

生活方式

癌症的获得性风险因素包括生活方式因素以及职业和其他环境暴露于致癌物质。主要的生活方式风险因素包括烟草、酒精和其他饮食因素，以及缺乏体育活动（表2.3）。

烟草

烟草制品是目前全球癌症发病率和死亡率的最主要原因。与不吸烟者相比，吸烟者的癌症发病风险要高出20倍甚至更多。烟草在美国导致了1/3的癌症病例，而全球范围内，每年因烟草引发的癌症死亡人数超过百万。绝大多数肺癌可归因于吸烟，而接触二手烟会增加不吸烟者患肺癌的风险。吸烟、吸雪茄以及咀嚼烟草是头部、颈部、口腔和食管癌症的主要风险因素，还与胃癌、胰腺癌、肾癌、膀胱癌和宫颈癌的发生有关。虽然美国在过去20年中烟草使用有所下降，但其水平之高仍令人无法接受，尤其是在年轻女性中，并且在许多发展中国家，烟草使用量仍在上升。

营养

饮食和体重似乎在癌症的发生中扮演着重要角色。过量饮酒显然是肝脏、头颈部、食管和乳腺癌的显著风险因素。肥胖和膳食脂肪摄入与结肠和乳腺癌有关，但两者之间的确切关系仍在研究中。男性和女性的中心性或内脏脂肪沉积与一些癌症发病率和死亡率增加有关，包括子宫内膜癌、绝经后妇女乳腺癌、肾癌、胆囊癌、胰腺癌、食管癌、结肠癌和前列腺癌在内的多种癌症。

感染

几种慢性感染，包括细菌、病毒和寄生虫感染，均与不同类型癌症的风险增加有关。在某些发展中国家，血吸虫感染是膀胱鳞状细胞癌的主要病因。DNA

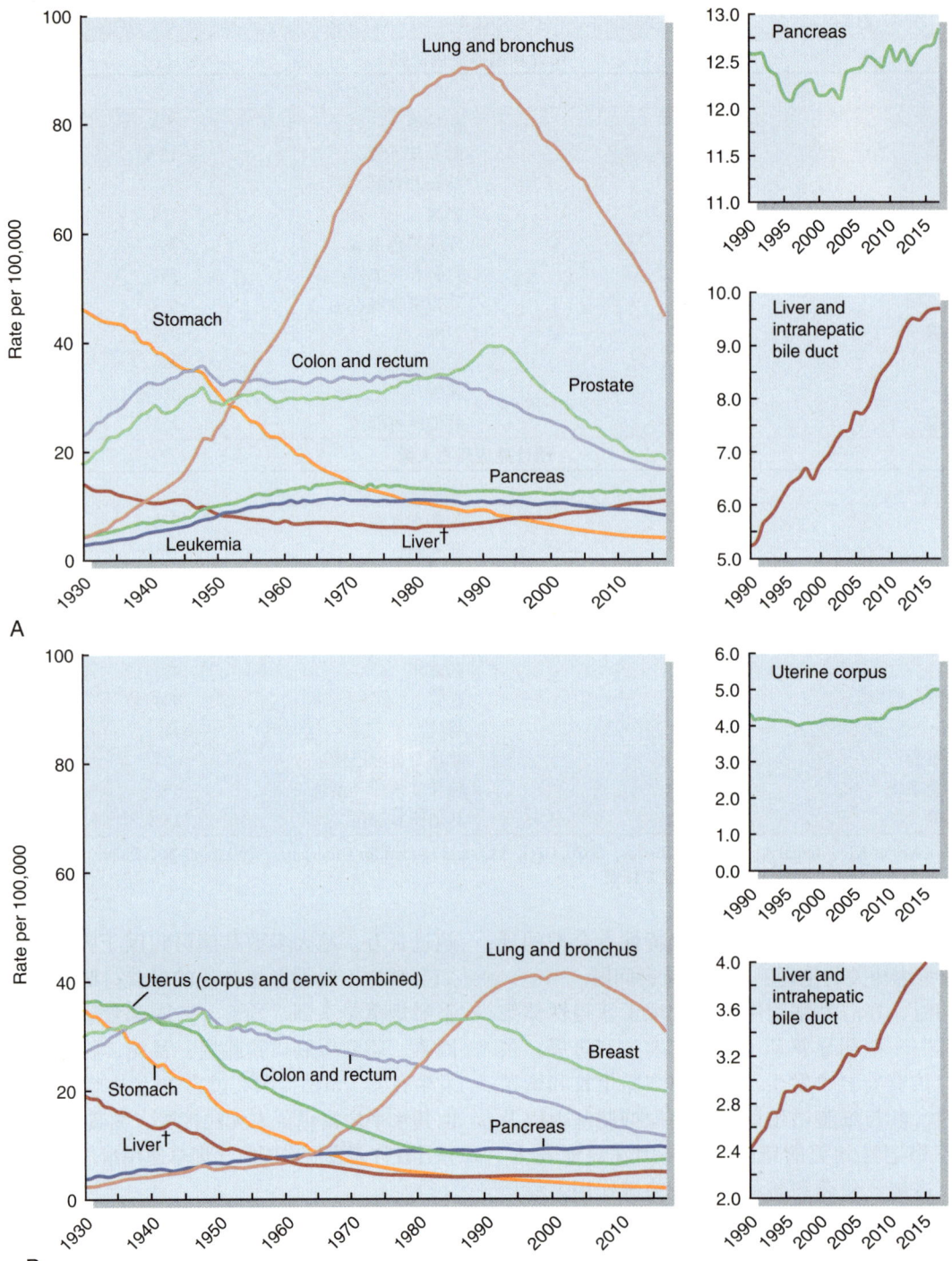

Fig. 2.1 US cancer mortality rates, 1930-2017. (A) Males. (B) Females. †Includes intrahepatic bile duct, gall bladder, and other biliary. (From Siegel RL, Miller KD, Jemal A: Cancer statistics, 2020, CA: A Cancer Journal for Clinicians [70]1:7-30, 2020.)

Both DNA and RNA viruses have been associated with human cancers. Viruses associated with human malignancies include the Epstein-Barr virus (EBV) (nasopharyngeal cancer and Burkitt lymphoma) and human T-cell leukemia virus type I (HTLV-1). Patients with the acquired immunodeficiency syndrome (AIDS) associated with the human immunodeficiency virus (HIV) are at increased risk of Kaposi's sarcoma, non-Hodgkin lymphoma, and anogenital squamous cell carcinoma. Chronic hepatitis B and C viral infections have been linked with the development of hepatocellular carcinoma. Human papillomaviruses 16 and 18 have been linked with cervical cancer, with vaccines against these virus strains and those causing genital warts, both on the market.

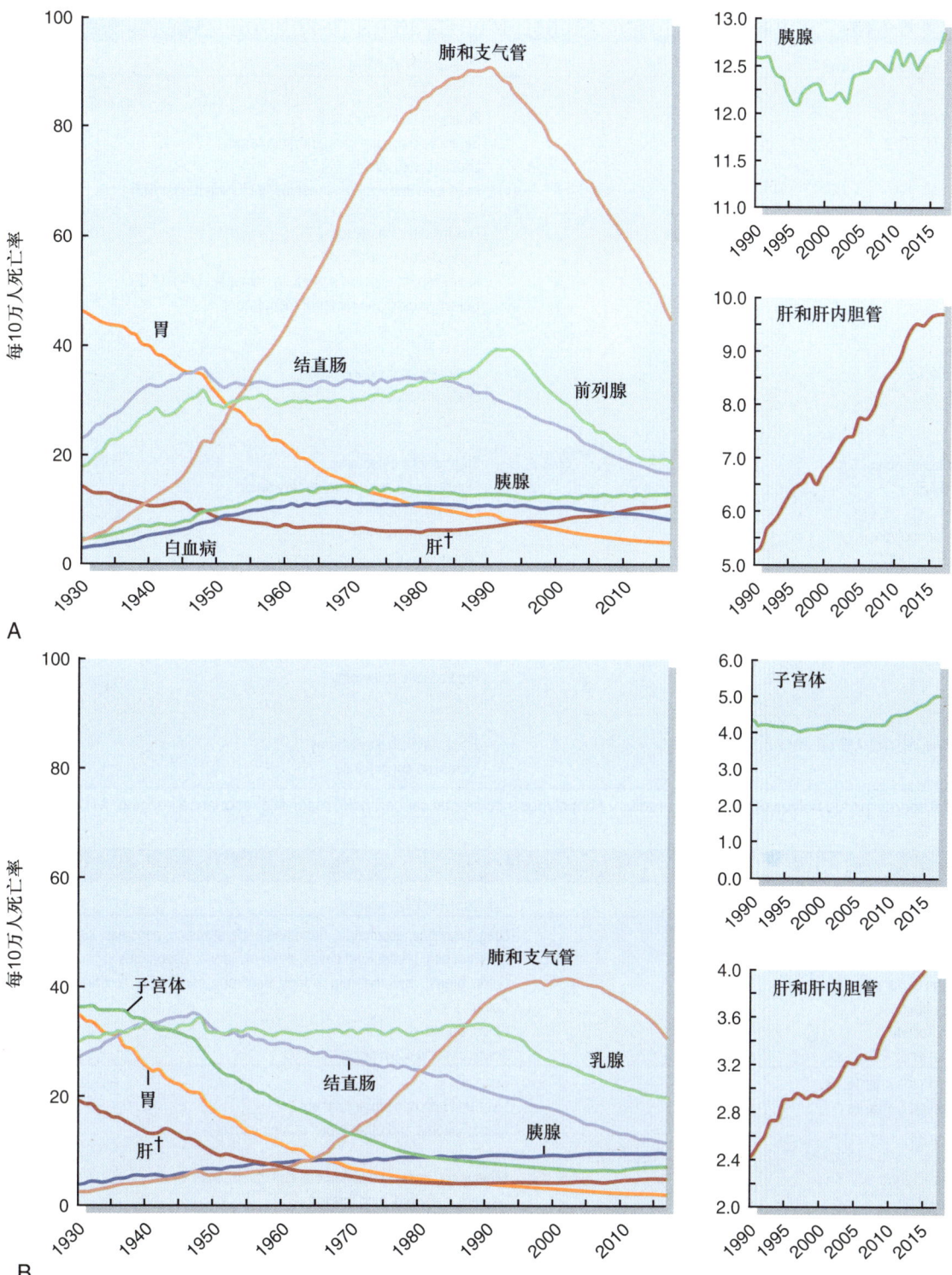

图 2.1 1930—2017 年美国癌症死亡率。（**A**）男性。（**B**）女性。† 包括肝内胆管、胆囊和其他胆道［引自 Siegel RL，Miller KD，Jemal A：Cancer statistics，2020，CA：A Cancer Journal for Clinicians（70）1：7-30，2020.］

病毒和 RNA 病毒均已被证实与人类癌症相关。与人类恶性肿瘤相关的病毒包括：埃博拉病毒（EBV）（与鼻咽癌和伯基特淋巴瘤相关）和人类 T 细胞白血病病毒 1 型（HTLV-1）。与人类免疫缺陷病毒（HIV）相关的获得性免疫缺陷综合征（AIDS）患者患卡波西肉瘤、非霍奇金淋巴瘤和外阴鳞状细胞癌的风险增加。慢性乙型和丙型肝炎病毒感染与肝细胞癌的发生有关。人乳头瘤病毒 16 和 18 与宫颈癌有关，目前市场上已有针对这些病毒株以及导致尖锐湿疣的病毒株的疫苗。

TABLE 2.2 Genetic Testing for Selected Hereditary Cancer Syndromes

Cancer: Involved Genes	Prevention Measures
Breast BRCA-1, BRCA-2 PTEN, STK-11, TP53	Prophylactic mastectomy Selective estrogen receptor modulators Lifestyle measures Increased intensity of screening, including breast MRI
Lobular Breast Cancer and Gastric Cancer CDH-1 (E-cadherin)	Prophylactic mastectomy Prophylactic gastrectomy Increased intensity of screening, including breast MRI Selective estrogen receptor modulators
Ovarian BRCA-1, BRCA-2	Prophylactic oophorectomy Oral contraceptives
Colon Familial adenomatous Polyposis (FAP) APC Hereditary nonpolyposis Colon cancer (HNPCC) MLH-1, MSH-2 MSH-6, PMS-2 MYH-associated polyposis MYH	Prophylactic colectomy Nonsteroidal anti-inflammatory drugs Lifestyle measures Lifestyle measures Nonsteroidal anti-inflammatory drugs Increased surveillance Prophylactic total abdominal hysterectomy and oophorectomy Lifestyle measures Nonsteroidal anti-inflammatory drugs Prophylactic colectomy
Uterine PTEN, MLH-1, MSH-2, MSH-6, PMS-2	Prophylactic hysterectomy Increased surveillance

FAP, Familial adenomatous polyposis; *HNPCC*, hereditary nonpolyposis colorectal cancer; *MRI*, magnetic resonance imaging; *MYH*, mutY homologue.

TABLE 2.3 Cancer Risk Factors

Lifestyle Factor	Associated Cancers
Tobacco	Lung, bronchus, esophagus, head and neck, stomach, pancreas, kidney, bladder, cervix
High alcohol consumption	Liver, rectum, breast, oral cavity, pharynx, larynx, esophagus
Obesity, high dietary fat	Colon, breast, endometrium, kidney, pancreas, esophagus, prostate
Low dietary fiber	Colon
Sedentary lifestyle	Colon, breast
Environmental Exposures	**Associated Cancers**
Human papillomavirus:16,18	Cervical
Hepatitis B and C viruses	Liver and hepatocellular cancers
Asbestos	Mesothelioma and other types of lung cancer
Radon	Lung
Ultraviolet radiation	Melanoma, basal and squamous cell carcinomas
Ionizing radiation	Leukemia, thyroid, lung, breast

Cancer and the Severe Acute Respiratory Syndrome Coronavirus 2 (SARS-Cov-2)

The 2020 pandemic from SARS-Cov-2 has placed patients with cancer at disproportionately greater risk of contracting COVID-19, as well as greater risk of serious medical complications including hospitalization, need for intensive care and ventilator support, and a greater risk for mortality. The reason for this impact is multifactorial and includes greater exposure to the health care system and infected patients and staff as well as greater risk from the immunosuppression resulting from disease and cancer therapies. Other factors that lead to greater risk include older age, one or more serious medical comorbidities, and concurrent complications from other infectious agents and a range of demographic and geographic disparities.

Given the sudden and urgent crisis of this global pandemic, much of the epidemiologic information currently available has risen out of crowd-sourcing efforts to rapidly and broadly gather as much information as possible on the impact of COVID-19 on patients with cancer and their management. The major driving force has been the need to gather and disseminate this information as quickly as possible for both clinical and public heath purposes or containment and mitigation. While the resulting

表 2.2　针对特定遗传性癌症综合征的基因检测

癌症：相关基因	预防措施
乳腺癌	
BRCA-1，BRCA-2	预防性乳腺切除术
PTEN，STK-11，TP53	选择性雌激素受体调节剂
	生活方式措施
	增加筛查力度，包括乳腺 MRI
小叶性乳腺癌和胃癌	
	预防性乳腺切除术
	预防性胃切除术
CDH-1（E-钙黏蛋白）	增加筛查力度，包括乳腺 MRI
	选择性雌激素受体调节剂
卵巢癌	
BRCA-1，BRCA-2	预防性卵巢切除术
	口服避孕药
结肠癌	
家族性腺瘤性息肉病（FAP）	预防性结肠切除
	非甾体抗炎药
腺瘤性结肠息肉（APC）	生活方式措施
遗传性非息肉病性结直肠癌（HNPCC）	生活方式措施
	非甾体抗炎药
MLH-1，MSH-2	增加监测
MSH-6，PMS-2	预防性全子宫切除术和卵巢切除术
MYH 相关息肉病	生活方式措施
MYH	非甾体抗炎药
	预防性结肠切除
子宫癌	
PTEN，MLH-1，MSH-2，MSH-6，PMS-2	预防性子宫切除术
	增加监测

FAP：家族性腺瘤性息肉病；HNPCC：遗传性非息肉性结肠癌；MRI：磁共振成像；MYH：突变 Y 同源物。

表 2.3　癌症风险因素

生活方式因素	相关癌症
烟草	肺癌，支气管癌，食管癌，头颈癌，胃癌，胰腺癌，肾癌，宫颈癌
大量饮酒	肝癌，直肠癌，乳腺癌，口腔癌，喉癌，食管癌
肥胖，高脂饮食	结肠癌，乳腺癌，子宫内膜癌，肾癌，胰腺癌，食管癌，前列腺癌
低纤维饮食	结肠癌
久坐	结肠癌，乳腺癌
环境暴露	**相关癌症**
人乳头瘤病毒：16，18 型	宫颈癌
乙型和丙型肝炎	肝脏和肝细胞癌
失眠	间皮瘤和其他类型肺癌
氡	肺癌
紫外线辐射	黑色素瘤，基底和鳞状细胞癌
电离辐射	白血病，甲状腺癌，肺癌，乳腺癌

癌症与严重急性呼吸综合征冠状病毒 2（SARS-Cov-2）

2020 年由 SARS-Cov-2 引发的疫情使癌症患者患上 COVID-19 的风险显著增加，同时也使他们面临更严重的医疗并发症风险，包括住院、需要重症监护以及使用呼吸机的支持，以及更高的死亡风险。这种影响的原因是多方面的，包括对医疗系统和感染患者及医务人员的更大暴露，以及由疾病和癌症治疗导致的免疫抑制所带来的更大风险。其他导致风险增加的因素还包括年龄较大、具有一种或多种严重合并症、源自其他传染病病原体的共存并发症以及存在一系列人口统计学和地理差异。

鉴于全球疫情的突然性和紧迫性，目前可用的大部分流行病学信息都是通过群众努力迅速广泛地收集有关 COVID-19 对癌症患者及其治疗影响的信息而来的。主要推动力是尽快收集和传播这些信息，以满足临床和公共卫生目的或遏制和缓解的需要。案例研究和队列研究从全球各地提供了大量重要且及时的信息，但这也带来了分析和解读上的挑战。因适应证产生的

case experience and cohort studies have provided much important and timely information from across the globe, it has come with analytic challenges and interpretation. Confounding by indication has complicated the rush to evaluate both preventive and therapeutic interventions in these largely uncontrolled and non-randomized studies. In the meantime, large-scale conventional epidemiologic studies are under development that should provide longer-term and more reliable information about the risk of COVID-19 in patients with cancer. Such studies may also provide data about the concurrent factors that impact the most on the risk of infection in the critically ill patient and disease and treatment-related predictors of serious and even fatal outcomes, while we are awaiting the development of effect treatments and vaccines. Nevertheless, the essentially exponential spread of SARS-Cov-2 both globally and in multiple specific sites, and the apparent, albeit limited, success of mitigation measures such as social distancing and masking, have reminded us of epidemiologic and public health measures of the past, which are equally if not more relevant today and critically important for patients with cancer.

Radiation

Non-ionizing radiation. Excess to ultraviolet (UV) radiation is unquestionably associated with an increased risk of skin cancers including basal and squamous cell carcinomas as well as cutaneous melanoma, with observed rates increasing directly with the amount of daily sunlight exposure. Most of the harmful effects from sun exposure are thought to be related to direct DNA damage associated with exposure to intermediate wavelength UV-B. The use of tanning beds and other frequent exposures to sunlight are of particular concern given the rapid increase in rates of melanoma among younger individuals.

Ionizing radiation. Ionizing radiation is arguably the most extensively studied carcinogen and has been unequivocally associated with an increased risk of both hematologic malignancies and various solid tumors in humans. Radiation-induced malignancies including leukemia and solid tumors are most extensively studied in the occupational settings among radiation workers and miners, among survivors of the atomic weapons used in Hiroshima and Nagasaki in World War II, and among those exposed to radiation for various medical indications. Excess cancer risk from radiation exposure can be seen with a latency period ranging from a few years (leukemia) to decades (solid tumors) and correlates with the cumulative exposure dose. As the survivors of the atomic bombing of Japan age, estimates of the associated risk of cancer have continued to increase.

Natural sources account for at least 80% of human exposure to radiation, most notably from radon. It has been estimated that radon exposure is the second leading cause of lung cancer due to widespread low-level exposure in the residential setting. In the occupational setting, there is a strong interaction between smoking and radon such that most radon-induced lung cancers are among smokers. Medical exposure accounts for most of the remaining average annual radiation exposure in the United States. There is increasing evidence that repeated exposure to radiation from multiple imaging studies such as CT scans, especially at a young age, is associated with an increased risk of cancer later in life.

Chemicals

Various pharmacologic agents have been associated with an increased risk for specific cancers. As with radiation, these agents may be used in the occupational setting, for diagnostic or therapeutic medical use, as well as for various purposes in the home setting. Organic and inorganic chemical compounds linked to human cancers including benzene (leukemia), benzidine (bladder), arsenic, soot and coal tars (lung and skin), and wood dusts (nasal). Arguably, asbestos is probably the most common cause of occupational cancer because of its link with the development of mesothelioma and other types of lung cancer. Nearly all mesotheliomas diagnosed in the United States are associated with prior asbestos exposure. A strong interaction exists between asbestos exposure and cigarette smoking for lung cancer.

A range of medications are associated with an increased risk of cancer, including the alkylating agents, anthracyclines, and other classes of cancer chemotherapy and immunosuppressants. Estrogen use in postmenopausal women increases the risk of endometrial cancer, while the rates drop when combined with progesterone. Synthetic estrogens, such as diethylstilbestrol (DES), administered to mothers during pregnancy increase the risk of vaginal cancer in offspring. Lifestyle exposures to carcinogenic chemicals covered previously include multiple carcinogens in tobacco products and dietary factors including aflatoxins in many part of the world.

CANCER PREVENTION

Cancer prevention strategies can be thought of as primary or secondary based on whether they reduce risk of exposure or detect cancer at an early stage when intervention can change the natural history of the disease. Reasonable primary prevention strategies include reductions in lifestyle risks (smoking cessation; use of sunscreen; adherence to a low-fat, high-fiber diet), avoidance of occupational or environmental risks, and chemoprevention (see Table 55.3).

Lifestyle Changes

Smoking cessation is unquestionably the most direct and effective cancer prevention strategy available. More than 1 million people die from tobacco-induced cancers globally each year, and tobacco accounts for one third of all cancer diagnoses in the United States. Although tobacco prevention and control programs have resulted in a decline in smoking prevalence in the United States, tobacco use continues to be high and has been increasing in a number of countries. There is also evidence from epidemiologic studies that other lifestyle changes including regular exercise and dietary modification may also reduce the risk of cancer. Central adiposity is associated with increased incidence and mortality from a number of cancers, including breast and endometrium. Sufficient dietary intake of fruits and vegetables appears to reduce the risk for gastric and esophageal cancers. Avoidance of excessive sun exposure and the use of artificial tanning devices also is important to reversing recent upward trends in cutaneous malignancies. Reduction in exposures to known carcinogenic agents is an important goal in both the occupational and domestic setting. Evidence for an association between air pollution and lung cancer incidence illustrates how difficult that may be. However, prudent use of potentially carcinogenic chemicals and radiation in the medical setting will hopefully minimize exposures to settings where the benefit clearly outweighs the potential harms.

Chemoprevention

Chemopreventive agents are drugs, vaccines, or micronutrients (e.g., minerals, vitamins) used to prevent the development of cancer. Both randomized trials and epidemiologic studies have suggested that a number of strategies may be capable of reducing the risk of some common types of cancer. Recent data from multiple studies have provided suggestive evidence that daily aspirin use may reduce the risk of several types of cancer, including colon and melanoma. Evidence suggests that hepatitis B vaccination can reduce the incidence of hepatocellular cancer. The vaccine directed against specific strains of the human papillomavirus (HPV) offers the strong promise of preventing cervical cancer.

CANCER SCREENING

Cancer screening programs should be able to detect premalignant states or early-stage cancer before the onset of symptoms with relatively high sensitivity. Likewise, for cancer screening to be useful there

混杂因素使我们很难迅速评估这些很大程度上缺乏对照和未采用随机化方法的研究中的预防性和治疗性干预措施。与此同时，正在开展大规模的常规流行病学研究，将为癌症患者的 COVID-19 风险提供更长期和更可靠的信息。这些研究还可能提供对重症患者感染风险影响最大的并发因素数据，以及引发严重甚至致命后果的治疗相关预测因素数据，同时我们也在等待着有效治疗方法和疫苗的发展。然而，SARS-Cov-2 在全球和多个特定地区的几乎指数级传播，保持社交距离和戴口罩等缓解措施尽管有限但取得了明显成功，提醒我们注意过去的流行病学和公共卫生措施，这些措施同样有效并且对于癌症患者至关重要。

辐射

非电离辐射　过度的紫外线辐射无疑与皮肤癌的风险增加有关，包括基底细胞癌、鳞状细胞癌和黑色素瘤，其发病率直接与每日日照量成正比。大多数来自阳光照射的有害影响被认为与中波紫外线-B 照射引起的直接 DNA 损伤有关。在年轻个体中黑色素瘤发病率快速上升的情况下，使用日光浴床和其他频繁暴露于阳光的行为尤其令人担忧。

电离辐射　电离辐射可以说是研究最广泛的致癌物，已被明确与人类血液系统恶性肿瘤和各种实体肿瘤的风险增加有关。在职业环境中，对于辐射引起的恶性肿瘤，包括白血病和实体肿瘤，最广泛研究的对象是辐射工人和矿工、二战期间广岛和长崎原子弹幸存者，以及因医疗需要接受辐射暴露的人群。辐射暴露引起的癌症风险增加可有几年（如白血病）至几十年（如实体瘤）不等的潜伏期，并与累积暴露剂量相关。随着日本原子弹爆炸的幸存者年龄的增长，与癌症相关的风险估计也在不断增加。

自然来源的暴露至少占人类辐射暴露的 80%，其中氡是最显著的来源。据估计，由于在住宅环境中普遍存在低水平暴露，氡暴露是导致肺癌的第二大原因。在职业环境中，吸烟和氡之间存在很强的相互作用，因此大多数由氡引起的肺癌都发生在吸烟者中。医疗暴露占美国平均年度辐射暴露的大部分。越来越多的证据表明，反复接受多次影像学检查（如 CT 扫描）的辐射，尤其是在年轻时期，与晚年患癌症的风险增加有关。

化学物质

多种药物已被发现与癌症风险增加有关。与辐射一样，这些物质可能在职业环境中使用，用于诊断或治疗医学用途，以及家庭环境中的各种用途。与人类癌症相关的有机和无机化学化合物包括苯（白血病）、联苯胺（膀胱癌）、砷、烟尘和煤焦油（肺癌和皮肤癌）以及木屑（鼻癌）。可以说，石棉可能是最常见的职业癌症病因，因为它与间皮瘤和其他类型的肺癌的发展有关。在美国诊断出的几乎所有间皮瘤都与石棉有关。石棉暴露与吸烟之间存在强烈的相互作用，进一步增加肺癌的风险。

一系列药物与癌症风险增加有关，包括烷化剂、蒽环类药物和其他类型的癌症化疗药物和免疫抑制剂。绝经后女性使用雌激素会增加子宫内膜癌的风险，而同时使用黄体酮可降低这一风险。在妊娠期间给予母亲合成雌激素，如二乙基己烯雌酚（DES），会增加后代罹患阴道癌的风险。先前提到的生活方式中致癌化学物质暴露包括烟草制品中含有的多种致癌物质以及世界各地饮食中的有害物质，包括黄曲霉毒素。

癌症预防

癌症预防策略可以根据它们是减少暴露风险还是在早期发现癌症并进行干预来改变疾病的自然进程分为一级或二级预防两类。合理的一级预防策略包括降低生活方式风险（戒烟；使用防晒霜；遵守低脂肪和高纤维饮食），避免职业或环境风险以及化学预防（见表 55.3）。

生活方式改变

毫无疑问，戒烟是目前最有效的癌症预防策略。全球每年有超过 100 万人因烟草引发的癌症死亡，且烟草导致了美国 1/3 的癌症病例。虽然美国的烟草预防和控制项目导致吸烟率有所下降，但烟草使用率仍然很高，并且在一些国家呈上升趋势。流行病学研究还提供了其他生活方式改变（包括定期锻炼和饮食调整）可能降低癌症风险的证据。中心性肥胖与多种癌症的发病率和死亡率增加有关，包括乳腺癌和子宫内膜癌。足够的水果和蔬菜摄入似乎能降低胃癌和食管癌的风险。避免过度日晒和使用人工日光浴设备对于逆转近年来皮肤癌的上升趋势也很重要。减少已知致癌物暴露是职业和家庭环境中的一个重要目标。空气污染与肺癌发病率之间的关联使得实现这一目标尤为困难。然而，在医疗环境中谨慎使用潜在的致癌化学物质和辐射有望将暴露降至最低。在这些情况下，患者获益显然大于潜在的危害。

化学预防

化学预防剂是用于预防癌症发展的药物、疫苗或微量营养素（如矿物质和维生素）。随机对照试验和流行病学研究都表明，一些策略可能有助于降低某些常见癌症的风险。多项研究的最新数据提供了有说服力的证据，这些研究表明每日服用阿司匹林可降低包括结肠癌和黑色素瘤在内的多种癌症的风险，乙型肝炎疫苗接种可降低肝细胞癌的发病率。针对特定人乳头瘤病毒（HPV）株的疫苗在预防宫颈癌方面表现出强大的潜力。

癌症筛查

癌症筛查项目应该能够在症状出现之前，以相对较高的敏感度检测出癌前状态或早期癌症。同样，癌症筛查必须有可用的治疗方法，以改善癌前或早期患者的预

must be a treatment available that improves the outcome of patients with premalignant or early-stage disease. Such cancer screening programs should also, ideally, be noninvasive, inexpensive, and associated with high specificity (low false-positive rate). Identification of high-risk individuals can be of value to the effective and cost-effective application of genetic counseling and testing as well as cancer screening efforts.

Proper interpretation of the results of cancer screening studies must consider both *lead-time bias* and *length-time bias*. Lead time is the time between detection of disease by screening and the actual appearance of symptomatic disease. Diagnosing the disease earlier with screening may make it appear that the patient lived longer even when the survival of the patient from the onset of disease has not been altered. Length-time bias occurs when subsets of the cancer under study have different growth rates. Screening is more likely to detect cancers that grow slowly because of the greater prevalence of asymptomatic people with slow-growing tumors than with fast-growing tumors. Thus patients with cancer that is detected with screening appear to have longer survival as a result of screening, when in fact the longer course of their disease results from the behavior of the tumor itself. While randomized controlled trials of cancer screening programs require large numbers of participants and take years to complete, such trials are needed to accurately estimate screening performance and to address both lead-time and length-time bias.

It is important to note that screening tests may also be associated with false-negative and false-positive results. *False-negative results* fail to obtain a proper diagnosis and patients, therefore, are not provided the opportunity for effective early treatment. *False-positive results* may also cause harm by leading to unnecessary testing and treatment as well as contributing to patient costs and emotional stress.

A number of cancer screening tests are currently recommended, including clinical examination and mammography to detect breast cancer, Papanicolaou smears and HPV DNA tests to detect cervical dysplasia or cancer, colonoscopy to detect polyps or colon cancer, and digital rectal examination and serum PSA to detect prostate cancer. Low-dose CT scanning for screening appropriate high-risk individuals for lung cancer has recently been recommended based on several large randomized controlled trials.

SUGGESTED READINGS

Colditz GA, Sellers TA, Trapido E: Epidemiology-Identifying the causes and preventability of cancer, Nat Rev Cancer 6:75–83, 2006.

Dai M, Liu D, Liu M, Zhou F, Li G, Chen Z, et al: Patients with cancer appear more vulnerable to SARS-COV-2: a multicenter study during the COVID-19 Outbreak, Cancer Discov 10(6):783–791, 2020.

Desai A, Warner J, Kuderer N, Thompson M, Pinter C, Lyman G, Lopes G: Crowdsourcing a crisis response for COVID-19 in oncology, Nat Cancer Apr 21:1–4, 2020.

Detterbeck FC, Mazzone PJ, Naidich DP, et al: Screening for lung cancer: diagnosis and management of lung cancer, 3rd ed: American College of Chest Physicians evidence-based clinical practice guidelines, Chest 143:e78S–e92S, 2013.

Kuderer NM, Choureiri TK, Shah DP, et al: Clinical impact of COVID-19 on patients with cancer (CCC19): a cohort study, Lancet 395:1907–1918, 2020.

Kushi LH, Doyle C, McCullough M, et al: American Cancer Society Guidelines on nutrition and physical activity for cancer prevention: reducing the risk of cancer with healthy food choices and physical activity, CA Cancer J Clin 62:30–67, 2012.

Lyman GH, Dale DC, Wolff DA, et al: Acute myeloid leukemia or myelodysplastic syndrome in randomized controlled clinical trials of cancer chemotherapy with granulocyte colony-stimulating factor: a systematic review, J Clin Oncol 28:2914–2924, 2010.

Raaschou-Nielsen O, Andersen ZJ, Beelen R, et al: Air pollution and lung cancer incidence in 17 European cohorts: prospective analyses from the European Study of Cohorts for Air Pollution Effects (ESCAPE), Lancet Oncol 14:813–822, 2013.

Rivera DR, Peters S, Panagiotou OA, et al: Utilization of COVID-19 treatments and clinical outcomes among patients with cancer: a COVID-19 and Cancer Consortium (CCC19) cohort study, Cancer Discovery, 2020 (epub ahead of print July 22 2020).

Schottenfeld D, Beebe-Dimmer JL: Advances in cancer epidemiology: understanding causal mechanisms and the evidence for implementing interventions, Annu Rev Public Health 26:37–60, 2005.

Schottenfeld D, Beebe-Dimmer J: Alleviating the burden of cancer: a perspective on advances, challenges and future directions, Cancer Epidemiol Biomarkers Prev 15:2049–2055, 2006.

Siegel RL, Miller KD, Jemal AJ: Cancer statistics, CA Cancer J Clin 70:7–30, 2020, 2020.

Smith RA, Brooks D, Cokkinides V, et al: Cancer screening in the United States, 2013: a review of current American Cancer Society guidelines, current issues in cancer screening, and new guidance on cervical cancer screening and lung cancer screening, CA Cancer J Clin 63:88–105, 2013.

后。理想的癌症筛查项目还应是非侵入性、价格低廉且特异性高的（即假阳性率低）。识别高危人群对于有效且低成本地实施遗传咨询和检测以及癌症筛查工作也有价值。

对癌症筛查研究结果的正确解读必须考虑前导时间偏倚和长度时间偏倚。前导时间是指通过筛查发现疾病到实际出现症状性疾病之间的时间。通过筛查更早地诊断出疾病可能会让患者看起来活得更久，即使患者从疾病真正开始时的生存时间没有改变。长度时间偏倚在研究中的癌症亚群有不同的生长速度时发生。筛查更有可能检测到生长缓慢的癌症，因为相比于生长迅速的肿瘤，生长缓慢的肿瘤中存在无症状人群的概率更高。因此，通过筛查检测到癌症的患者似乎由于筛查而拥有更长的生存时间，但实际上，他们的疾病更长的病程是由肿瘤自身行为导致的。尽管癌症筛查项目的随机对照试验需要大量参与者并需要数年才能完成，但这些试验对于准确评估筛查效果以及解决前导时间和长度时间偏倚问题是必要的。

值得注意的是，筛查测试也可能出现假阴性和假阳性结果。假阴性结果无法获得正确的诊断，因此患者无法获得有效的早期治疗机会。假阳性结果也可能造成伤害，导致不必要的测试和治疗，增加患者的费用和精神压力。

目前推荐的癌症筛查测试包括：临床检查和乳房X线检查以检测乳腺癌，巴氏涂片和HPV DNA检测以检测宫颈病变或癌症，结肠镜检查以检测息肉或结肠癌，直肠指检和血清前列腺特异性抗原（PSA）检测以检测前列腺癌。根据几项大型随机对照试验的结果，最近还推荐对高危人群进行低剂量CT扫描以筛查肺癌。

推荐阅读

Colditz GA, Sellers TA, Trapido E: Epidemiology-Identifying the causes and preventability of cancer, Nat Rev Cancer 6:75–83, 2006.

Dai M, Liu D, Liu M, Zhou F, Li G, Chen Z, et al: Patients with cancer appear more vulnerable to SARS-COV-2: a multicenter study during the COVID-19 Outbreak, Cancer Discov 10(6):783–791, 2020.

Desai A, Warner J, Kuderer N, Thompson M, Pinter C, Lyman G, Lopes G: Crowdsourcing a crisis response for COVID-19 in oncology, Nat Cancer Apr 21:1–4, 2020.

Detterbeck FC, Mazzone PJ, Naidich DP, et al: Screening for lung cancer: diagnosis and management of lung cancer, 3rd ed: American College of Chest Physicians evidence-based clinical practice guidelines, Chest 143:e78S–e92S, 2013.

Kuderer NM, Choureiri TK, Shah DP, et al: Clinical impact of COVID-19 on patients with cancer (CCC19): a cohort study, Lancet 395:1907–1918, 2020.

Kushi LH, Doyle C, McCullough M, et al: American Cancer Society Guidelines on nutrition and physical activity for cancer prevention: reducing the risk of cancer with healthy food choices and physical activity, CA Cancer J Clin 62:30–67, 2012.

Lyman GH, Dale DC, Wolff DA, et al: Acute myeloid leukemia or myelodysplastic syndrome in randomized controlled clinical trials of cancer chemotherapy with granulocyte colony-stimulating factor: a systematic review, J Clin Oncol 28:2914–2924, 2010.

Raaschou-Nielsen O, Andersen ZJ, Beelen R, et al: Air pollution and lung cancer incidence in 17 European cohorts: prospective analyses from the European Study of Cohorts for Air Pollution Effects (ESCAPE), Lancet Oncol 14:813–822, 2013.

Rivera DR, Peters S, Panagiotou OA, et al: Utilization of COVID-19 treatments and clinical outcomes among patients with cancer: a COVID-19 and Cancer Consortium (CCC19) cohort study, Cancer Discovery, 2020 (epub ahead of print July 22 2020).

Schottenfeld D, Beebe-Dimmer JL: Advances in cancer epidemiology: understanding causal mechanisms and the evidence for implementing interventions, Annu Rev Public Health 26:37–60, 2005.

Schottenfeld D, Beebe-Dimmer J: Alleviating the burden of cancer: a perspective on advances, challenges and future directions, Cancer Epidemiol Biomarkers Prev 15:2049–2055, 2006.

Siegel RL, Miller KD, Jemal AJ: Cancer statistics, CA Cancer J Clin 70:7–30, 2020, 2020.

Smith RA, Brooks D, Cokkinides V, et al: Cancer screening in the United States, 2013: a review of current American Cancer Society guidelines, current issues in cancer screening, and new guidance on cervical cancer screening and lung cancer screening, CA Cancer J Clin 63:88–105, 2013.

3

Principles of Cancer Therapy

Davendra P.S. Sohal, Alok A. Khorana

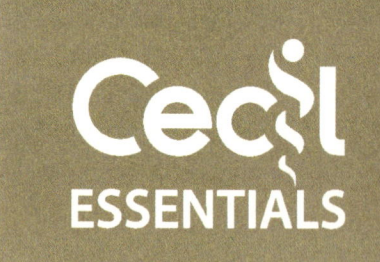

INTRODUCTION

The treatment of cancer includes a rapidly growing portfolio of modalities and agents: locoregional therapies (surgery, radiation), systemic therapies (chemotherapy, targeted therapies, immunotherapies), and supportive care agents. Surgery and radiation therapy are safe and effective treatments for localized cancers, and techniques continue to be refined. In most settings (particularly advanced stages), however, cancer is a systemic disease and requires systemic treatment. Chemotherapy—the "first generation" of cancer drugs—is the current mainstay of systemic treatment. The explosive increase in our knowledge of cancer biology and genomics has allowed the development of both specific targeted agents and drugs harnessing the immune system to fight cancer. Many new drugs have been approved, and many more are in clinical trials—more than for any other class of medicine. Moreover, cancer treatment incurs many side effects. Symptom control, therefore, is a very important component of cancer therapy. All these modalities make it imperative that patients with cancer be treated by multidisciplinary teams at dedicated cancer centers. This chapter reviews the principles of the various components of cancer therapy.

DIAGNOSIS AND STAGING

Definitive treatment for cancer usually requires histologic diagnosis. This typically involves an invasive biopsy to obtain sufficient material to evaluate the morphology and invasiveness of the tumor and the expression of various molecular markers. Noninvasive tests such as radiologic imaging are seldom substitutes for tissue diagnosis. (There are occasional exceptions, such as an elevated α-fetoprotein level along with imaging evidence in a patient with cirrhosis, which can be used to make a diagnosis of hepatocellular carcinoma.)

Once the diagnosis of cancer has been made, for most solid-organ tumors, the next step is to systematically determine the extent of tumor spread, a process called *staging*. Tumor staging can be clinical or pathologic. *Clinical staging* involves physical examination and imaging studies, including targeted ultrasound (percutaneous or using invasive endoscopy devices), computed tomography scans, magnetic resonance imaging, whole-body positron-emission tomography scans, and radionuclide scans, usually in some combination, depending on the propensity of particular tumors to spread to particular organs. *Pathologic staging* is more definitive and follows the tumor-node-metastasis (TNM) method developed by the American Joint Committee on Cancer and the International Union against Cancer. This system requires a careful evaluation of the primary resection specimen for three measurements: (1) the size and extent of invasion of the primary tumor (the T score), (2) the number and location of histologically involved regional lymph nodes (the N score), and (3) the presence or absence of distant metastases (the M score). The M score is based on information derived from both clinical and pathologic staging. TNM scores are then grouped into a pathologic stage, typically from I through IV, reflecting an increasing burden of disease. The final TNM stage has both prognostic and therapeutic implications. For instance, a resected colon cancer that invades the muscularis propria, involves 2 of 16 lymph nodes, but shows no evidence of distant metastases is staged as a T2 N1 M0 (stage III) colon cancer. The likelihood of tumor recurrence is 40% to 50%; and patients are recommended 3 to 6 months of chemotherapy after surgery. On the other hand, if no lymph nodes are involved (T2 N0 M0, stage I), the likelihood of recurrence is less than 10%, and chemotherapy is usually not recommended.

Biomarkers provide additional prognostic information, such as the absence of hormone receptors or expression of HER2 in breast cancer, which are indicative of a poor prognosis. Such markers can also be predictive; for instance, overexpression of HER2 in breast cancer predicts response to trastuzumab. Similarly, *KRAS* mutations in colorectal cancer predict lack of response to antibodies (e.g., cetuximab, panitumumab) that are directed against the epidermal growth factor receptor (EGFR) (Fig. 3.1). Both prognostic and predictive biomarkers provide important information in addition to the formal TNM stage. With an increasing array of biomarkers being identified, a panel of them are now usually tested, using next-generation sequencing (NGS) platforms that can sequence hundreds of relevant genes to identify point mutations, translocations, copy number alterations, and expression level changes. All of this information is compiled into a final assessment of whether the cancer is curable or not.

The next step is to evaluate the patient's overall clinical condition with respect to comorbidities affecting major organ function and the patient's functional ability, termed *performance status*. Performance status is assessed with the use of various history-based methods, such as the Eastern Cooperative Oncology Group (ECOG) or Karnofsky performance score. Patients with poor performance status or major comorbid conditions may not derive a benefit from cancer-directed therapy and are at greater risk for adverse events. This comprehensive assessment—diagnosis, stage, prognostic and predictive markers, and patient condition—dictates the management plan: either curative or palliative.

PRINCIPLES OF CANCER SURGERY

Surgery can prevent cancer by removal of precancerous lesions or organs that are at high risk for cancer (e.g., bilateral mastectomy in those with hereditary defects that can lead to breast cancer). Surgery can also make the diagnosis of cancer by biopsy; assist in staging by sampling lymph nodes; provide definitive treatment by removing the primary tumor; reconstruct the limb or organ sacrificed; and provide palliative treatment of cancer (e.g., intestinal bypass for obstruction, spinal cord decompression, or orthopedic procedures to prevent or

癌症治疗原则

何焱 译　王志杰 仲佳 审校　王洁 通审

引言

癌症治疗领域发展迅速，涵盖局部治疗（外科手术、放射治疗）、全身治疗（化疗、靶向治疗、免疫治疗）以及支持性治疗药物等。手术和放射治疗作为局部治疗的有效手段，技术不断精进。鉴于癌症在多数情况下（尤其是晚期）为全身性疾病，全身治疗尤为重要。化疗作为"第一代"抗肿瘤药物，仍是全身治疗的核心。随着肿瘤的分子生物学以及基因组学研究日新月异，抗肿瘤药物临床试验层出不穷，免疫治疗和靶向治疗药物相继问世，目前抗肿瘤药物数量激增，远超其他药物类别。此外，癌症治疗常伴随诸多副作用，因此症状控制已成为癌症治疗中的重要环节。所有治疗方法均要求患者在专业的肿瘤中心接受来自多学科团队的综合治疗。本章将探讨癌症治疗各环节的原则。

诊断和分期

癌症的精准治疗依赖于组织学诊断，往往需要通过侵入性活检获取肿瘤组织样本，以评估其形态、侵袭性及分子标志物表达特征。尽管非侵入性检查如放射影像学在某些情况下可作为辅助诊断方法，但通常无法替代组织学诊断（偶尔会有例外，例如对于肝硬化患者，α-甲胎蛋白水平升高伴随影像学证据时，可用于诊断肝细胞癌）。

对于大多数实体肿瘤，一旦被确诊，则需要进行分期评估，以明确肿瘤的扩散程度。肿瘤分期包括临床分期和病理分期。其中，临床分期基于体格检查和影像学检查，包括靶向超声（经皮或使用侵入性内窥镜设备）、计算机断层成像、磁共振成像、全身正电子发射断层成像和放射性核素扫描。以上检查通常会根据特定类型的肿瘤及其转移到相应器官的倾向性联合使用。病理分期则更为明确，基于美国癌症联合委员会和国际抗癌联盟制定的肿瘤-淋巴结-转移（TNM）分期系统。该系统要求对原发肿瘤切除标本进行仔细评估，以确定三项指标：①原发肿瘤的大小和侵袭范围（T分期），②组织学受累的区域淋巴结的数量和位置（N分期），③有无远处转移（M分期），其中M分期基于临床信息和病理结果。根据TNM分期划分病理分期（从Ⅰ期到Ⅳ期），精准地反映了疾病负担的逐步加剧与肿瘤恶化过程。此外，TNM分期也为临床治疗方案的制订提供了不可或缺的指导依据，更是预测患者预后的关键工具。例如，切除的结肠癌侵犯了固有肌层，受累淋巴结数量为2/16，无远处转移迹象，则分期为T2N1M0（Ⅲ期），肿瘤复发的可能性为40%～50%，建议患者在手术后进行3～6个月的化疗。反之，如果不存在淋巴结受累则分期为T2N0M0（Ⅰ期），肿瘤复发的可能性小于10%，通常不建议进行术后化疗。

生物标志物可提供额外的预后信息，例如乳腺癌中激素受体阴性或人表皮生长因子受体-2（HER2）过表达提示预后不良。同时这些标志物还具有预测意义，例如，乳腺癌中HER2的过表达提示曲妥珠单抗治疗有效。结直肠癌中的*KRAS*突变提示患者对表皮生长因子受体（EGFR）抗体（如西妥昔单抗、帕尼单抗）的治疗缺乏应答（图3.1）。目前临床上常使用二代测序（NGS）平台对其中的一组生物标志物进行检测，以及对数百个相关基因进行测序，以确定点突变、易位、拷贝数变化和基因表达水平变化。综合以上信息来最终评估肿瘤是否可以治愈。

评估患者的整体临床状况同样重要，包括影响主要器官功能的合并症与患者的体力状态。常用的评估方法包括东部肿瘤协作组（ECOG）或Karnofsky评分。体力状态差或有严重合并症的患者可能无法从抗肿瘤治疗中获益，并且出现不良反应的风险更高。综合评估诊断、分期、预后和预测标志物以及患者体力状态后，决定对患者采取根治性或姑息性的治疗方案。

手术治疗的原则

手术可以通过切除具有癌变风险或已发生癌前病变的器官来预防肿瘤的发生。例如，对存在高乳腺癌遗传风险的患者进行双侧乳房切除术。手术还可以通过活检来进行确诊；通过淋巴结取样来辅助分期；通过切除原发肿瘤提供根治性治疗；重建因疾病或创伤而丧失的肢体或器官；并为患者提供姑息性治疗（如针对肠道梗阻的肠旁路术、脊髓减压术，或预防和治疗病理性骨折的骨科手

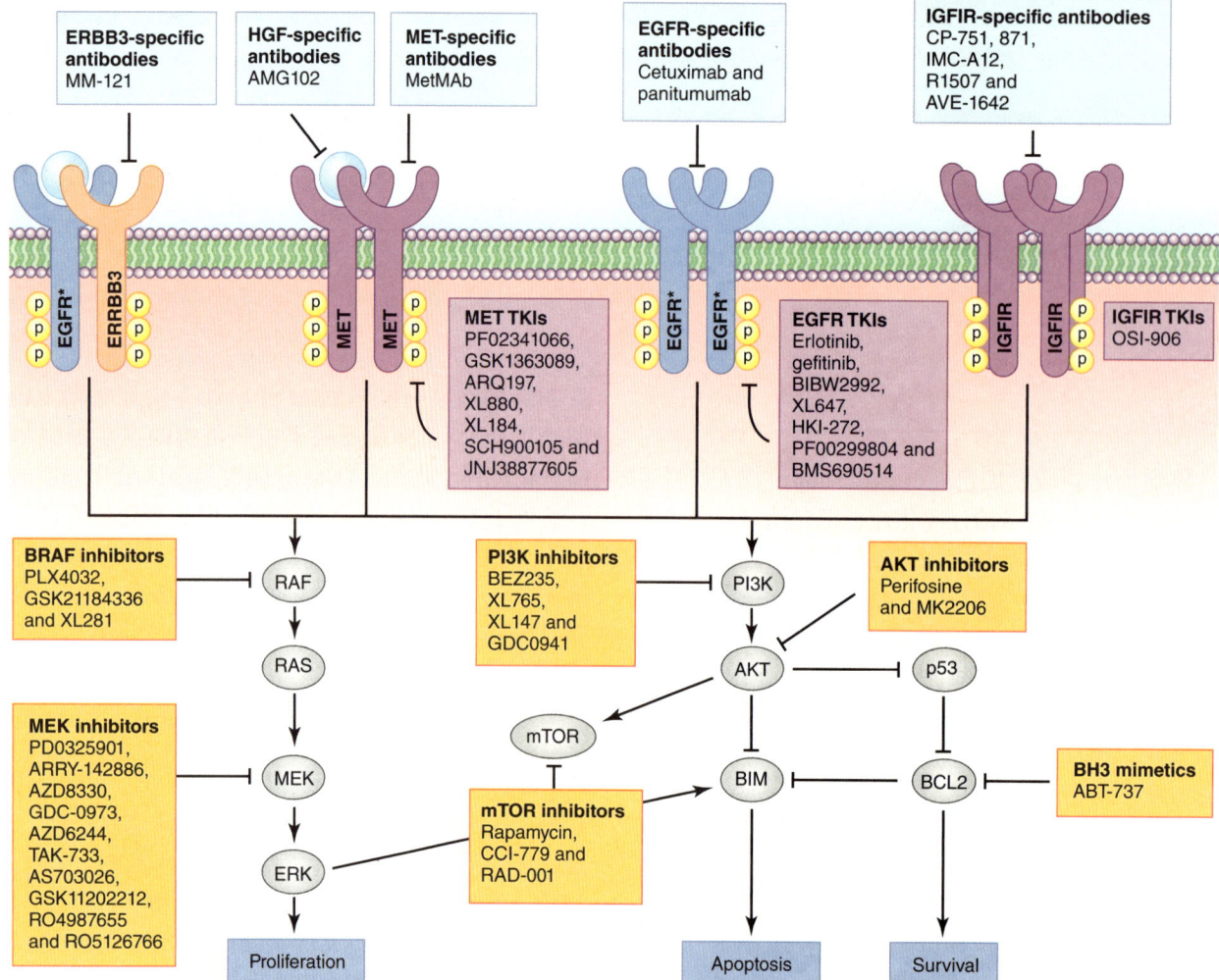

Fig. 3.1 The epidermal growth factor receptor (EGFR) pathway and related therapeutic targets. This figure depicts the transmembrane receptors of the EGFR family and the molecules involved in downstream signal transduction that ultimately lead to control of key proteins affecting cell survival, growth, and proliferation.

treat pathologic fractures). Invasive procedures, such as biopsies and the insertion of various access devices, tubes, stents, catheters, and drains, are also performed by interventional specialists, such as radiologists, gastroenterologists, and pulmonologists.

When a solid organ cancer is localized, surgery is the most effective curative treatment available. The intent is to completely remove the tumor, regional lymph nodes, and adjacent involved tissue, along with a safe margin of normal tissue. At surgery, the tumor is isolated and is almost never opened during the procedure. Refinements in cancer surgery include increasing use of minimally invasive methods in selected cancers and the identification of a sentinel lymph node by injection of a dye during surgery, which avoids a full lymph node dissection if the sentinel node is uninvolved by cancer.

PRINCIPLES OF RADIATION THERAPY

Radiation therapy can sometimes be used as definitive treatment, either alone or in combination with systemic therapy. Unlike surgery, local or regional treatment with radiation can preserve organ structure and function, improving quality of life for patients. For example, use of radiation with chemotherapy for treatment of localized laryngeal cancer has outcomes similar to those of surgery but allows preservation of the larynx. Radiation therapy is also effective in the palliative setting, where it is used to control various cancer-related problems such as pain, mechanical obstruction of a luminal organ, and bleeding.

Ionizing radiation damages cellular DNA directly or indirectly through free radical intermediates. Cells are most susceptible to radiation during the M and G_2 phases of the cell cycle. The aim of radiation therapy is to deliver the highest dose possible to the tumor with minimal toxicity to adjacent normal tissues. Dividing the total planned radiation dose into small daily fractions takes advantage of the difference in repair capability between normal and malignant tissue and improves the tolerance of normal tissue. The biologic effects of radiation can be modified by numerous factors, including the amount of oxygen in the irradiated tissue and the use of chemotherapy for sensitizing tissue to radiation.

The goal of treatment planning for radiation therapy is to precisely define the dose and volume to be irradiated. The dose of radiation is measured in units of absorbed dose, Gray (Gy), which has replaced the older unit, rad (1 Gy = 100 rad). Conventional radiation treatments deliver 1.8 to 2 Gy/day on 5 days per week, over a period of 5 to 6 weeks. For palliative treatment, higher doses per fraction may be used to deliver an effective dose over a shorter period.

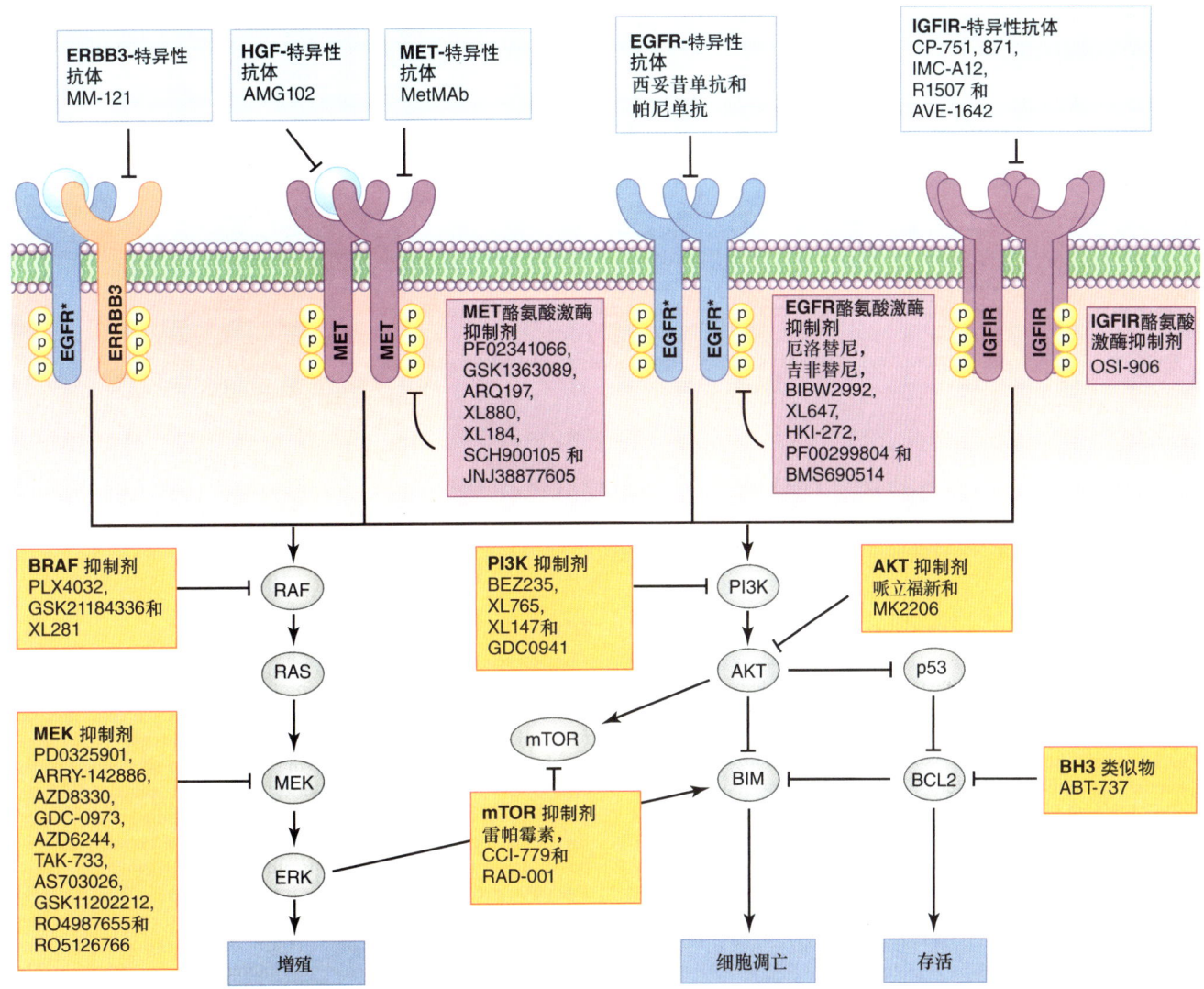

图 3.1 表皮生长因子受体（EGFR）通路及相关治疗靶点。图中描述了 EGFR 家族的跨膜受体及参与下游信号传导的分子，最终对影响细胞存活、生长和增殖的关键蛋白进行调控

术）。此外，侵入性手术，如组织活检以及插入各类通路设备（支架、导管和引流管）等，通常由有介入经验的专家操作，包括放射科医师、消化科医师和呼吸科医师等。

对于较为局限的实体肿瘤，手术是最有效的根治性治疗手段。其核心目的在于彻底清除肿瘤病灶、区域淋巴结和邻近受累组织，同时确保切除一定范围的正常组织作为安全切缘。在手术过程中，肿瘤会被严格隔离以保证在手术中不被切开。目前，肿瘤手术的改进不断取得新进展，这包括在特定肿瘤中更多地选择微创术式，以及在手术过程中通过注射特殊染料来识别前哨淋巴结。如果前哨淋巴结没有受累，则可以避免进行全面的淋巴结清扫，从而减少对患者的创伤。

放射治疗的原则

放射治疗有时可以作为肿瘤根治性治疗手段，既可单独使用，也可与全身治疗相结合。与手术不同，局部或区域性放射治疗可以保留器官结构和功能，进而提高患者的生活质量。例如，在治疗局限性喉癌时，采用放射治疗和化疗相结合的方法，其疗效与手术相似，但可以同时保留喉部功能。此外，放射治疗在姑息治疗中也是有效的，可用于控制肿瘤相关的疼痛、空腔脏器的机械性梗阻和出血等。

电离辐射通过自由基中间体对细胞 DNA 造成直接或间接的损伤。细胞在细胞周期的 M 期和 G2 期对辐射最为敏感。放射治疗的主要目标是向肿瘤组织提供高剂量的辐射，同时尽量降低对邻近正常组织的毒性。为实现这一目标，通常将计划的总辐射剂量分割成每日小剂量进行，利用正常组织和肿瘤组织在修复能力上的差异，提高正常组织的耐受性。辐射的生物学效应受多种因素的影响，包括受辐射组织中的氧含量以及是否通过化疗来增强组织对辐射的敏感性。

放射治疗计划的核心在于精准地确定辐射剂量和辐射体积。辐射剂量以吸收剂量的单位——戈瑞（Gray, Gy）进行衡量，Gy 已取代旧单位拉德（rad）（1 Gy = 100 rad）。常规放射治疗的总疗程为 5～6 周，每周治疗 5 日，单日剂量为 1.8～2 Gy。对于姑息性治疗，可以在较短时间内通过提高单次剂量来提供有效剂量。

TABLE 3.1 Commonly Used Chemotherapy Agents

Drug	Cancers Treated	Specific Class or Mechanism of Action	Common Side Effects
Cell Cycle–Specific			
5-Fluorouracil	Gastrointestinal, head and neck, breast	Antimetabolite, inhibits thymidylate synthase	Myelosuppression, mucositis, diarrhea
Gemcitabine	Pancreas, lung, breast, bladder	Antimetabolite, deoxycytidine analogue	Myelosuppression, nausea, emesis
Methotrexate	ALL, choriocarcinoma, bladder, lymphoma	Antimetabolite, folic acid antagonist	Myelosuppression, mucositis, acute renal failure
Doxorubicin	Breast, lung, NHL	Anthracycline, intercalates into DNA	Myelosuppression, nausea, emesis, cardiomyopathy
Irinotecan	Colorectal, lung	Camptothecin, topoisomerase I inhibitor	Myelosuppression, diarrhea
Paclitaxel	Breast, lung, Kaposi's sarcoma, ovarian	Plant alkaloid, inhibits microtubule formation	Myelosuppression, hypersensitivity reaction, neuropathy
Vincristine	ALL, lymphomas, myeloma, sarcoma	Plant alkaloid, disrupts microtubule assembly	Peripheral neuropathy, constipation
Cell Cycle–Nonspecific			
Cyclophosphamide	Breast, NHL, CLL, sarcoma	Alkylating agent, cross-links DNA	Myelosuppression, hemorrhagic cystitis, nausea, emesis
Cisplatin	Lung, bladder, ovarian, testicular, head and neck	Alkylating agent, cross-links DNA	Nephrotoxicity, nausea, emesis, ototoxicity, sensory neuropathy

ALL, Acute lymphoblastic leukemia; *CLL,* chronic lymphocytic leukemia; *NHL,* non-Hodgkin's lymphoma.

Ionizing radiation can be administered as external-beam therapy with the use of a linear accelerator to generate electrons or high-energy radiographs. Electrons have a limited depth of penetration and are useful for superficial tumors. High-energy radiographs deliver the radiation deep into the body while reducing the dose to the skin as they enter. Brachytherapy uses radioactive sources to deliver ionizing radiation (gamma rays) directly to the tumor. An example is the implantation of iodine-125 seeds into the prostate as definitive therapy for early prostate cancer. Current approaches to improving radiation therapy include the use of advanced technology that allows delivery of a higher dose of radiation to specific areas of the tumor and sparing of normal tissue (conformal and intensity-modulated radiation therapy).

Injury to normal tissue from radiation therapy can be either acute or late. Acute effects occur within days to weeks after irradiation and are seen primarily in rapidly proliferating tissues such as skin and gastrointestinal mucosa. The severity depends on the total dose, but the damage can usually be repaired. Late effects, such as necrosis, fibrosis, or organ failure, appear months or years after irradiation and are dependent on fraction size. Another late complication of radiation therapy is the development of secondary malignancies of organs in the radiation field, sometimes decades after radiation.

PRINCIPLES OF MEDICAL THERAPY

The term *chemotherapy* refers to the use of cytotoxic agents, singly or in combination, for the systemic treatment of cancer. Most such agents are general antiproliferative agents that are more effective against rapidly growing tumors and have significant adverse effects on normal tissues that also divide rapidly, such as bone marrow and digestive tract mucosa. Newer agents, including monoclonal antibodies and signal transduction inhibitors, are directed against targets that are relatively specific to tumor cells and therefore may have less toxicity. These drugs are classified separately from chemotherapy as *targeted therapy* agents. The newest class of anticancer drugs is *immunotherapy*. These drugs stimulate the T cell cytotoxic machinery to allow cancer cell kill by native immunologic mechanisms. Related to these immunotherapy drugs is the use of the T-cell arsenal from a donor (stem cell transplantation) or self (chimeric antigen receptor–T cells).

Mechanisms of Chemotherapy

Chemotherapeutic agents can be cell cycle–specific or cell cycle–nonspecific. Cell cycle–nonspecific agents have a greater effect on cells traversing the cell cycle but also affect noncycling cells; cell cycle–specific agents affect only cycling cells. Chemotherapy agents are further classified according to their mechanism of action into alkylating agents, antimetabolites, antitumor antibiotics, and mitotic spindle inhibitors (Table 3.1). Most chemotherapy agents suppress the bone marrow, increasing the risk of neutropenic infections, anemia, and exacerbated bleeding. For most drugs, treatment schedules involve successive doses every 2 to 4 weeks. This interval between successive doses, the *cycle* of chemotherapy, allows recovery of blood counts and other side effects before administration of the next dose. The concept of *dose intensity* is also important. Cellular killing with chemotherapy follows first-order kinetics: A given dose of drug kills only a fraction of tumor cells. The dose-response curve for chemotherapy drugs is steep. Therefore, the greater the dose administered, the greater the kill: A 2-fold increase in dose can lead to a 10-fold increase in tumor cell kill. This also means that dose reductions may adversely affect the eventual cure rate. Shortening of the duration of cycles of chemotherapy using growth factor support—a "dose-dense" approach—has been shown to improve survival in selected patients when compared with traditional chemotherapy for breast cancer.

Single chemotherapy agents seldom cure cancer. Combination chemotherapy regimens have therefore been developed for a variety of cancers. Combination therapy provides maximal cell kill and broader coverage of resistant cells; it may also prevent or slow the development of resistant cells. Drugs used in a combination are chosen because they have known efficacy as single agents but have differing mechanisms of action and non-overlapping toxicity profiles. These regimens are commonly referred to by acronyms, such as CHOP (cyclophosphamide, doxorubicin, vincristine, and prednisone) for lymphoma or FOLFOX (5-fluorouracil, leucovorin, and oxaliplatin) for colorectal cancer.

Indications for Chemotherapy

Chemotherapy outcomes in general for localized or advanced cancers are summarized in Table 3.2. *Adjuvant* chemotherapy refers to its use after the primary tumor has been resected. Here, chemotherapy is

表 3.1 常用化疗药物

药物名称	适用的肿瘤	作用机制类别	常见副作用
细胞周期特异性			
5-氟尿嘧啶	胃肠道肿瘤，头颈癌，乳腺癌	抗代谢药物，抑制胸苷酸合酶	骨髓抑制，黏膜炎，腹泻
吉西他滨	胰腺癌，肺癌，乳腺癌，膀胱癌	抗代谢药物，脱氧胞苷类似物	骨髓抑制，恶心，呕吐
甲氨蝶呤	ALL，绒毛膜癌，膀胱癌，淋巴瘤	抗代谢药物，叶酸拮抗剂	骨髓抑制，黏膜炎，急性肾衰竭
多柔比星	乳腺癌，肺癌，NHL	蒽环类，嵌入 DNA	骨髓抑制，恶心，呕吐，心肌病
伊立替康	结直肠癌，肺癌	喜树碱，拓扑异构酶 I 抑制剂	骨髓抑制，腹泻
紫杉醇	乳腺癌，肺癌，卡波西肉瘤，卵巢癌	植物生物碱，抑制微管形成	骨髓抑制，超敏反应，神经病变
长春新碱	ALL，淋巴瘤，骨髓瘤，肉瘤	植物生物碱，破坏微管组装	周围神经病，便秘
细胞周期非特异性			
环磷酰胺	乳腺癌，NHL，CLL，肉瘤	烷化剂，交联 DNA	骨髓抑制，出血性膀胱炎，恶心，呕吐
顺铂	肺癌，膀胱癌，卵巢癌，睾丸癌，头颈癌	烷化剂，交联 DNA	骨髓抑制，恶心，呕吐，耳毒性，感觉神经病变

注：ALL，急性淋巴细胞白血病；CLL，慢性淋巴细胞白血病；NHL，非霍奇金淋巴瘤。

电离辐射可以通过使用直线加速器产生电子或高能射线进行外照射治疗。由于电子的穿透深度有限，特别适用于浅表肿瘤的治疗。而高能射线则可以将辐射传送到体内深处，同时减少对皮肤的照射剂量。另一种治疗方法是近距离放射治疗，它使用放射源将电离辐射（伽马射线）直接传送到肿瘤部位。例如，将碘-125粒子植入前列腺，可以作为早期前列腺癌的根治性治疗手段。目前，放射治疗的新进展包括使用先进技术，使得能够向肿瘤特定区域提供更高剂量的辐射，同时保护正常组织（适形放疗和调强放射治疗）。

然而，经放射治疗的正常组织可能会发生急性或迟发性损伤。急性损伤发生在辐射后数天至数周内，主要见于快速增殖的组织，如皮肤和胃肠黏膜。其严重程度取决于放射治疗的总剂量，但这类损伤通常具有可修复性。相比之下，迟发性损伤如坏死、纤维化或器官衰竭，则在辐射后数月或数年出现，其出现时间取决于单次辐射剂量大小。放射治疗的另一个迟发性并发症是辐射野内的器官出现继发性恶性肿瘤，有时在辐射后数十年才出现。

内科治疗的原则

化疗是指单独或联合使用细胞毒性药物对肿瘤进行全身治疗。此类药物多为抗增殖药物，对快速生长的肿瘤更为有效，但同时也会对同样快速分裂的正常组织（如骨髓和消化道黏膜）产生明显的副作用。近年来，新型药物如单克隆抗体和信号转导抑制剂相继出现，它们直接靶向肿瘤细胞的特异性靶点。相较于传统化疗药物，该类药物毒性可能较小，被称为靶向治疗药物。新型抗肿瘤药物还包括免疫治疗药物，这些药物通过激活细胞毒性 T 细胞，利用自身免疫细胞杀伤肿瘤细胞。与免疫治疗相关的还包括使用来自供体（干细胞移植）或自体（嵌合抗原受体-T 细胞）的 T 细胞库治疗。

化疗机制

化疗药物可分为细胞周期特异性或非特异性药物。细胞周期非特异性药物对处于细胞周期的细胞影响更大，但同时也会影响 G_0 期细胞；而细胞周期特异性药物仅影响处于周期的细胞。根据其作用机制的不同，可将化疗药物进一步分为烷化剂、抗代谢药物、抗肿瘤抗生素和有丝分裂纺锤体抑制剂等几大类（表3.1）。大多数化疗药物会抑制骨髓功能，从而增加中性粒细胞减少所引起的感染、贫血和出血风险。对于大多数化疗药物而言，治疗方案为每 2～4 周连续给药 1 次，连续给药之间的间隔即为化疗周期。血细胞计数和其他副作用在下次给药前得以恢复。剂量强度的概念也非常重要，因为化疗药物的细胞杀伤效果遵循一级动力学原理：即一定剂量的药物仅能杀死一部分肿瘤细胞，且化疗药物的剂量-反应曲线陡峭。这意味着给予化疗药物的剂量越大，其杀伤力越强：剂量增加 2 倍可以使得对肿瘤细胞的杀伤力增加 10 倍。因此，减少剂量可能不利于最终的治疗效果和治愈率。与传统的乳腺癌化疗相比，使用生长因子支持下的"剂量密集"法可以缩短化疗周期，改善某些患者的生存。

在化疗的应用中，单药化疗很少能够完全治愈肿瘤。因此，在多种肿瘤的治疗中已开发多种联合化疗方案。联合化疗可以最大程度地杀死肿瘤细胞，更广泛地覆盖耐药细胞；同时还可能预防或延缓耐药细胞的发展。之所以选择联合化疗，是因为这些单药化疗的疗效已明确，但它们的作用机制不同，且毒性不重叠。联合化疗方案通常以首字母缩略词表示，如治疗淋巴瘤的 CHOP 方案（环磷酰胺、多柔比星、长春新碱和泼尼松），或用于结直肠癌的 FOLFOX 方案（5-氟尿嘧啶、亚叶酸和奥沙利铂）。

化疗适应证

局部或晚期肿瘤的化疗疗效总结见表 3.2。辅助化疗是指在原发肿瘤切除后进行的化疗。在这种情况下，

TABLE 3.2 Efficacy of Medical Therapy in Selected Cancers

Cure Possible Even in Advanced Disease
Testicular cancer
Acute leukemia: lymphocytic, promyelocytic, selected myelocytic
Lymphomas: Hodgkin's lymphoma, selected non-Hodgkin's lymphomas
Childhood solid tumors: rhabdomyosarcoma, Ewing sarcoma, Wilms tumor
Choriocarcinoma
Small cell lung cancer

Cure Likely in Locoregional Disease
Breast cancer
Colorectal cancer
Prostate cancer
Renal cancer
Head and neck cancer

Long-Term Control Possible in Advanced Disease
Melanoma
Non-small cell lung cancer
Chronic myeloid leukemia

directed against presumed systemic micrometastases in patients who are at high risk for recurrence. In the example of stage III colon cancer (described earlier), 3 to 6 months of adjuvant chemotherapy after primary tumor resection can reduce the patient's likelihood of developing recurrent cancer from 50% to 25%. Adjuvant chemotherapy has been shown to increase cure rates in many other cancers.

Neoadjuvant or *preoperative* chemotherapy refers to the use of chemotherapy before surgery, sometimes in combination with radiation therapy. If successful, neoadjuvant therapy can reduce the size of the tumor and consequently permit less removal of normal tissue, such as a lumpectomy instead of a mastectomy in breast cancer or limb-sparing surgery instead of amputation in extremity sarcoma.

Chemotherapy can be curative on its own in cancers such as germ cell tumors, lymphomas, and leukemias. Most often, chemotherapy is employed in the treatment of metastatic disease for which surgery or radiation therapy is ineffective. Even when it is not curative, chemotherapy often extends survival and improves cancer-related symptoms and quality of life.

Limitations of Chemotherapy

Chemotherapy is curative only under certain circumstances, because it is inherently limited by side effects (i.e., the dose ceiling). There are several reasons for the inability of standard doses of chemotherapy to cure cancer. First, tumor cell kinetics naturally protect against chemotherapy. When chemotherapy was initially developed, it was believed that tumors contained a percentage of cells traversing the cell cycle. However, most human tumors display Gompertzian growth kinetics—that is, the rate of tumor cell doubling *slows* progressively as tumor size increases. Therefore, the growth fraction of tumors is greatest when a tumor is clinically undetectable. By the time the patient is symptomatic and has clinically evident disease, the growth fraction of tumors can be less than 5%. Chemotherapy can be successful in the adjuvant setting (when the burden of disease is minimal), but it rarely results in cure in the metastatic setting.

Second, cancer cells can become resistant to chemotherapy. One of the most important forms of resistance is intrinsic and is mediated by an evolutionarily conserved cell membrane efflux pump called *P-glycoprotein*. Resistance can also be acquired after a period of exposure to chemotherapy agents by a variety of mechanisms; for example, tumor cells can decrease the uptake of methotrexate by decreasing the expression of the folate transporter, or they can amplify expression of the target enzyme thymidylate synthase when treated with 5-fluorouracil.

Third, mutations in the *TP53* gene are common in various cancers. The TP53 protein causes cell-cycle arrest and mediates apoptosis when DNA damage occurs. In the absence of a functioning TP53, cancer cells are protected from chemotherapy-induced apoptosis.

Targeted Therapy

The limitations of chemotherapy, coupled with a greater understanding of cancer cell biology, has led to the development of a new class of drugs directed against targets that are relatively specific to cancer cells: growth factors and signaling molecules that are essential for proliferation of tumor cells; cell-cycle proteins; regulators of apoptosis; and molecules mediating host-tumor interactions such as angiogenesis and tumor immunity. These agents include monoclonal antibodies directed against cell surface antigens or growth factors, specific or multitargeted receptor tyrosine kinase inhibitors, specific pathway signal transduction inhibitors, antisense oligonucleotides, and gene therapies. Additional agents are under development. The usual side effects of chemotherapy, such as myelosuppression, nausea, emesis, diarrhea, and alopecia, are not necessarily observed with these drugs. However, other target-specific toxicities require careful monitoring and management (Table 3.3).

The best-known targeted therapy agent is imatinib, which inhibits both BCR-ABL, the constitutively active fusion product arising from the Philadelphia chromosome of CML, and KIT (c-kit, CD117), which is overexpressed in gastrointestinal stromal tumors (GIST). The daily oral administration of imatinib results in complete hematologic responses in more than 90% of patients in chronic-phase CML and partial responses in more than 50% of patients with metastatic GIST. Ibrutinib is another novel agent, targeting Bruton tyrosine kinase, with excellent efficacy in CLL and Waldenström's macroglobulinemia.

In many other malignancies, there are multiple redundant signaling pathways that are dysregulated. Increasingly, tyrosine kinase inhibitors with multiple (as opposed to specific) targets have been developed to treat such cancers. Sorafenib and sunitinib are two examples of such agents that inhibit various pathways, including vascular endothelial growth factor (VEGF), platelet-derived growth factor (PDGF), and KIT. Studies have shown these drugs to be effective in renal and liver cancers.

Targeted therapy drugs can also increase the efficacy of chemotherapy, through various mechanisms. For instance, the EGFR antagonists cetuximab and panitumumab increase the efficacy of irinotecan-based chemotherapy in colorectal cancer and that of definitive radiation therapy in oropharyngeal cancers. The availability of these agents has increased the number of drug combinations that can be used in particular cancers. As multiple combinations of chemotherapy and targeted therapy have become available for the treatment of advanced colon cancer the median survival time of patients with this disease has more than doubled. Targeted therapy agents are also increasingly being used in the adjuvant setting—imatinib in patients with resected GIST or trastuzumab in patients with resected HER2-positive breast cancer have substantially improved outcomes for these malignancies.

Endocrine Therapy

Cancers originating from organs that are regulated by hormones, such as breast and prostate, may be susceptible to hormonal control mechanisms even when metastatic. Endocrine therapy includes the use of both hormonal and antihormonal agents that work as antagonists or partial agonists.

表 3.2 部分肿瘤的化疗疗效
晚期可能治愈的肿瘤
睾丸癌
急性白血病：淋巴细胞白血病，早幼粒细胞白血病，部分粒细胞白血病
淋巴瘤：霍奇金淋巴瘤，部分非霍奇金淋巴瘤
儿童实体肿瘤：横纹肌肉瘤，尤因肉瘤，肾母细胞瘤
绒毛膜癌
小细胞肺癌
局部治愈可能性大的肿瘤
乳腺癌
结直肠癌
前列腺癌
肾癌
头颈癌
晚期可长期控制的肿瘤
黑色素瘤
非小细胞肺癌
慢性髓系白血病

化疗针对的是高复发风险患者体内可能存在的全身微小转移病灶。在前面提到的Ⅲ期结肠癌案例中，原发肿瘤切除后进行 3～6 个月的辅助化疗，可以将肿瘤复发的概率由 50% 降低到 25%。此外，在其他多种肿瘤中也显示辅助化疗可提高其治愈率。

新辅助化疗是指在手术前进行的化疗，有时会与放射治疗联合使用。如果有效，新辅助化疗可以缩小肿瘤的大小，从而减少对正常组织的切除。例如，在乳腺癌中进行肿块切除术代替乳房切除术，或在肢端肉瘤中进行保肢手术代替截肢术。

化疗本身对于某些肿瘤类型，如生殖细胞肿瘤、淋巴瘤和白血病等，具有治愈潜力。化疗通常多用于治疗手术或放射治疗无效的转移性疾病。即使无法根治肿瘤，化疗通常也能延长患者的生存期，改善肿瘤相关症状和生活质量。

化疗的局限性

化疗并非在所有情况下都能治愈肿瘤，这主要受到其副作用（即剂量上限）的限制。标准剂量的化疗无法治愈肿瘤的原因有几个方面。首先，肿瘤细胞本身会对化疗产生抵抗。在化疗应用之初，人们认为肿瘤中含有一定比例的跨越细胞周期的肿瘤细胞。然而，大多数人类肿瘤具有 Gompertzian 生长动力学特征，即随着肿瘤体积的增加，肿瘤细胞倍增的速度逐渐减慢。因此，当临床上检测不到肿瘤时，肿瘤的生长分数最大。当患者出现症状并有临床证据显示疾病存在时，肿瘤的生长分数可能低于 5%。化疗在辅助治疗（疾病负担很小时）中可能会取得成功，但很少能治愈转移性疾病。

其次，肿瘤细胞可以发生化疗耐药，包括先天性耐药和获得性耐药。先天性耐药，主要由一种进化保守的细胞膜外排泵——P-糖蛋白介导。此外，肿瘤细胞也可以在接触化疗药物一段时间后，通过多种机制发生获得性耐药；例如，肿瘤细胞可以通过降低叶酸转运蛋白的表达来减少对甲氨蝶呤的摄取，或者在接受 5-氟尿嘧啶治疗时增加靶标胸苷酸合酶的表达。

不仅如此，在多种肿瘤中常见 *TP53* 基因突变。当发生 DNA 损伤时，TP53 蛋白会导致细胞周期停滞，介导细胞凋亡。而在 TP53 功能缺失时，肿瘤细胞能够避免发生化疗诱导的细胞凋亡。

靶向治疗

化疗具有一定的局限性，随着对肿瘤细胞生物学的深入研究，针对肿瘤细胞相对特异性靶点的新药层出不穷。这些药物针对的靶点包括：对肿瘤细胞增殖至关重要的生长因子和信号分子；细胞周期蛋白；细胞凋亡调节因子；以及介导宿主与肿瘤相互作用（如血管生成和肿瘤免疫）的分子。具体药物包括：针对细胞表面抗原或生长因子的单克隆抗体、特异性或多靶点受体酪氨酸激酶抑制剂、特异性通路的信号转导抑制剂、反义寡核苷酸和基因治疗药物，其他药物正在研发中。靶向治疗药物可能不会发生化疗常见的副作用，如骨髓抑制、恶心、呕吐、腹泻和脱发，但靶点特异性毒性仍需严格监测和管理（表 3.3）。

靶向治疗药物已经取得了显著的疗效。例如，伊马替尼可以同时抑制 BCR-ABL（慢性髓系白血病患者的费城染色体的组成型活性融合产物）和 KIT（c-kit，CD117），后者在胃肠道间质瘤（GIST）中过表达。每日口服伊马替尼，90% 以上的慢性期慢性髓系白血病患者达到血液学完全缓解，50% 以上的转移性 GIST 患者获得部分缓解。伊布替尼是另一种新型药物，靶向布鲁顿酪氨酸激酶，对慢性粒细胞白血病和 Waldenström 巨球蛋白血症疗效可观。

在许多其他恶性肿瘤中，存在多条信号通路失调。越来越多的多靶点（而非单一靶点）酪氨酸激酶抑制剂已被开发用于治疗此类肿瘤。作为代表药物，索拉非尼和舒尼替尼可以抑制多条通路，包括血管内皮生长因子（VEGF）、血小板源性生长因子（PDGF）和 KIT。研究表明，这类药物对肾癌及肝癌有效。

除了单独使用外，靶向治疗药物还可以通过多种机制提高化疗的疗效。如 EGFR 抑制剂西妥昔单抗和帕尼单抗可以提高结直肠癌中以伊立替康为基础的化疗疗效，并增强口腔癌中根治性放射治疗的疗效。这些药物的可及性使得某些肿瘤中可用药物组合的数量增加。在晚期结肠癌中，随着多种化疗和靶向治疗联合方案的出现，患者的中位生存时间已得到显著延长。同时，靶向治疗药物也越来越多地用于辅助治疗，如伊马替尼用于 GIST 切除后患者，曲妥珠单抗用于 HER2 阳性乳腺癌切除后患者。此类药物改善了这些恶性肿瘤的预后。

内分泌治疗

起源于受激素调控器官（如乳腺和前列腺）的肿瘤，即使在转移时也可能对激素调控机制敏感。内分泌治疗包括使用激素和抗激素类药物，它们作为抑制剂或部分激动剂发挥作用。

TABLE 3.3 Examples of Targeted Therapy Agents

Drug	Cancers Treated	Targets	Common Side Effects
Monoclonal Antibodies			
Alemtuzumab	CLL	CD52	Myelosuppression, fever, rash
Bevacizumab	Colorectal, renal, lung	VEGF	Hypertension, proteinuria, bleeding, thromboembolism
Cetuximab	Colorectal	EGFR	Rash
Ipilimumab	Metastatic melanoma	CTLA4	Cytokine release storm
Ofatumumab	CLL	CD20	Rash, diarrhea, respiratory tract infections
Panitumumab	Colorectal	EGFR	Rash
Pertuzumab	Breast	HER2	Rash, diarrhea
Rituximab	NHL	CD20	Infusional reaction, skin reactions
Trastuzumab	Breast	HER2/Neu	Infusional reaction, congestive heart failure
Signal Transduction Inhibitors			
Axitinib	Renal	VEGF, PDGF, KIT	Hypertension, hand-foot syndrome, diarrhea
Crizotinib	Lung	EML4-ALK	Edema, diarrhea
Dasatinib	CML	BCR-ABL	Myelosuppression, pleural effusions
Imatinib	CML, GIST	BCR-ABL	Diarrhea, fluid retention, myelosuppression
Erlotinib	Lung, pancreas	EGFR tyrosine kinase	Rash, diarrhea
Gefitinib	Lung	EGFR tyrosine kinase	Rash, hypertension
Ibrutinib	CLL, Waldenström's macroglobulinemia	Bruton tyrosine kinase	Bacterial infections
Imatinib	CML, GIST	BCR-ABL	Diarrhea, fluid retention, myelosuppression
Lapatinib	Breast	HER2, EGFR	Rash, diarrhea
Regorafenib	GIST, colorectal	VEGF	Hypertension, hepatotoxicity, dysphonia
Sunitinib	Renal, GIST	VEGF, PDGF, KIT	Rash, diarrhea, fatigue
Sorafenib	Liver, renal	VEGF, PDGF, KIT	Hypertension, fatigue, diarrhea, hand-foot syndrome
Vandetanib	Medullary thyroid	VEGF, EGFR, RET	Rash, abdominal pain, diarrhea
Vemurafenib	Melanoma	BRAF	Rash, skin lesions, arthralgia
Others			
All-*trans*-retinoic-acid	Acute promyelocytic leukemia	Differentiating agent	Vitamin A toxicity, retinoic acid syndrome, hyperlipidemia
Azacitidine	Myelodysplasia	Hypomethylating agent	Myelosuppression, injection site reactions
Bortezomib	Lymphoma, myeloma	Proteasome inhibitor	Rash, nausea, emesis, neuropathy
Everolimus	Renal, breast, neuroendocrine	mTOR inhibitor	Hyperglycemia, diarrhea, fatigue

CLL, Chronic lymphocytic leukemia; *CML*, chronic myelogenous leukemia; *CTLA4*, cytotoxic T lymphocyte–associated protein 4; *EGFR*, epidermal growth factor receptor; *GIST*, gastrointestinal stromal tumor; *mTOR*, mammalian target of rifampin; *NHL*, non-Hodgkin's lymphoma; *VEGF*, vascular endothelial growth factor.

Many patients with metastatic breast cancer express hormone receptors (estrogen or progesterone) in tumor cells. Most of these patients respond either to tamoxifen, an estrogen receptor modulator, or to aromatase inhibitors (letrozole, anastrozole, or exemestane), which inhibit adrenal steroid production. Similar responses are observed in men with metastatic prostate cancer treated with the luteinizing hormone–releasing hormone agonists leuprolide or goserelin, which decrease testosterone to castrate levels.

In selected breast and prostate cancer patients, metastatic disease can be controlled for years with only endocrine therapy. Tamoxifen and the aromatase inhibitors are also highly effective adjuvant treatments after breast cancer resection. Furthermore, tamoxifen has been shown to reduce the incidence of breast cancer by 50% in healthy women who are at high risk for developing breast cancer.

Personalized Medicine

These targeted therapies—kinase inhibitors, antibodies, hormones—work only when their specific targets are present in the cancer cells. The paradigm of evaluation of tissue specimens for such targets to allow the use of drugs impinging on those targets is referred to as *precision* or *personalized medicine/oncology*. The time and costs involved in analyzing genomic alterations from a patient's tumor are now much reduced. In addition to DNA, transcriptomic (RNA), epigenomic (DNA methylation), and single-nucleotide polymorphism (SNP array) analyses can also be performed. Several cancers have already been sequenced completely. Such work creates "reference libraries" against which a patient's tumor can be tested. Based on findings from such analyses, specific drugs or regimens can be recommended for individual patients. Most of the targeted therapies, and even immunotherapies, have predictive molecular markers: microsatellite instability, tumor mutation burden, *NTRK* and *FGFR* fusions, *KRAS* and *BRAF* mutations, HER2 and cMET overexpression being prominent examples. A prominent success story has been lung cancer, where therapies targeting EGFR mutations, ALK fusions, MET alterations, and others are now front-line treatments with much greater clinical benefit than traditional cytotoxic agents.

Immunotherapy

Immunotherapy agents act by altering the host immune response to the tumor. They either stimulate the cytotoxic T-cell machinery directly

表 3.3 靶向治疗药物示例

药物名称	适用的肿瘤	靶点	常见副作用
单克隆抗体			
阿仑单抗	CLL	CD52	骨髓抑制，发热，皮疹
贝伐珠单抗	结直肠癌，肾癌，肺癌	VEGF	高血压，蛋白尿，出血，血栓栓塞
西妥昔单抗	结直肠癌	EGFR	皮疹
伊匹木单抗	转移性黑色素瘤	CTLA4	细胞因子释放风暴
奥法木单抗	CLL	CD20	皮疹，腹泻，呼吸道感染
帕尼单抗	结直肠癌	EGFR	皮疹
培妥珠单抗	乳腺癌	HER2	皮疹，腹泻
利妥昔单抗	NHL	CD20	输液反应，皮肤反应
曲妥珠单抗	乳腺癌	HER2/Neu	输液反应，充血性心力衰竭
信号转导抑制剂			
阿昔替尼	肾癌	VEGF，PDGF，KIT	高血压，手足综合征，腹泻
克唑替尼	肺癌	EML4-ALK	水肿，腹泻
达沙替尼	CML	BCR-ABL	骨髓抑制，胸腔积液
伊马替尼	CML，GIST	BCR-ABL	腹泻，液体潴留，骨髓抑制
厄洛替尼	肺癌，胰腺癌	EGFR 酪氨酸激酶	皮疹，腹泻
吉非替尼	肺癌	EGFR 酪氨酸激酶	皮疹，高血压
伊布替尼	CLL，Waldenström 巨球蛋白血症	布鲁顿酪氨酸激酶	细菌感染
伊马替尼	CML，GIST	BCR-ABL	腹泻，体液潴留，骨髓抑制
拉帕替尼	乳腺癌	HER2，EGFR	皮疹，腹泻
瑞戈非尼	GIST，结直肠癌	VEGF	高血压，肝毒性，发声困难
舒尼替尼	肾癌，GIST	VEGF，PDGF，KIT	皮疹，腹泻，疲劳
索拉非尼	肝癌，肾癌	VEGF，PDGF，KIT	高血压，疲劳，腹泻，手足综合征
凡德他尼	甲状腺髓样癌	VEGF，PDGF，KIT	皮疹，腹痛，腹泻
维莫非尼	黑色素瘤	BRAF	皮疹，皮肤病变，关节痛
其他类			
全反式维甲酸	急性早幼粒细胞白血病	分化诱导剂	维生素 A 毒性，视黄酸毒性，高脂血症
阿扎胞苷	骨髓增生异常综合征	低甲基化剂	骨髓抑制，注射部位反应
硼替佐米	淋巴瘤，骨髓瘤	蛋白酶体抑制剂	皮疹，恶心，呕吐，神经毒性
依维莫司	肾癌，乳腺癌，神经内分泌癌	mTOR 抑制剂	高血糖，腹泻，疲劳

注：BRAF，B-Raf 原癌基因；CLL，慢性淋巴细胞白血病；CML，慢性粒细胞白血病；CTLA4，细胞毒性 T 细胞相关蛋白 4；EGFR，表皮生长因子受体；GIST，胃肠道间质瘤；KIT，KIT 原癌基因；mTOR，哺乳动物雷帕霉素靶蛋白；NHL，非霍奇金淋巴瘤；VEGF，血管内皮生长因子；PDGF，血小板源性生长因子。

许多转移性乳腺癌患者的肿瘤细胞中表达激素（雌激素或孕激素）受体。此类患者大多数对他莫昔芬（一种雌激素受体调节剂）或抑制肾上腺类固醇生成的芳香化酶抑制剂（来曲唑、阿那曲唑或依西美斯坦）治疗有效。在转移性前列腺癌中，接受促黄体素释放激素激动剂亮丙瑞林或戈舍瑞林治疗的患者也观察到类似的反应，可以将睾酮降低至去势水平。

在部分乳腺癌和前列腺癌患者中，仅使用内分泌治疗就可以控制转移性疾病达数年。他莫昔芬和芳香化酶抑制剂也是乳腺癌切除术后非常有效的辅助治疗手段。此外，他莫昔芬可使乳腺癌高危健康妇女的乳腺癌发病率降低 50%。

个性化医疗

靶向治疗包括激酶抑制剂、抗体和激素，仅在癌细胞中存在其特异性靶点时有效。对组织样本中的靶点进行评估，进而使用针对这些靶点的药物的模式被称为精准或个性化医疗。目前，分析患者肿瘤的基因组变异所需的时间和成本大大降低。除了 DNA 测序，还可进行转录组（RNA）、表观基因组（DNA 甲基化）和单核苷酸多态性（SNP 阵列）分析。某些肿瘤已完成全部测序工作，创建了可用于测试患者肿瘤的"参考文库"。根据这些分析结果，可以为每一位患者推荐具体的药物或方案。大多数靶向治疗，甚至包括免疫疗法，都有预测性的分子标志物，其中最具有代表性的包括：微卫星不稳定性、肿瘤突变负荷、*NTRK* 和 *FGFR* 融合、*KRAS* 和 *BRAF* 突变、HER2 和 cMET 过表达。以肺癌为例，针对 *EGFR* 突变、*ALK* 融合、*MET* 突变等靶点的靶向治疗已成为一线治疗选择，相比传统的细胞毒性药物能带来更大的临床获益。

免疫治疗

免疫治疗药物通过改变宿主对肿瘤的免疫应答来发挥作用。它们通过直接刺激细胞毒性 T 细胞，或解除 T 细胞免疫抑制，从而激活 T 细胞识别和杀灭癌细胞。肿瘤疫苗利用特异性肿瘤抗原，作为活化 T 细胞的靶点

or counter the inhibitory mechanisms keeping these cells quiescent, the result being that T cells get primed to recognize and kill cancer cells. Cancer vaccines, such as the dendritic cell vaccine sipuleucel-T for prostate cancer, exploit the presence of specific tumor antigens that can serve as targets of the stimulated T cells. Their use is so far limited to a handful of scenarios.

More recently, antibodies targeting CTLA4 and PD1, which are inhibitory receptors on the surface of cytotoxic T-cells (or PD-L1, the ligand on tumor cells that corresponds to PD1), have achieved great success in the treatment of various malignancies. These checkpoint inhibitors—so called because they block the molecular "checkpoints" that normally inhibit cytotoxic T-cells—unleash the body's immune response to recognize cancer cells as "foreign" and kill them. This is akin to the graft-versus-tumor response used in allogeneic hematopoietic stem cell transplantation; only here, the body's native immune system is primed to achieve the desired effect, with much less toxicity. A major toxicity observed with this approach is the possibility of "autoimmune" reaction whereby uncontrolled T-cell cytotoxicity damages normal cells and tissues. These drugs are now routinely used to treat melanoma, kidney cancer, and lung cancer, and achieve remarkably durable clinical responses.

The ability of these checkpoint inhibitors to work is dependent largely on their ability to see the cancer cells as "different" from the normal cells. Because cancer cells frequently have mutations that lead to the production of abnormal proteins, these neopeptides serve as neoantigens for the T cells, allowing differential identification and targeting of cancer cells. Therefore, the higher the tumor mutation burden, the more likely the efficacy of these drugs. This is clearly evident in high mutational load tumors such as ultraviolet light–associated melanoma, smoking-associated lung cancer, and cancers with high microsatellite instability, which respond very well to these drugs.

Stem Cell Transplantation

The traditional model of using T-cell immunity to counter cancer has been allogeneic stem cell transplantation. By using harvested stem cells (typically from the bone marrow of an HLA-matched donor), the immunologic response mounted by the donor cells, termed *graft-versus-tumor* effect, can lead to durable cures in various leukemias. However, allogeneic transplantations can be offered only to a minority of patients because of the limited availability of matched donors (particularly in ethnic minority populations) and the inability of older patients and those with comorbid illnesses to tolerate this procedure. To increase the availability of donors, umbilical cord blood is being studied as a source of stem cells.

The complications of stem cell transplantation are primarily related to the toxicity of chemotherapy and radiation therapy to vital organs, including lungs and liver. Long-term morbidity and mortality after allogeneic transplantation can result from *graft-versus-host disease* and from complications of immunosuppressive agents used to treat it.

CAR-T Cell Therapy

The newest advance in the field of using T cell cytotoxicity to kill cancer cells is chimeric antigen receptor–T (CAR-T) cells. This involves extracting a cancer patient's T cells and then modifying them using retroviral, lentiviral, or CRISPR/Cas9 gene editing methods. This editing process attaches a chimeric receptor on the surface of these T cells: the chimeric receptor combines a cancer cell–specific antigen binding site and a T cell activating site. These primed T cells are then infused back into the patient after depleting native T cells using chemotherapy. Extensive cytotoxic T cell activity leads to a "cytokine storm" that requires aggressive supportive care, but eventually, durable clinical responses in leukemias and lymphomas have been achieved. The efficacy of this approach in patients with solid organ malignancies is currently being tested.

EVALUATION OF RESPONSE

The efficacy of cancer-directed therapies is gauged by various methods and has been granted its own vocabulary. In patients with metastatic disease, all known sites of disease are monitored by physical examinations and serial radiologic imaging. Responses are judged according to the internationally accepted Response Evaluation Criteria in Solid Tumors (RECIST) rules. Disappearance of all known lesions is called a *complete response*, whereas a 30% or greater reduction in size is called a *partial response*. Appearance of new lesions or an increase in the size of known lesions by 20% is termed *progression of disease* and implies failure of treatment. A tumor that is neither responding nor progressing is termed *stable disease*.

The percentage of patients who experience a response is called the *response rate* to the agent or agents being administered. New drugs are often evaluated on the basis of response rates. However, a response does not imply cure. Even a drug with a 100% response rate is not curative if all patients relapse. Therefore, the "gold standard" for measuring the efficacy of a drug is considered to be an improvement in *overall survival*, or its surrogate, *disease-free survival*—the time interval during which the patient is alive without disease. The use of effective second-line therapies may minimize the survival differences between two treatments prescribed as initial therapy, and in this context, disease-free survival can serve as an important end point in evaluating new regimens. Increasingly, quality-of-life end points such as use of pain medications or patient-reported outcomes are also being used to assess the efficacy of drugs in palliation.

SUPPORTIVE CARE

Supportive care interventions can improve the safety and tolerability of cancer treatments. Many drugs can mitigate chemotherapy-related side effects. Serotonin receptor antagonists and neurokinin-1 receptor antagonists, in combination with older antiemetic drugs, may control chemotherapy-induced nausea and vomiting. Granulocyte colony-stimulating factor (filgrastim) and granulocyte-macrophage colony-stimulating factor (sargramostim) stimulate the proliferation and differentiation of myeloid progenitor cells and can prevent or minimize the duration of chemotherapy-induced neutropenia and reduce the likelihood of neutropenic fever. These agents are also used to mobilize and collect stem cells for transplantation.

Supportive care is an integral part of the treatment of cancer, particularly in noncurative settings. Palliative aspects of treating cancer address not only physical symptoms in particular pain syndromes but also psychosocial and spiritual concerns. Chemotherapy and radiation therapy are often used with palliative intent and can improve quality of life.

Acknowledgments

Dr. Khorana would like to acknowledge support from the Sondra and Stephen Hardis Endowed Chair in Oncology Research and the National Institutes of Health (U01-HL143402).

SUGGESTED READINGS

DeVita VT, Rosenberg SA: Two hundred years of cancer research, N Engl J Med 366:2207–2214, 2012.

Khalil DN, Smith EL, Brentjens RJ, Wolchok JD: The future of cancer treatment: immunomodulation, CARs and combination immunotherapy, Nat Rev Clin Oncol 13:273–290, 2016.

Mardis ER: The impact of next-generation sequencing on cancer genomics: from discovery to clinic, Cold Spring Harb Perspect Med 3:a036269, 2019.

（如用于前列腺癌的树突状细胞疫苗 sipuleucel-T）。然而，到目前为止，肿瘤疫苗的应用仍然有限。

近年来，靶向 CTLA4 和 PD-1（细胞毒性 T 细胞表面的抑制性受体）的抗体或针对 PD-L1（肿瘤细胞上 PD1 的配体）的药物，在治疗多种恶性肿瘤方面取得显著成效。由于这些药物能阻断抑制细胞毒性 T 细胞的分子"检查点"，从而激活机体的免疫应答，使免疫系统将肿瘤细胞视为"异物"并将其消灭，因此被称为免疫检查点抑制剂。这种机制类似于同种异体造血干细胞移植中的移植物抗肿瘤反应，但在这里，是机体的固有免疫系统被激活以达到治疗效果，且毒性相对较小。然而，这种治疗方法的主要毒性是可能引发"自身免疫"反应，即失控的 T 细胞毒性可能损害正常细胞和组织。目前，这些药物常规用于治疗黑色素瘤、肾癌和肺癌，取得显著持久的临床疗效。

这些免疫检查点抑制剂能否发挥作用，很大程度上取决于它们能否将肿瘤细胞视为与正常细胞"不同"的细胞。由于肿瘤细胞经常发生突变，导致异常蛋白质的生成，这些新生成的肽段可作为 T 细胞识别的新抗原，使得肿瘤细胞能够被特异性地识别和靶向。因此，肿瘤突变负荷越高，这些药物的疗效就可能越好。在高突变负荷肿瘤中，这一效果尤为明显，例如在紫外线相关的黑色素瘤、吸烟相关的肺癌以及具有高度微卫星不稳定性的肿瘤中，这类药物的疗效较为显著。

干细胞移植

利用 T 细胞免疫进行抗肿瘤治疗的经典手段是异体干细胞移植。该方法通过采集的 HLA 匹配供体的骨髓中的干细胞，利用供体细胞产生的免疫应答（即移植物抗肿瘤效应）来实现对多种白血病的持久治疗。然而，由于配型相合的供体有限（尤其是在少数民族人群中），且老年患者及有合并症的患者无法耐受这一过程，因此同种异体移植的应用范围相对有限。为了提高供体的可及性，目前正在研究将脐带血作为干细胞的来源。

干细胞移植的并发症主要与化疗和放疗对肺和肝等重要器官的毒性有关。异体移植后长期的发病和死亡可由移植物抗宿主病和用于治疗该病的免疫抑制剂并发症引起。

CAR-T 细胞治疗

在利用 T 细胞的细胞毒性杀灭肿瘤细胞方面，最新的进展为嵌合抗原受体 -T（CAR-T）细胞治疗。该过程涉及从肿瘤患者提取 T 细胞，然后使用逆转录病毒、慢病毒或 CRISPR/Cas9 技术对其进行基因编辑。这种编辑过程使嵌合受体在这些 T 细胞表面表达。嵌合受体同时具有肿瘤细胞特异性抗原结合位点和 T 细胞激活位点。在化疗清除原有的 T 细胞后，将这些 CAR-T 细胞回输到患者体内。尽管细胞毒性 T 细胞大量激活会导致"细胞因子风暴"，需要积极的支持性治疗，但 CAR-T 治疗在白血病和淋巴瘤中已观察到持续性的临床获益。目前，CAR-T 细胞治疗在实体器官恶性肿瘤患者中的疗效仍在探索中。

疗效评估

肿瘤疗效的评估方法多样。在转移性疾病患者中，通过体格检查和连续影像学检查监测所有已知的病灶。根据国际公认的实体瘤疗效评估标准（RECIST）规则进行疗效评估。具体内容包括：所有已知病灶消失称为完全缓解，病灶缩小达 30% 或以上称为部分缓解。出现新病灶或已知病灶增大达 20% 称为疾病进展，意味着治疗失败。肿瘤既没有缓解也没有进展的称为疾病稳定。

患者发生应答的比例被称为药物的应答率，这一指标通常用于新药评估。然而，应答并不等同于治愈。即使一种药物的应答率达到 100%，但如果所有患者都最终复发，那么也不能称为治愈。因此，总生存期或其替代指标——无病生存期（指患者在没有疾病的状态下存活的时间间隔）的提高被视为评估药物疗效的"金标准"。有效的二线治疗可能会缩小两种初始疗法之间的生存差异，在这种情况下，无病生存期可以作为评估新方案的重要终点。越来越多的生活质量终点，如止痛药物的使用或患者报告的结果也用于评估药物缓解的疗效。

支持性治疗

支持性治疗干预措施在肿瘤治疗中具有重要作用，可以提高治疗的安全性和耐受性。许多药物可以减轻化疗相关的副作用。例如，5- 羟色胺受体拮抗剂和神经激肽 -1 受体拮抗剂与传统止吐药联合使用，可以控制化疗诱发的恶心和呕吐。粒细胞集落刺激因子（如非格司亭）和粒细胞 - 巨噬细胞集落刺激因子（如沙格司亭）可以刺激髓系祖细胞的增殖和分化，从而预防化疗诱发的中性粒细胞减少症或缩短其持续时间，并降低发生中性粒细胞减少性发热的概率。这些药物还可以动员和收集干细胞用于移植。

支持性治疗是肿瘤治疗的一个重要组成部分，尤其在无法治愈的情况下更为关键。肿瘤治疗中的缓和医疗不仅要解决躯体症状，尤其是疼痛综合征的缓解，还包括社会心理和精神方面的全面治疗。化疗和放疗通常具有缓和医疗的目的，旨在改善患者的生活质量。

致谢

Khorana 博士谨感谢肿瘤学教授 Sondra 和 Stephen Hardis 以及美国国立卫生研究院（U01-HL143402）的支持。

推荐阅读

DeVita VT, Rosenberg SA: Two hundred years of cancer research, N Engl J Med 366:2207–2214, 2012.

Khalil DN, Smith EL, Brentjens RJ, Wolchok JD: The future of cancer treatment: immunomodulation, CARs and combination immunotherapy, Nat Rev Clin Oncol 13:273–290, 2016.

Mardis ER: The impact of next-generation sequencing on cancer genomics: from discovery to clinic, Cold Spring Harb Perspect Med 3:a036269, 2019.

4

Lung Cancer

Zoe G.S. Vazquez, Jason M. Aliotta, Christopher G. Azzoli

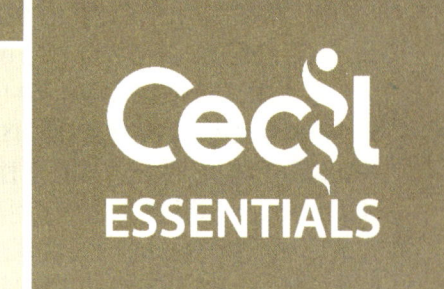

DEFINITION AND EPIDEMIOLOGY

Lung cancer is the second most common cancer in the United States and the leading cause of cancer death. Worldwide, an estimated 1 million people die of lung cancer each year. Despite recent advances in understanding of the biology and genetics of lung cancer and the advent of novel therapeutic agents for its treatment, the 5-year survival rate for patients with lung cancer is below 20%. The relatively poor long-term survival partly stems from the fact that most patients with lung cancer have an advanced stage of the disease at the time of diagnosis.

Historically, lung cancer has been divided into two major types: *small cell lung carcinoma* (SCLC) and *non–small cell lung carcinoma* (NSCLC). It is increasingly important to recognize the subtypes of NSCLC (based on histologic, or genetic differences), and it is essential to do so when selecting drug therapy for stage IV (metastatic) NSCLC. Histologic subtypes of NSCLC include adenocarcinoma (40% of lung cancers), squamous cell carcinoma (30% of lung cancers), large cell carcinoma (10% of lung cancers), and some more poorly differentiated histologic subtypes not otherwise specified (NOS).

A current or prior history of cigarette smoking remains the leading known risk factor for the development of lung cancer. SCLC, in particular, is so causally linked to tobacco smoking that its prevalence (currently <15% of all lung cancers) is falling as smoking prevalence falls. Still, up to 15% of newly diagnosed NSCLCs (usually adenocarcinoma) are seen in never-smokers. In recent years, it has been recognized that lung cancer in smokers is a different disease from lung cancer in never-smokers and impacts prognosis, genetic underpinnings, and response to immune therapy.

The risk for lung cancer is generally proportional to the number of cigarette pack-years smoked (packs per day × years smoked), and the incidence peaks in the sixth and seventh decades of life. Former-smokers have a persistent risk for lung cancer throughout life. Second-hand smoking is also a risk factor for lung cancer in a portion of nonsmokers who develop the disease. Nonsmokers who live with smokers have a more than 30% increased risk of developing lung cancer than those who live with nonsmokers. Other risk factors for lung cancer include environmental hazards such as asbestos and petroleum exposure. Smoking is considered an important cofactor of lung cancer in the setting of asbestos exposure. Radon exposure also increases the risk for developing lung cancer (see Chapter 2).

An ever-growing list of genetic alterations have been identified in terms of both proto-oncogenes and tumor suppressor genes. Unique molecular-genomic subgroups of lung cancer have been recognized, including those harboring (1) mutated epidermal growth factor receptor *(EGFR/ERBB1)*, (2) mutated Kirsten rat sarcoma viral oncogene homolog *(KRAS)*, and (3) anaplastic lymphoma kinase *(ALK)* 2p23 chromosomal rearrangement, more commonly known as *EML4-ALK*, a fusion with echinoderm microtubule-associated protein-like 4 *(EML4)*. Importantly, these oncogenic alterations inform gene-targeted drug selection in that the cancer is dependent upon a single oncogenic pathway for sustained proliferation and/or survival (oncogene addiction).

Several targeted therapies have been approved by the US Food and Drug Administration (FDA) for the treatment of advanced NSCLCs containing mutated *EGFR* (gefitinib, erlotinib, afatinib, osimertinib) or the *ALK* 2p23 rearrangement (crizotinib, ceritinib, alectinib, brigatinib, lorlatinib). Lung cancers with *EGFR* mutations are more frequently identified in never-smokers or in those with a light smoking history. They are more often of the adenocarcinoma subtype and more commonly found in women and in patients of East Asian descent. *KRAS*-mutated lung cancers are found primarily in patients with a more extensive smoking history. Lung cancers with mutated *EGFR* and those with the *ALK* 2p23 rearrangement are typically seen in younger patient populations, with a median age at diagnosis of approximately 55 years.

PATHOLOGY

Histologic Subgroups

Non–Small Cell Lung Carcinomas

Most lung cancers fall under the major histologic subgroup of NSCLC. Of these, *adenocarcinomas* and *squamous cell carcinomas* are the most common.

Adenocarcinomas. Adenocarcinoma is the most commonly diagnosed subtype of lung cancer, accounting for approximately 40% of lung cancer diagnoses and 65,000 deaths each year in the United States. It is the histologic subtype most commonly diagnosed in never-smokers. Primary lung adenocarcinomas are usually found in the periphery of the lung (75%), in contrast to squamous cell carcinomas that may arise in central airways.

Histologically, adenocarcinomas typically form glandular structures and produce mucin. *EGFR* mutations are more commonly associated with nonmucinous lung adenocarcinoma, whereas the mucinous subtype is more commonly associated with mutated *KRAS*. The tumor cells typically stain positive for cytokeratin 7 (CK7) and thyroid transcription factor 1 (TTF-1) and stain negative for cytokeratin 20 (CK20). *Lepidic adenocarcinomas* (previously known as bronchioloalveolar carcinomas) grow along alveolar spaces and allow air to enter the tumor. These adenocarcinomas manifest as translucent *ground-glass* lung infiltrates on computed tomography (CT) scan. Mucinous adenocarcinomas can cause dense lung consolidation and can be accompanied by copious sputum production, known as *bronchorrhea*.

Squamous cell carcinomas. Squamous cell carcinomas arise from the epithelial layer of the bronchial wall. Normal columnar

肺 癌

庄威 译　段建春 万蕊 审校　王洁 通审

定义和流行病学

肺癌是美国第二常见的癌症，也是癌症相关死亡的首要病因。全世界每年约有一百万人死于肺癌。尽管近年来对肺癌的生物学和基因特征研究取得了进展，并且研发出新型治疗药物，但肺癌患者的5年生存率仍低于20%。长期生存率相对较低的部分原因是大多数肺癌患者在确诊时已处于进展期。

历史上，肺癌主要分为两种类型：小细胞肺癌（SCLC）和非小细胞肺癌（NSCLC）。（基于组织病理学或基因差异）识别NSCLC的亚型十分重要，且在为Ⅳ期（转移性）NSCLC选择药物治疗时更为重要。NSCLC的病理亚型包括腺癌（约占40%）、鳞状细胞癌（约占30%）、大细胞癌（约占10%），以及一些分化较差的非特指病理亚型（NOS）。

当前或既往吸烟史是肺癌发生、发展的主要危险因素。尤其是SCLC，其发病率（目前占所有肺癌的15%以下）随着吸烟率的下降而下降。但是高达15%的新诊断NSCLC（通常为腺癌）见于从不吸烟者。近年来，人们认识到吸烟者的肺癌与从不吸烟者的肺癌截然不同，吸烟影响预后、基因基础结构和对免疫治疗的响应。

肺癌的风险通常与吸烟包-年（包/天×吸烟年数）的数量成正相关，发病率在60岁到70岁时达到峰值。既往吸烟者患肺癌的风险终身持续存在。二手烟也是部分非吸烟者患肺癌的危险因素。与吸烟者生活在一起的非吸烟者患肺癌的风险比与非吸烟者生活在一起的人增加30%。肺癌的其他危险因素包括环境因素，如石棉和石油接触。在石棉暴露环境中，吸烟被认为是肺癌的一个重要辅助因素。氡暴露也会增加罹患肺癌的风险（见第2章）。

越来越多的原癌基因和抑癌基因变异被发现。已经识别多种肺癌独特的分子-基因组亚群，包括：①表皮生长因子受体（*EGFR/ERBB1*）突变，②克尔斯顿大鼠肉瘤病毒癌基因同源物（*KRAS*）突变，和③间变性淋巴瘤激酶（*ALK*）2p23染色体重排，多为*EML4-ALK*，即棘皮动物微管相关蛋白样4（*EML4*）与*ALK*的融合。重要的是，由于癌症依赖于单一致癌通路来实现持续增殖和（或）生存（癌基因成瘾），所以这些致癌突变为基因靶向药物的选择提供了信息。

美国食品药品监督管理局（FDA）已批准多种靶向药物用于治疗具有*EGFR*突变的晚期NSCLC（吉非替尼、厄洛替尼、阿法替尼、奥希替尼）或*ALK* 2p23重排的晚期NSCLC（克唑替尼、色瑞替尼、阿来替尼、布格替尼、洛拉替尼）。*EGFR*突变的肺癌更常见于从不吸烟者或轻度吸烟者；更常见于腺癌亚型，女性和东亚裔患者。*KRAS*突变肺癌主要见于有较长吸烟史的患者。*EGFR*突变和*ALK* 2p23重排的肺癌通常见于较年轻的患者人群，诊断时的中位年龄约为55岁。

病理学

病理亚型

非小细胞肺癌

大多数肺癌归类在NSCLC的主要病理亚型中。其中，腺癌和鳞状细胞癌最为常见。

腺癌　腺癌是最常见的肺癌亚型，约占确诊肺癌的40%，导致美国每年65 000例患者死亡。这是不吸烟者中最常见的病理亚型。原发性肺腺癌通常为周围型（75%），而鳞状细胞癌则可能发生于中央气道。

组织学上，腺癌通常形成腺体结构并产生黏蛋白。*EGFR*突变多与非黏液型腺癌相关，而黏液型腺癌多与*KRAS*突变相关。腺癌细胞的免疫组化特征通常为细胞角蛋白7（CK7）、甲状腺转录因子1（TTF-1）阳性，细胞角蛋白20（CK20）阴性。附壁型腺癌（既往称为细支气管肺泡癌）沿肺泡腔生长，并允许空气进入肿瘤，计算机断层成像（CT）上表现为半透明的磨玻璃状肺浸润。黏液腺癌可引起致密的肺实变，并可伴有大量痰液产生，即支气管溢液。

鳞状细胞癌　鳞状细胞癌（鳞癌）起源于支气管壁的上皮层。正常的柱状上皮细胞经历化生、不典型

epithelial cells undergo metaplasia, dysplasia, and then localized carcinoma formation *(carcinoma in situ)*, which can then further extend and invade beyond the bronchial mucosa as it acquires a full malignant invasive phenotype. Most squamous cell carcinomas arise within central airways. Therefore, the airway lumen may become obstructed, leading to collapse of the lung or postobstructive pneumonia. Although necrosis and cavity formation can occur in any lung tumor, this feature is more common in squamous cell carcinomas. Squamous lung cancers have a lower potential for metastatic spread compared to invasive adenocarcinomas. Histologically, squamous cell carcinomas can be distinguished from other NSCLCs by the presence of keratinization, pearl formation, intercellular bridging, and staining positive for p40 and/or p63.

Adenosquamous carcinomas. Adenosquamous carcinomas constitute between 0.4% and 4% of all lung cancers and have a worse prognosis. They have components of both adenocarcinoma and squamous cell carcinoma, each comprising at least 10% of the tumor. It is important to recognize intratumor heterogeneity and mixed histology NSCLCs, especially when the diagnosis is based on a single needle biopsy. Most molecular pathology guidelines recommend genetic analysis of small biopsy specimens so as not to miss the druggable gene mutations that are more common to adenocarcinoma.

Sarcomatoid carcinomas. Sarcomatoid carcinomas, also known as *giant cell* or *pleiotropic carcinomas*, are high-grade lung cancers with a poor prognosis but that may harbor druggable oncogene drivers (especially MET exon 14 skipping) or may be particularly susceptible to immune checkpoint inhibitors.

NSCLC not otherwise specified. These NSCLCs are poorly differentiated tumors that defy specific classification based on their histology and immunophenotyping profile, but they may still be subtyped based on gene mutation analyses.

Small Cell Lung Carcinoma

SCLC cells are of pulmonary neuroendocrine cell origin and are often associated with paraneoplastic syndromes (Table 4.1). SCLCs typically are perihilar in location. They often originate from the main bronchi and have associated malignant adenopathy. These tumors have a high propensity for metastasis, most commonly to the thoracic lymph nodes, bones, liver, adrenal glands, and brain. Most patients are already affected with metastatic disease at the time of presentation. SCLC is an aggressive lung tumor. In fact, without treatment, the median survival time of patients with SCLC is less than 5 months. The overall survival for all patients is 5% at 5 years and has not improved over the past several decades.

Molecular-Genomic Subtypes

Lung cancer is now increasingly regarded as a disease with distinct genetic subgroups (Table 4.2). Many of these molecular-genomic alterations can inform the use of targeted therapeutics and predict responses.

Mutant *EGFR*

EGFR mutation testing and targeted therapy are essential to the care of patients with stage IV (metastatic) NSCLC. Specific somatic *EGFR* activating-sensitizing mutations predict clinical response to *EGFR* tyrosine kinase inhibitors (gefitinib, erlotinib, afatinib, osimertinib). These mutations are usually found in never-smokers with adenocarcinoma. *EGFR* mutations are more prevalent in women and patients of Asian race (30%, compared with 7% to 10% in Caucasians).

ALK 2p23 Rearrangement

The *EML4-ALK* fusion is an oncogenic driver that occurs in 3% to 7% of NSCLCs and is often found in light smokers (<10 pack-years) or never-smokers. In most cases, *EML4-ALK* fusions do not overlap with other oncogenic mutations of *EGFR* or *KRAS*. Patients with *ALK* rearrangements can be treated with *ALK* inhibitors (crizotinib, ceritinib, alectinib, brigatinib, lorlatinib).

ROS-1 Rearrangement

ROS-1 is a receptor tyrosine kinase of the insulin receptor family. *ROS-1* gene rearrangements are found in approximately 2% of NSCLCs. There is protein homology between the *ALK* and *ROS-1* kinase domain, such that the lists of active drugs overlap. FDA-approved drugs for *ROS-1* include crizotinib and entrectinib. Other *ALK*-inhibitors (ceritinib, lorlatinib) are effective against both *ALK* and *ROS-1*.

Mutant *KRAS*

KRAS gene mutations are uncommon in squamous cell carcinomas but are present in 15% to 25% of lung adenocarcinomas. *KRAS* mutations are more commonly seen in former or current cigarette smokers than in never-smokers or light smokers. There is currently no FDA-approved treatment for mutated *KRAS*, but covalent modifiers of the *KRAS G12C* oncoprotein show promise and have moved into phase 2 clinical testing.

TABLE 4.1 Paraneoplastic Syndromes Associated With Lung Cancer

Syndrome	Cell Type	Mechanism
Hypertrophic pulmonary osteoarthropathy and clubbing	All except small cell	Unknown
Hyponatremia	Small cell most common; may be any type	SIADH, ectopic antidiuretic hormone production by tumor
Hypercalcemia	Usually squamous cell	Bone metastases, osteoclast-activating factor, parathyroid hormone–like hormone, prostaglandins
Cushing syndrome	Usually small cell	Ectopic ACTH production
Eaton-Lambert myasthenic syndrome	Usually small cell	Voltage-sensitive calcium-channel antibodies in >75%; affects presynaptic neuronal calcium channel activity
Other neuromyopathic disorders	Small cell most common; may be any type	Antineuronal nuclear antibodies, also known as anti-Hu; others unknown
Thrombophlebitis	All types	Unknown

ACTH, Adrenocorticotropic hormone; *SIADH,* syndrome of inappropriate secretion of antidiuretic hormone.

增生，然后形成局限性癌（原位癌），然后进一步浸润并侵犯到支气管黏膜之外，随之获得完全恶性侵袭表型。大多数鳞癌起源于中央气道。因此，气道管腔可能阻塞，导致肺萎陷或阻塞性肺炎。尽管坏死和空洞形成可发生于任何肺部肿瘤，但这种特征在肺鳞癌中更常见。与浸润性腺癌相比，肺鳞癌转移扩散的可能性较低。在组织学上，鳞癌可以通过角化、角化珠形成、细胞间桥以及 p40 和（或）p63 阳性来与其他 NSCLC 鉴别。

<u>腺鳞癌</u> 腺鳞癌占所有肺癌的 0.4%～4%，预后差。腺鳞癌同时含有腺癌和鳞癌的成分，每种成分至少占 10%。认识瘤内异质性和混合性病理类型对 NSCLC 的诊断具有重要意义，尤其是基于单次针吸活检取材时。大多数分子病理学指南建议对小活检标本进行基因检测，以免遗漏在腺癌中更常见的可药物治疗的基因突变。

<u>肉瘤样癌</u> 肉瘤样癌也称为巨细胞癌或多形性癌，是预后不良的高级别肺癌，但可能携带有靶向药物的驱动基因突变（尤其是 MET14 外显子跳跃突变），或者可能对免疫检查点抑制剂响应较好。

<u>非特指型 NSCLC</u> 这些 NSCLC 是分化较差的肿瘤，无法根据其组织学和免疫表型进行特定分类，但仍可根据基因突变分析进行分型。

小细胞肺癌

SCLC 细胞起源于肺神经内分泌细胞，常伴有副肿瘤综合征（表 4.1）。SCLC 通常位于肺门周围。它们通常起源于主支气管并伴有恶性淋巴结肿大。这类型肿瘤有很高的转移倾向，最常转移到胸部淋巴结、骨、肝、肾上腺和脑。大多数患者在就诊时已经发生转移。SCLC 是一种侵袭性肺肿瘤。事实上，未经治疗的 SCLC 患者的中位生存时间不到 5 个月。所有患者的 5 年总生存率为 5%，在过去数十年中均未得到改善。

分子基因亚型

现在越来越多的证据表明肺癌是一组具有不同基因分型的疾病（表 4.2）。其中许多分子-基因变异可指导靶向治疗并能预测疗效。

EGFR 突变

EGFR 突变检测和靶向治疗对于 Ⅳ 期（转移性）NSCLC 患者至关重要。体细胞 *EGFR* 激活致敏突变可预测 *EGFR* 酪氨酸激酶抑制剂（吉非替尼、厄洛替尼、阿法替尼、奥希替尼）的临床疗效。*EGFR* 突变通常发生在不吸烟、腺癌患者，女性和亚裔患者中更为普遍（30%，而高加索裔中为 7%～10%）。

ALK 2p23 重排

EML4-ALK 融合是一种致癌驱动基因，发生于 3%～7% 的 NSCLC，常见于轻度吸烟（<10 包-年）或不吸烟患者。在大多数情况下，*EML4-ALK* 融合与 *EGFR* 或 *KRAS* 等其他致癌突变互斥。*ALK* 重排患者可使用 *ALK* 抑制剂（克唑替尼、色瑞替尼、阿来替尼、布格替尼、洛拉替尼）治疗。

ROS-1 重排

ROS-1 是胰岛素受体家族的一种受体酪氨酸激酶。约 2% 的 NSCLC 存在 *ROS-1* 基因重排。*ALK* 和 *ROS-1* 激酶结构域之间存在蛋白同源性，因此活性药物重叠。FDA 批准用于治疗 *ROS-1* 重排的药物包括克唑替尼和恩曲替尼。其他 *ALK* 抑制剂（色瑞替尼、洛拉替尼）对 *ALK* 和 *ROS-1* 重排均有效。

KRAS 突变

KRAS 基因突变在肺鳞癌中不常见，但在 15%～25% 的肺腺癌中存在。*KRAS* 突变在既往或当前吸烟者中相较不吸烟或轻度吸烟者中更为常见。目前尚无 *KRAS* 突变疗法获得美国 FDA 批准，但 *KRAS* G12C 癌蛋白的共价修饰剂显示出前景，并已进入 2 期临床试验。

表 4.1　与肺癌相关的副肿瘤综合征		
症状	病理类型	机制
肥厚性肺骨关节病和杵状指	除小细胞癌以外	未知
低钠血症	小细胞癌最常见；也可能是任何类型	SIADH，肿瘤产生异位抗利尿激素
高钙血症	通常是鳞状细胞癌	骨转移，破骨细胞活化因子，甲状旁腺素样激素，前列腺素
库欣综合征	通常小细胞癌	异位 ACTH 产生
伊顿-兰伯特肌无力综合征	通常小细胞癌	电压敏感性钙通道抗体 >75%；影响突触前神经元钙通道活性
其他神经肌病	小细胞癌最常见；可能是任何类型	抗神经元核抗体，又称抗 Hu 抗体；其他未知
血栓性静脉炎	各种类型	未知

ACTH，促肾上腺皮质激素；SIADH，抗利尿激素分泌失调综合征。

TABLE 4.2 Selected Molecular-Genomic Subtypes of NSCLC

Oncogene	Class of Molecular-Genomic Alterations	Characteristics
EGFR-mutant	Somatic missense mutations (most common with L858R in exon 21) and exon 19 deletions	More frequent in Asians, females, never-smokers or light smokers; most frequently adenocarcinoma subtype Sensitizing to EGFR inhibitors gefitinib, erlotinib, afatinib, osimertinib T790M mutation in EGFR is resistant to gefitinib, erlotinib, afatinib
EML4-ALK	ALK 2p23 chromosomal translocation	3-7% of NSCLCs More common in light smokers (<10 pack-years) or never-smokers Sensitizing to ALK inhibitors crizotinib, ceritinib, alectinib, brigatinib, lorlatinib
KRAS-mutant	Somatic mutations	Found in 15-25% lung adenocarcinomas More commonly seen in former or current cigarette smokers No effective targeted treatment at present but covalent inhibitors of G12C are in phase 2 development
BRAF-mutant	Somatic mutations	Belong to a family of serine-threonine protein kinases Identified in 1-3% of cases Only BRAF V600E is sensitive to trametinib, dabrafenib
HER2-mutant	Exon 20 insertion	HER2 alterations were identified in ≈2-4% of NSCLCs In the selected population of EGFR/KRAS/ALK-mutation–negative patients, HER2 mutations can reach up to 6% Predominantly found in females, nonsmokers; predominantly adenocarcinoma subtype May be associated with sensitivity to HER2-targeting drugs (trastuzumab, lapatinib, pertuzumab, and T-DM1)
STK11/LKB1	Inactivating mutations, deletion	A tumor suppressor gene Mutational frequency about 17-35% of NSCLCs, associated with resistance to immune checkpoint inhibition
RET-fusion	Chromosomal translocations	Occur in lung adenocarcinomas (1-2%). Respond to vandetanib, cabozantinib with off-target toxicity. On-target TKIs with fewer side effects are in late-phase development.
ROS-1-fusion	Chromosomal translocations	ROS-1 is a receptor tyrosine kinase of the insulin receptor family ROS-1-fusions were identified in ≈2% of NSCLCs More commonly found in younger people, more likely in never-smokers, and Asian patients are overrepresented Similar protein structure to other RTKs leads to overlapping active drug list (crizotinib, entrectinib, ceritinib, lorlatinib)
MET	Alternative spliced variant, mutations, amplification, receptor overexpression	The MET proto-oncogene is a receptor tyrosine kinase that binds to hepatocyte growth factor MET gene amplification can be found in 2-4% of NSCLCs, whereas overexpression of its receptor protein is much more common. May respond to crizotinib. MET exon 14 skipping results in lung cancers that respond to crizotinib. Several more potent MET inhibitors are in late-phase development.
NTRK	Chromosomal translocations	Rare, <1%. The NTRK genes encode the tropomyosin receptor kinases, which are receptors for nerve growth factors. When detected in lung cancer, patients respond to TKIs larotrectinib, entrectinib.

EGFR, Epithelial growth factor receptor; *FDA*, US Food and Drug Administration; *NSCLC*, non–small cell lung cancer; *RTK*, receptor tyrosine kinase.

The Lung Cancer Genome

In the last decade, The Cancer Genome Atlas (TCGA) project has provided a more comprehensive understanding of lung cancer by defining many of its nuances on a genomic level. The TCGA analysis of lung adenocarcinoma identified a relatively high exonic somatic mutation rate (mean, 12.0 events per megabase), similar to the rate found in squamous cell lung carcinoma. Three distinct expression subtypes of lung adenocarcinoma were identified from RNA-sequencing data: bronchioid, magnoid and squamoid. In addition, multiple gene fusions were found to be expressed in lung adenocarcinomas and multiple mechanisms for inactivation of the tumor suppressor gene *CDKN2A* were discovered.

For squamous cell NSCLCs, a most unexpected finding in the TCGA study was the identification of loss-of-function mutations in the *HLA-A* gene, which plays an important role in tumor cell surface antigen presentation and immune recognition. This is regarded as the first evidence of somatic cancer genome alterations evading the immune system by changing their surface antigens. Potential therapeutic targets were identified in most tumors, offering new therapeutic avenues of investigation for targeted therapy in lung cancer.

CLINICAL PRESENTATION

Initial symptoms of lung cancer are usually nonspecific (cough, dyspnea, sputum production, chest pain, weight loss) and are often attributed to bronchitis or pneumonia. The cancer has often invaded adjacent structures or metastasized when first recognized, causing symptoms that reflect the site of involvement. For example, destruction of blood vessels can cause hemoptysis, and tumor invasion of the pleura or chest wall can cause pleuritic chest pain. Involvement of

表 4.2　NSCLC 特定分子基因亚型

癌基因	分子基因亚型	特点
EGFR 突变	体细胞错义突变（最常见的是 21 外显子 *L858R*）和 19 外显子缺失	在亚洲人、女性、不吸烟者或轻度吸烟者中更常见；是最常见的腺癌亚型。对 *EGFR* 抑制剂吉非替尼、厄洛替尼、阿法替尼、奥希替尼敏感。*EGFR T790M* 突变患者对吉非替尼、厄洛替尼、阿法替尼耐药
EML4-ALK	*ALK 2p23* 染色体易位	3%～7% 的 NSCLC 更常见于轻度吸烟者（＜10 包-年）或不吸烟者 对 *ALK* 抑制剂克唑替尼、色瑞替尼、阿来替尼、布格替尼、洛拉替尼敏感
KRAS 突变	体细胞突变	15%～25% 的肺腺癌 多见于既往或当前吸烟者 目前尚无有效的靶向治疗药物，但 *G12C* 共价抑制剂正处于 2 期开发阶段
BRAF 突变	体细胞突变	属于丝氨酸-苏氨酸蛋白激酶家族 在 1%～3% 的病例中发现 仅 *BRAF V600E* 对曲美替尼、达拉非尼敏感
HER2 突变	20 外显子插入	在约 2%～4% 的 NSCLC 中发现了 *HER2* 改变 在 *EGFR/KRAS/ALK* 突变阴性患者人群中，*HER2* 突变率可达 6% 主要见于女性、非吸烟者；以腺癌为主 可能与 HER2 靶向药物（曲妥珠单抗、拉帕替尼、帕妥珠单抗、T-DM1）的敏感性相关
STK11/LKB1	失活突变，缺失	抑癌基因 NSCLC 中的突变频率约为 17%～35%，与免疫检查点抑制剂耐药相关
RET 融合	染色体易位	发生于肺腺癌（1%～2%）。凡德他尼和卡博替尼对其有效，但二者均有脱靶毒性。副作用较少的针对靶点的 TKI 正处于后期研发阶段
ROS-1 融合	染色体易位	*ROS-1* 是胰岛素受体家族的一种受体酪氨酸激酶 *ROS-1* 融合，在约 2% 的 NSCLC 中发现 在年轻人中更常见，更多为从未吸烟者，并且亚裔患者占比较高 与其他 RTK 蛋白结构相似导致活性药物重叠（克唑替尼、恩曲替尼、色瑞替尼、洛拉替尼）
MET	可变剪接变异体，突变，扩增，受体过表达	*MET* 原癌基因是一种与肝细胞生长因子结合的受体酪氨酸激酶 *MET* 基因扩增见于 2%～4% 的 NSCLC，而其受体蛋白的过表达更为常见。克唑替尼可能有效 克唑替尼对 *MET* 外显子 14 跳跃突变肺癌治疗有效。数种更强效的 *MET* 抑制剂正处于后期开发阶段
NTRK	染色体易位	罕见，＜1%。*NTRK* 基因编码原肌球蛋白受体激酶，这是神经生长因子的受体。当在肺癌患者中检测到时，患者对 TKI 有反应，如拉罗替尼、恩曲替尼

EGFR，表皮生长因子受体；FDA，美国食品药物监督管理局；NSCLC，非小细胞肺癌；RTK，受体酪氨酸激酶；TKI，酪氨酸激酶抑制剂。

肺癌基因组

在过去的十年中，癌症基因组图谱（the Cancer Genome Atlas，TCGA）项目在基因组水平上定义了肺癌的许多细微差别，使人们对肺癌有了更全面的了解。肺腺癌的 TCGA 数据分析发现了相对较高的体细胞外显子突变率（平均，12.0 起事件/兆碱基），与肺鳞癌的突变率相似。从 RNA 测序数据中鉴定出 3 种不同的肺腺癌亚型：细支气管型、大结节型和鳞状细胞型。此外，我们发现了多种基因融合在肺腺癌中表达，并且发现了抑癌基因 *CDKN2A* 失活的多种机制。

对于鳞癌，TCGA 数据分析中最意想不到的发现是识别了在肿瘤细胞表面抗原提呈和免疫识别中起重要作用的 *HLA-A* 基因的失活突变。这被认为是体细胞癌症基因组变异通过改变其表面抗原逃避免疫系统的首个证据。在大多数肿瘤组织中发现了潜在的治疗靶点，为肺癌的靶向治疗提供了新的研究方向。

临床表现

肺癌的初始症状通常缺乏特异性（咳嗽、呼吸困难、咳痰、胸痛、体重减轻），常被归因为支气管炎或肺炎。通常以肿瘤侵犯邻近结构或转移引起受累部位的症状为首发表现，例如，破坏血管引起咯血，肿瘤侵犯胸膜或胸壁引起胸膜炎性胸痛。左侧喉返神经或食管受累分别引起声音嘶哑或吞咽困难。胸腔积液

the left recurrent laryngeal nerve or esophagus can cause hoarseness or dysphagia, respectively. Pleural effusions can develop either due to direct tumor involvement of the pleura or obstruction of lymph flow from the mediastinal nodes. By a similar mechanism, malignant pericardial effusions can form, which can progress to *cardiac tamponade*. Patients might develop focal neurologic deficits due to spinal cord compression or brain metastasis. Superior vena cava obstruction may result in the *superior vena cava syndrome*, with edema of the face and upper extremities due to impaired venous return. Tumors in the apex of the lung (called *Pancoast tumors or superior sulcus tumors*) can invade adjacent chest wall structures and compress the brachial plexus, resulting in ipsilateral upper extremity weakness and/or pain. Tumor erosion into the cervical sympathetic chain causes *Horner syndrome*, with ptosis, miosis, and anhidrosis over the face and forehead.

Physical examination can be normal but may reveal changes in the lungs that reflect the impact of the tumor, such as crackles (e.g., postobstructive pneumonia); inspiratory wheezes, suggestive of airway obstruction; dullness to percussion at the lung bases from underlying pleural effusion; and lymph node enlargement in the supraclavicular or cervical and axillary areas. The most common sites of metastases are the lymph nodes, liver, brain, adrenal glands, kidneys, and lungs.

DIAGNOSIS AND DIFFERENTIAL DIAGNOSIS

Prevention and Screening

The most effective lung cancer prevention strategy is smoking cessation. In addition, the United States Preventive Services Task Force (USPSTF) recommends lung cancer screening by yearly, low-dose, noncontrast CT scan in patients between the ages of 55 and 80 years who are either current smokers or former smokers who quit less than 15 years ago, with a smoking history of 1 pack per day for 30 years (or 30 pack-year equivalent). This recommendation is based on a prospective clinical trial showing a 20% reduction in lung cancer–specific mortality in a CT-screened population of heavy smokers.

Diagnostic and Staging Work-Up

Early diagnosis of lung cancer is essential and can potentially lead to cure in the case of a malignant tumor. Diagnostic evaluation should consider the patient's age, sex, smoking history, family history of lung and other types of cancer, and other relevant risk factors.

When lung cancer is suspected, either incidentally or because of symptoms, a tissue diagnosis is essential unless the patient is not eligible for treatment because of comorbidity. After assessment for metastases, the site of biopsy should be chosen to determine the highest stage of the tumor, if this is feasible. If the apparent tumor is confined to the chest, bronchoscopy is appropriate for central masses and transthoracic needle aspiration for peripheral lesions. Pleural effusion should be sampled to assess for malignant cells, which would indicate stage IV (metastatic) disease.

Contrast-enhanced chest CT, including images of the abdomen, is useful to delineate the location and size of the primary tumor and to examine for mediastinal lymph nodes, pleural disease, and adrenal or liver metastases. CT has limited ability to distinguish benign from malignant lymphadenopathy in the mediastinum. Positron emission tomography (PET) using 18-fluorodeoxyglucose (FDG) is more sensitive and more specific than CT in the detection of mediastinal lymph node metastases and may also detect unexpected metastases elsewhere. In principle, any suspected mediastinal or extrathoracic metastases identified by imaging alone should be confirmed with tissue sampling before the patient is excluded from being considered an operative candidate. Techniques for invasive staging of the mediastinal lymph nodes include endobronchial ultrasound (EBUS)–guided needle aspiration and/or mediastinoscopy. EBUS is best for ruling in lymph node metastases. Mediastinoscopy can assess mediastinal spread of disease in patients without definite imaging evidence of lymph node involvement and is used to rule out lymph node metastases prior to surgery. PET scanning is limited in its ability to detect brain lesions, and magnetic resonance imaging (MRI) of the brain with intravenous contrast (or CT scanning if MRI cannot be done) should be performed if brain metastases are suspected or prior to surgery for stage IB or higher. Bone scans are useful for suspected symptomatic bony metastases.

Once a diagnosis of lung cancer is established, staging is necessary for prognostication and treatment. Staging of NSCLC determines whether surgical resection for cure, radiation, and/or chemotherapy is indicated. The tumor-node-metastasis (TNM) system is used to stage NSCLCs (Table 4.3). Using the TNM staging system, patients are classified as having stage I to IV disease (Table 4.4). For staging of SCLC, the Veterans Administration Lung Study Group designations of limited-stage (confined to one hemithorax) and extensive-stage (beyond one hemithorax) are used. Combined chemoradiation therapy with curative intent is considered for limited-stage SCLC, whereas extensive-stage SCLC is treated with palliative chemotherapy.

Metastatic NSCLC is subdivided into disease that is confined to the chest (M1a)—malignant pleural/pericardial effusion or separate tumor nodule(s) in the contralateral lung—which has a better prognosis compared to patients with disseminated disease in liver, bone, brain, or adrenal gland (M1b/M1c). Of patients with widely disseminated disease, there is a better prognosis in patients with a single site of metastasis in a single organ (M1b) compared to multiple metastases (M1c).

Solitary Pulmonary Nodule

A *solitary pulmonary nodule* (SPN) is a single, rounded lesion in the lung that is 3 cm in diameter or smaller. Although these lesions are commonly lung cancers in certain patient populations, the differential diagnosis of SPN includes many other malignant and benign processes. In addition to primary lung cancer (adenocarcinoma), other possible causes include bronchial carcinoid tumors and metastases from extrapulmonary malignancies (e.g., malignant melanoma, sarcoma, colon, kidney, breast, and testicular cancers). Benign etiologies include benign tumors of the lung (hamartomas), infectious granulomas (from fungal diseases, including histoplasmosis and coccidioidomycosis, and mycobacterial disease), lung abscess, vascular abnormalities (arteriovenous malformation), rounded atelectasis, and pseudotumor (pleural fluid trapped within a fissure).

Radiographic features of an SPN can be helpful diagnostically. Larger lesions are more likely to be malignant. Lesions 4 to 7 mm in diameter in patients without a history of cancer have a 0.9% chance of being malignant; this probability rises to 18% for lesions 8 mm to 2 cm in diameter and 50% for those larger than 2 cm. Benign tumors are more likely to have smooth, discrete borders, whereas malignant tumors often have irregular or spiculated borders. Central, popcorn, diffuse and laminated (onion-skin) calcification patterns are associated with benign tumors. Conversely, lesions with eccentric (asymmetrical) or stippled calcifications are more likely to be malignant. It is important to assess the rate of progression of an SPN or its stability by comparing imaging studies with previous scans whenever available. An SPN that has not changed in size for more than 2 years is unlikely to be malignant, with the exception of ground-glass nodules that might represent slowly growing adenocarcinoma in situ.

的发生既可能是由于肿瘤直接累及胸膜，也可能是由于纵隔淋巴结肿大引起淋巴回流受阻。通过类似机制，可形成恶性心包积液，并可进展为心脏压塞。患者可因脊髓压迫或脑转移而出现局灶性神经功能障碍。上腔静脉阻塞可导致上腔静脉综合征，并因静脉回流障碍而出现面部和上肢水肿。位于肺尖部的肿瘤（称为肺上沟瘤或上沟瘤）可侵犯邻近胸壁结构，压迫臂丛神经，导致同侧上肢无力和（或）疼痛。肿瘤侵犯颈交感神经链引起霍纳综合征，表现为上睑下垂、瞳孔缩小、面部和前额无汗。

体格检查可能正常，但可能显示出由肿瘤导致的肺部改变，如爆裂音（可由阻塞性肺炎引起）；吸气相喘鸣提示气道阻塞；胸腔积液可引起肺基底部叩诊浊音；触诊可发现锁骨上、颈部和腋窝区域淋巴结肿大。最常见的转移部位是淋巴结、肝、脑、肾上腺、肾和肺。

诊断和鉴别诊断

预防和筛查

肺癌最有效的预防策略是戒烟。此外，美国预防服务工作组（United States Preventive Services Task Force，USPSTF）建议对 55～80 岁的当前吸烟者或戒烟不到 15 年、有 30 年每日 1 包（30 包-年）吸烟史的既往吸烟者进行每年 1 次的低剂量平扫 CT 筛查。这一建议是基于一项前瞻性临床研究，该研究结果显示，在接受 CT 筛查的重度吸烟人群中，肺癌特异性死亡率降低了 20%。

诊断和分期检查

肺癌的早期诊断至关重要，即使恶性肿瘤在早期也仍有治愈机会。诊断评估应考虑患者的年龄、性别、吸烟史、肺癌及其他类型肿瘤家族史等相关危险因素。

当偶然发现或由于症状而怀疑肺癌时，病理诊断至关重要，除非患者因合并症不适合抗肿瘤治疗。评估转移情况后，如果可行，应选择合适的活检部位以确定肿瘤的最高分期。如果肿瘤局限于胸部，中央型肿块可采用支气管镜检查，周围型病变可采用经胸针吸活检。还应对胸腔积液进行检验，评估是否存在恶性细胞，如有恶性细胞将提示患者为Ⅳ期（转移性）肺癌。

胸部增强 CT（包括腹部）有助于确定原发肿瘤的位置和大小，并有助于判断纵隔淋巴结、胸膜以及肾上腺或肝脏转移情况。CT 鉴别纵隔良恶性淋巴结病变的能力有限。使用 18-氟脱氧葡萄糖（FDG）的正电子发射断层成像（PET）在判断纵隔淋巴结转移方面比 CT 更敏感、更特异，也可能意外发现其他部位的转移。原则上，通过影像学检查发现的任何疑似纵隔或胸外转移灶都应通过组织活检进行确认，然后才能排除患者根治性手术的可能性。纵隔淋巴结的侵入性分期检查技术包括支气管内超声（EBUS）引导下的针吸活检和（或）纵隔镜检查。EBUS 是判断淋巴结转移的最佳方法。纵隔镜检查可在影像学无明确淋巴结受累证据的患者中评估疾病的纵隔淋巴结转移，并用于手术前除外淋巴结转移。PET 扫描检出脑部病变的能力有限，如果怀疑脑转移，或者ⅠB 期及以上分期患者接受手术之前，应对脑部进行增强磁共振成像（MRI）（如果无法进行 MRI，则进行 CT 扫描）。骨扫描对于疑似有症状的骨转移具有意义。

一旦确诊肺癌，分期对于判断预后和治疗是必需的。NSCLC 的分期决定了是否需要根治性手术、放疗和（或）化疗。TNM（肿瘤原发灶-淋巴结-远处转移，tumor-node-metastasis）系统用于 NSCLC 分期（表 4.3）。根据 TNM 分期系统，患者被分为Ⅰ～Ⅳ期（表 4.4）。对于 SCLC 的分期，美国退伍军人管理局肺研究组（Veterans Administration Lung Study Group）将其分为局限期（局限于一侧胸腔内）和广泛期（超过一侧胸腔）。局限期 SCLC 可考虑根治性同步放化疗，而广泛期 SCLC 可采用姑息性化疗。

转移性 NSCLC 被细分为局限于胸部的疾病（M1a）——恶性胸腔/心包积液或对侧肺的分散肿瘤结节，和出现远处转移如肝、骨、脑或肾上腺转移的 NSCLC（M1b/M1c）。M1a 的患者与 M1b/M1c 的患者相比有更好的预后。在全身广泛转移的患者中，单一器官单个部位转移（M1b）患者的预后优于多部位转移（M1c）患者。

孤立性肺结节

孤立性肺结节（SPN）是肺内单个的、直径≤3 cm 的圆形病变。虽然这些病变在某些患者人群中通常是肺癌，但 SPN 的鉴别诊断还包括许多其他的恶性和良性疾病。除了原发性肺癌（腺癌），其他可能的病因包括支气管类癌和肺外恶性肿瘤（如恶性黑色素瘤、肉瘤、结肠癌、肾癌、乳腺癌和睾丸癌）的转移。良性病因包括肺良性肿瘤（错构瘤）、感染性肉芽肿（真菌病，包括组织胞浆菌病、球孢子菌病和分枝杆菌病）、肺脓肿、血管异常（动静脉畸形）、圆形肺不张和假瘤（胸腔积液包裹在肺叶间隙内）。

SPN 的影像学特征有助于诊断。病灶越大，恶性可能性越大。在无肿瘤病史的患者中，直径 4～7 mm 的病变恶性的可能性为 0.9%；对于直径为 8 mm 至 2 cm 的病变，这一概率升至 18%，对于直径大于 2 cm 的病变，这一概率升至 50%。良性肿瘤更可能有光滑、不连续的边界，而恶性肿瘤往往有不规则或毛刺的边界。中央型、爆米花型、弥漫性和层状（洋葱皮）钙化模式与良性肿瘤相关。相反，有偏心（不对称）或点状钙化的病变更有可能是恶性的。重要的是通过比较以往的影像学检查，评估 SPN 的发展速度或其稳定性。除磨玻璃结节（代表缓慢生长的原位腺癌）外，2 年以上大小不变的 SPN 不太可能是恶性的。

TABLE 4.3 TNM Staging System for Lung Cancer (2018)

T (Primary Tumor)

TX	Primary tumor cannot be assessed
	Or tumor proven by the presence of malignant cells in sputum or bronchial washings but not visualized by imaging or bronchoscopy
T0	No evidence of primary tumor
Tis	Carcinoma in situ
T1	Tumor ≤3 cm in greatest dimension, surrounded by lung or visceral pleura, without bronchoscopic evidence of invasion more proximal than the lobar bronchus (i.e., not in the main bronchus)
T1a	Tumor ≤1 cm in greatest dimension
T1b	Tumor >1 cm but ≤2 cm in greatest dimension
T1c	Tumor >2 cm but ≤3 cm in greatest dimension
T2	Tumor >3 cm but ≤5 cm or tumor with any of the following features (T2 tumors with these features are classified T2a if ≤4 cm): • Involves main bronchus • Locally invades visceral pleura • Locally invades the diaphragm • Associated with obstructive atelectasis (either partial or whole lung)
T2a	Tumor >3 cm but ≤4 cm in greatest dimension
T2b	Tumor >4 cm but ≤5 cm in greatest dimension
T3	Tumor >5 cm or tumor with local invasion to any of the following structures: • Chest wall (including superior sulcus tumors) • Phrenic nerve • Parietal pericardium OR If tumor is associated with a satellite nodule in the same lobe
T4	Tumor of any size that invades any of the following: • Mediastinum • Heart or great vessels • Trachea • Recurrent laryngeal nerve • Esophagus • Vertebrae • Carina OR If tumor is associated with an ipsilateral satellite nodule in a different lobe

N (Regional Lymph Nodes)

NX	Regional lymph nodes cannot be assessed
N0	No regional lymph node metastases
N1	Metastasis in ipsilateral peribronchial and/or ipsilateral hilar lymph nodes and intrapulmonary nodes, including involvement by direct extension
N2	Metastasis in ipsilateral mediastinal and/or subcarinal lymph node(s)
N3	Metastasis in contralateral mediastinal, contralateral hilar, ipsilateral or contralateral scalene, or supraclavicular lymph node(s)

M (Distant Metastasis)

MX	Distant metastasis cannot be assessed
M0	No distant metastasis
M1	Distant metastasis
M1a	Separate tumor nodule(s) in a contralateral lobe; tumor with pleural nodules or malignant pleural (or pericardial) effusion
M1b	Single extrathoracic metastasis or involvement of single distant lymph node
M1c	Multiple extrathoracic metastases

TABLE 4.4 Staging Using TNM Score (AJCC 8th Edition)

	N0	N1	N2	N3
T1a	Early (Stage I-II)		Locally Advanced (Stage IIIa)	
T1b				
T1c				
T2a				
T2b				
T3			Locally Advanced (Stage IIIb)	
T4				
M1a/b/c	Metastatic (Stage IV)			

TREATMENT

Small Cell Lung Cancer

SCLCs can occasionally be resected if no evidence of metastasis is found, but most SCLCs are treated with chemotherapy for systemic disease. Limited-stage SCLC is treated with combination chemoradiation with curative intent. Extensive-stage SCLC is treated with chemotherapy alone with palliative intent. Carboplatin plus etoposide has the lowest rate of side effects and best survival, making it the chemotherapy of choice for extensive-stage disease. Recent phase 3 data demonstrate an improvement in overall survival with the addition of the immune checkpoint inhibitor (ICPI), atezolizumab, to first-line carboplatin plus etoposide. Previously treated patients can benefit

表 4.3　肺癌的 TNM 分期系统（2018）

T（原发肿瘤）

TX	原发肿瘤不可评估 或痰脱落细胞、支气管灌洗液中找到癌细胞但影像学或支气管镜未发现原发肿瘤
T0	无原发肿瘤证据
Tis	原位癌
T1	最大径 ≤ 3 cm 的肿瘤，被肺和（或）脏层胸膜包绕，支气管镜下没有比叶段支气管更近端的浸润证据（即，不位于主支气管内）
T1a	原发肿瘤最大径 ≤ 1 cm
T1b	原发肿瘤最大径 > 1 cm，≤ 2 cm
T1c	原发肿瘤最大径 > 2 cm，≤ 3 cm
T2	原发肿瘤 > 3 cm，≤ 5 cm 或肿瘤具有以下任何特征（具有这些特征的 T2 期肿瘤如果 ≤ 4 cm 被归类为 T2a）： ● 累及主支气管 ● 累及脏层胸膜 ● 侵犯膈肌 ● 伴有阻塞性肺不张（部分或全肺）
T2a	原发肿瘤最大径 > 3 cm，≤ 4 cm
T2b	原发肿瘤最大径 > 4 cm，≤ 5 cm
T3	肿瘤 > 5 cm 或肿瘤局部侵犯以下任何结构： ● 胸壁（包括肺上沟瘤） ● 膈神经 ● 心包壁 或 原发肿瘤同一肺叶出现卫星结节
T4	任何大小的肿瘤侵犯以下任一结构： ● 纵隔 ● 心脏或大血管 ● 气管 ● 喉返神经 ● 食管 ● 椎体 ● 隆突 或 原发肿瘤同侧不同肺叶出现卫星结节

N（区域淋巴结）

NX	淋巴结转移无法评估
N0	无区域淋巴结转移
N1	同侧支气管周围和（或）同侧肺门淋巴结和肺内淋巴结转移，包括直接侵犯
N2	同侧纵隔和（或）隆突下淋巴结转移
N3	对侧纵隔、对侧肺门、同侧或对侧斜角肌或锁骨上淋巴结转移

M（远处转移）

MX	远处转移无法评估
M0	无远处转移
M1	有远处转移
M1a	对侧肺叶内孤立的肿瘤结节；伴有胸膜结节或恶性胸腔（或心包）积液的肿瘤
M1b	单个胸外转移或累及单个远处淋巴结
M1c	多发胸外转移

表 4.4　TNM 分期（AJCC 第 8 版）

	N0	N1	N2	N3
T1a	早期（Ⅰ～Ⅱ期）		局部晚期（Ⅲa 期）	
T1b				
T1c				
T2a				
T2b				
T3				局部晚期（Ⅲb 期）
T4				
M1a/b/c	转移期（Ⅳ期）			

治疗

小细胞肺癌

如果没有发现转移的证据，部分 SCLC 可以切除，但大多数 SCLC 采用化疗治疗这种全身性疾病。局限期 SCLC 采用以治愈为目的的同步放化疗。广泛期小细胞肺癌采用姑息性化疗。卡铂联合依托泊苷具有最小的不良反应和最佳的生存率，使其成为广泛期 SCLC 的首选化疗方案。近年的 3 期临床研究数据表明，在卡铂+依托泊苷一线治疗的基础上加用免疫检查点抑制剂阿替利珠单抗可改善总生存。既往接受过卡铂和依托泊苷治疗的患者，如果之前通过一线治疗达到至少 6 个月的疾病控制，那么其在疾病进展后仍可能获益于卡铂联合依托泊

from re-treatment with carboplatin plus etoposide if they achieve at least 6 months of disease control with initial therapy. Second-line therapies include topotecan or alternative immune checkpoint inhibitors (nivolumab or pembrolizumab) for patients who did not receive first-line atezolizumab. Durable responses to both chemotherapy and radiation therapy and long-term survival are possible. However, relapse with progressive therapeutic resistance is usual despite initial treatment response. Prophylactic cranial irradiation (PCI) improves overall survival in limited-stage disease after completion of chemoradiation. PCI is also favored for patients with extensive-stage disease following good response to primary chemotherapy, but recent evidence allows for active surveillance as a reasonable alternative.

Non–Small Cell Lung Cancer
Early-Stage Disease (Stages I and II)
Surgery is potentially curative for early-stage NSCLC and is indicated for patients with stage I or II disease who are eligible as operative candidates. Anatomic resection (lobectomy or pneumonectomy) is favored to remove the primary tumor as well as its draining lymph nodes (N1 disease). Lesser resections (wedge resections or segmentectomies) are favored to spare lung for clinically N0 peripheral tumors that are 2 cm or smaller, radiographically noninvasive cancers (ground glass), in patients with limited pulmonary function, or for multiple primary lung cancers. Stereotactic body radiation therapy (SBRT) or needle-directed thermal ablation may be used to cure stage I NSCLCs that are not amenable to surgery due to medical comorbidities. Once spread to lymph nodes is suspected, patients unable to tolerate anatomic resection are best treated as locally advanced.

Locally Advanced Disease (Stages IIIA and IIIB)
Stage III NSCLC is a heterogeneous disease and the optimal treatment strategy is unclear. For stage IIIA/N2 disease, "tri-modality" therapy with neoadjuvant chemotherapy or chemoradiation followed by surgery may be offered. Most patients with stage III NSCLC are not surgical candidates and are treated with chemoradiation followed by immune checkpoint blockade.

Advanced Metastatic Disease (Stage IV)
Molecular testing of diagnostic biopsy material is essential for optimal palliative drug selection for patients with stage IV NSCLC. Tumors that do not have any targetable mutations ("wild-type" patients) should be treated with immune checkpoint inhibitor therapy, either alone or in combination with chemotherapy. Prospective, randomized (phase 3) trials have shown that gene-targeted therapy is superior to chemotherapy for stage IV NSCLC with *EGFR* activating-sensitizing mutations or *ALK* gene rearrangement. In addition, single-arm (phase 2) studies have shown durable responses to targeted therapy for patients with *BRAF V600E*, rare *EGFR*, *HER2* mutations, or *ROS-1*, *RET*, *MET* or *NTRK* gene rearrangements with outcomes superior to chemotherapy.

These targeted drugs provide durable disease control but do not cure patients. Acquired drug resistance inevitably leads to disease progression and death. A repeat biopsy can be used to determine the molecular mechanism of acquired resistance to targeted therapy, which can be used to inform subsequent drug selection. Patterns of resistance have been used to refine first-line drug selection. For example, the predominant mechanism of gefitinib/erlotinib/afatinib resistance is the emergence of the *EGFR T790M* mutation (located on exon 20), which accounts for about half of all resistant cases. Patients who have progression of disease despite gefitinib/erlotinib/afatinib therapy are routinely tested for *T790M* mutation, and, if present, are candidates for osimertinib therapy. First-line osimertinib proved to be superior to gefitinib/erlotinib in a randomized phase 3 trial.

Acquired genetic changes may occur in "off target" genes, shifting oncogenic signal to so-called "bypass tracts." These include druggable targets such as *BRAF*, or *HER2* mutations, *RET* rearrangements, and *MET* amplification. Adenocarcinomas may undergo histologic transformation to squamous histology or SCLC. Patterns of primary sensitivity and acquired resistance may guide multiple lines of therapy in patients with *EGFR*, *ALK*, and *ROS-1* genetic changes, keeping their management pathway distinct compared to wild-type patients.

In wild-type patients, the decision whether or not to use chemotherapy is based on measurement of programmed death-ligand 1 (PD-L1) expression. PD-L1 expressed on cancer cells or nearby immune cells binds with the PD-1 receptor on T cells and blocks anticancer immunity. Patients with PD-L1 expression on more than 50% of cancer cells are candidates for single-agent pembrolizumab, an ICPI that is a monoclonal IgG antibody against PD-L1. In a phase 3 trial, pembrolizumab was associated with improved survival and fewer adverse events than chemotherapy in patients with metastatic NSCLC without *EGFR* or *ALK* mutations and high PD-L1 expression.

Cytotoxic chemotherapy plus pembrolizumab is used for wild-type patients with low PD-L1 expression. Cytotoxic drugs include platinum (carboplatin or cisplatin), which cause DNA double-strand breaks, combined with drugs that block DNA synthesis (pemetrexed, gemcitabine) or cellular mitosis (paclitaxel, docetaxel, *nab*-paclitaxel, vinorelbine). Cytotoxic chemotherapy lowers the neutrophil count, which can lead to septicemia. ICPIs cause autoimmune side effects, most commonly dermatitis, colitis, or thyroiditis, but also vital organ inflammation (pneumonitis, hepatitis, nephritis), which requires stopping the ICPI and consideration of corticosteroids. Targeted drug therapy is not without difficult or dangerous side effects, including skin rash, diarrhea, gastrointestinal side effects, and rarely cardiac or lung toxicity.

PROGNOSIS

The most important prognostic factor in lung cancer is the TNM stage of the disease at the time of initial diagnosis. Poor performance status and weight loss are negative prognostic factors for survival of patients with lung cancer.

For a deeper discussion on this topic, please see Chapter 182, ❖ "Lung Cancer and Other Pulmonary Neoplasms," in *Goldman-Cecil Medicine*, 26th Edition.

SUGGESTED READINGS

Gandhi L, Rodriguez-Abreau D, Gadgeel S, et al: Pembrolizumab plus chemotherapy in metastatic non-small-cell lung cancer, N Engl J Med 378(22):2078–2092, 2018.

Hirsch FR, Jänne PA, Eberhardt WE, et al: Epidermal growth factor receptor inhibition in lung cancer: status 2012, J Thorac Oncol 8:373–384, 2013.

Imielinski M, Berger AH, Hammerman PS, et al: Mapping the hallmarks of lung adenocarcinoma with massively parallel sequencing, Cell 150:1107–1120, 2012.

National Lung Screening Trial Research Team, Aberle DR, Adams AM, et al: Reduced lung-cancer mortality with low-dose computed tomographic screening, N Engl J Med 365:395–409, 2011.

Reck M, Rodriguez-Abreu D, Robinson AG, et al: Pembrolizumab versus chemotherapy for PD-L1-positive non-small-cell lung cancer, N Engl J Med 375(19):1823–1833, 2016.

Rosell R, Bivona TG, Karachaliou N: Genetics and biomarkers in personalization of lung cancer treatment, Lancet 382:720–731, 2013.

Sequist LV, Waltman BA, Dias-Santagata D, et al: Genotypic and histological evolution of lung cancers acquiring resistance to EGFR inhibitors, Sci Transl Med 3(75):75ra26, 2011.

苷的再挑战治疗。对于未接受阿替利珠单抗一线治疗的患者，二线治疗包括托泊替康或其他免疫检查点抑制剂（纳武利尤单抗或帕博利珠单抗）。经化疗和放疗获得持久缓解和长期生存是可能的。然而，尽管初始治疗有效，但复发和治疗耐药的情况很常见。预防性脑照射（PCI）可改善完成放化疗后局限期 SCLC 患者的总生存。对于初次化疗后应答良好的广泛期 SCLC 患者，PCI 也更受青睐，但近期证据支持积极监测作为合理的替代方案。

非小细胞肺癌

早期（Ⅰ～Ⅱ期）

手术可能治愈早期 NSCLC，适用于符合手术条件的Ⅰ期或Ⅱ期 NSCLC 患者。解剖性切除术（肺叶切除术或全肺切除术）是切除原发肿瘤及其引流淋巴结（N1）的首选方法。对于临床 N0、直径 ≤ 2 cm 的周围型肿瘤、影像学检查提示非浸润性癌（磨玻璃癌）、肺功能受限的患者或多发原发肺癌，范围较小的切除（楔形切除或肺段切除）有利于保留肺组织。立体定向放射治疗（SBRT）或细针定向热消融可用于治疗因内科合并症而不适合手术的Ⅰ期 NSCLC。一旦怀疑转移至淋巴结，不能耐受解剖性切除的患者最好视为局部晚期进行治疗。

局部晚期（ⅢA 和 ⅢB 期）

Ⅲ期 NSCLC 是一种异质性极大的疾病，最佳治疗策略尚不明确。对于Ⅲ A/N2 期疾病，可提供"三联疗法"，即新辅助化疗或放化疗，然后进行手术。大多数Ⅲ期 NSCLC 患者不适合手术，应先接受放化疗，随后接受免疫检查点抑制剂治疗。

晚期转移性疾病（Ⅳ期）

诊断性活检组织的分子检测对于Ⅳ期 NSCLC 患者的最佳姑息治疗药物选择至关重要。无任何驱动基因突变的肿瘤（"野生型"）患者应接受免疫检查点抑制剂单药或与化疗联合治疗。前瞻性、随机（3 期）试验表明，对于有 EGFR 激活致敏突变或 ALK 基因重排的Ⅳ期 NSCLC，靶向治疗优于化疗。此外，单臂（2 期）研究表明，携带 BRAF V600E、罕见 EGFR、HER2 突变或 ROS-1、RET、MET 或 NTRK 基因重排的患者接受靶向治疗后可达到持久缓解，疗效优于化疗。

这些靶向药物可带来持久的疾病控制，但不能治愈患者。获得性耐药不可避免地导致疾病进展和死亡。二次活检可用于确定靶向治疗获得性耐药的分子机制，可用于指导后续药物选择。耐药机制已被用于完善一线药物选择。例如，吉非替尼/厄洛替尼/阿法替尼耐药的主要机制是 EGFR T790M 突变（位于第 20 外显子）的出现，约占所有耐药病例的一半。吉非替尼/厄洛替尼/阿法替尼治疗后发生疾病进展的患者常规接受 T790M 突变检测，如果有 T790M 突变，则适合接受奥希替尼治疗。在一项随机 3 期试验中，奥希替尼一线治疗被证明优于吉非替尼/厄洛替尼。

获得性基因突变可发生在"脱靶"基因中，将致癌信号转移到所谓的"旁路通道"。包括有靶向药物的基因突变，如 BRAF 或 HER2 突变、RET 重排和 MET 扩增。腺癌也可以发生鳞癌或小细胞癌的组织学类型转化。原发敏感但出现获得性耐药的机制可指导 EGFR、ALK 和 ROS-1 基因突变患者的多线治疗模式，使其治疗策略与野生型患者不同。

在野生型患者中，是否使用化疗取决于程序性死亡受体配体 1（PD-L1）表达水平。肿瘤细胞或附近免疫细胞表达的 PD-L1 与 T 细胞上的 PD-1 受体结合，阻断抗肿瘤免疫。肿瘤细胞 PD-L1 表达超过 50% 的患者可采用帕博利珠单抗（抗 PD-1 的单克隆 IgG 抗体）单药治疗。在一项 3 期试验中，在无 EGFR 或 ALK 突变且 PD-L1 高表达的转移性 NSCLC 患者中，与化疗相比，帕博利珠单抗显著延长生存期，且不良反应较少。

细胞毒性化疗联合帕博利珠单抗适用于 PD-L1 低表达的野生型患者。细胞毒性药物包括引起 DNA 双链断裂的铂类（卡铂或顺铂）与干扰 DNA 合成的药物（培美曲塞、吉西他滨）或干扰细胞有丝分裂的药物（紫杉醇、多西他赛、白蛋白结合型紫杉醇、长春瑞滨）联用。细胞毒性化疗降低中性粒细胞计数，可导致感染中毒症。免疫检查点抑制剂可引起自身免疫不良反应，最常见的是皮炎、结肠炎或甲状腺炎，但也可引起重要器官炎症（肺炎、肝炎、肾炎），这需要停用免疫检查点抑制剂并考虑使用激素。靶向药物治疗并非不会遇到困难或出现严重的不良反应，可引起皮疹、腹泻、胃肠道不良反应，以及罕见的心脏或肺毒性在内的多种不良反应。

预后

肺癌最重要的预后因素是初诊时的 TNM 分期。体能状态差和体重减轻是影响肺癌患者生存的不良预后因素。

有关此专题的深入讨论，请参阅 *Goldman-Cecil Medicine* 第 26 版第 182 章"肺癌和其他肺肿瘤"。

推荐阅读

Gandhi L, Rodriguez-Abreau D, Gadgeel S, et al: Pembrolizumab plus chemotherapy in metastatic non-small-cell lung cancer, N Engl J Med 378(22):2078–2092, 2018.

Hirsch FR, Jänne PA, Eberhardt WE, et al: Epidermal growth factor receptor inhibition in lung cancer: status 2012, J Thorac Oncol 8:373–384, 2013.

Imielinski M, Berger AH, Hammerman PS, et al: Mapping the hallmarks of lung adenocarcinoma with massively parallel sequencing, Cell 150:1107–1120, 2012.

National Lung Screening Trial Research Team, Aberle DR, Adams AM, et al: Reduced lung-cancer mortality with low-dose computed tomographic screening, N Engl J Med 365:395–409, 2011.

Reck M, Rodriguez-Abreu D, Robinson AG, et al: Pembrolizumab versus chemotherapy for PD-L1-positive non-small-cell lung cancer, N Engl J Med 375(19):1823–1833, 2016.

Rosell R, Bivona TG, Karachaliou N: Genetics and biomarkers in personalization of lung cancer treatment, Lancet 382:720–731, 2013.

Sequist LV, Waltman BA, Dias-Santagata D, et al: Genotypic and histological evolution of lung cancers acquiring resistance to EGFR inhibitors, Sci Transl Med 3(75):75ra26, 2011.

Gastrointestinal Cancers

Khaldoun Almhanna

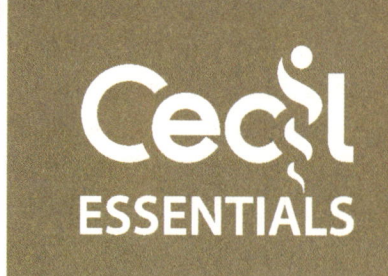

INTRODUCTION

Gastrointestinal (GI) cancers are among the most common cancers worldwide. In the United States, approximately 300,000 new cases of GI cancer were expected in 2018 with an estimated 150,000 deaths. Gastrointestinal cancers are typically epithelial malignancies—carcinomas—with well-defined pathologic patterns of neoplastic transformation. The incidence of GI malignancies is increasing. Screening and early detection have been established for colon cancer and hepatocellular cancer. Asian populations should be screened for gastric and esophageal cancer. Risk factors, presentations, and management of GI malignancies are site specific. Management usually involves advanced diagnostic procedures and multidisciplinary treatment including advanced endoscopy, chemotherapy, radiation, and surgical intervention. Complications of advanced disease including bowel and biliary obstruction, liver failure, bleeding, and impaired nutrition play a significant role in the prognosis and mortality of these diseases. Recent advances in immunotherapy and checkpoint inhibitors, although promising, have not yet significantly improved the overall outcome of these diseases.

ESOPHAGEAL CANCER

Epidemiology

The incidence rates of esophageal cancer vary by geographic region with the highest incidence in Asia and Eastern Africa and the lowest in Western countries. The incidence of squamous cell carcinoma in the United States is decreasing while the incidence of adenocarcinoma, mostly in the gastroesophageal junction, is increasing in part due to obesity, reflux disease, and Barrett esophagus.

Pathology

Squamous cell carcinoma (SCC) is commonly seen in the upper esophagus and is associated with smoking, alcohol use, and dietary intake. Consuming hot beverages in certain areas is thought to be responsible for a higher incidence of SCC (e.g., China, Iran). On the other hand, most adenocarcinomas arise in background of Barrett esophagus. Interestingly, only 50% of patients with Barrett esophagus report a history of chronic reflux. The risk of developing esophageal cancer is increased at least 30-fold in patients with Barrett esophagus and is higher in the presence of high-grade dysplasia.

Clinical Presentation

Progressive dysphagia and weight loss are the most common presenting symptoms in patients with esophageal cancer. Chronic blood loss leading to iron deficiency anemia is not an uncommon presentation as well. History of longstanding reflux disease is not as common as expected. Early stage tumors are usually asymptomatic and are diagnosed as part of GI bleeding work-up or Barrett esophagus follow-up.

Diagnosis and Staging

Upper endoscopy remains the preferred diagnostic test for esophageal cancer. The diagnosis of cancer will require a histologic examination of the primary tumor or, in case of advanced disease, of metastatic lesions. Endoscopic ultrasound (EUS) provides detailed images of the depth of invasion into the esophagus wall (T stage) and peri-esophageal lymphadenopathy (N stage). EUS also visualizes the left lobe of the liver and can identify metastatic lesions (M stage). Bronchoscopy is recommended in patients with tumors located at or above the carina. Contrast-enhanced computed tomography (CT) and 18-fluorodeoxyglucose positron emission tomography (FDG-PET) scans are helpful in detecting occult metastatic disease.

Treatment

Early stage esophageal cancer with negative lymph nodes (T1a: invasion into the mucosa) can be treated with endoscopic mucosal resection. T1b tumors (tumor invades the submucosa) should be treated with upfront surgery. For locally advanced disease, multimodality therapy is recommended. Neoadjuvant concurrent chemotherapy and radiation followed by surgical resection is the standard of care, at least in the United States. Definitive chemotherapy and radiation is an acceptable alternative for patients who are not surgical candidates. The combination of carboplatin and paclitaxel with radiation is currently the most commonly used neoadjuvant (chemotherapy administered before surgery) or definitive therapy. Esophagectomy can be performed with a transthoracic (Ivor-Lewis) or a transhiatal technique, with comparable clinical outcomes.

Advanced (stage IV) esophageal cancer is a highly lethal disease with poor outcome. The goals of treatment are to improve survival and quality of life. Several chemotherapeutic agents have shown benefits in patients with advanced esophageal cancer as a single agent or in combination including 5-fluorouracil (5-FU), platinum agents, irinotecan, and taxanes.

Two targeted agents, trastuzumab, a monoclonal antibody directed against human epidermal growth factor receptor 2 (HER2), and ramucirumab, a monoclonal antibody against vascular endothelial growth factor receptor 2 (VEGFR 2), have shown activity in metastatic esophageal cancer when combined with chemotherapy. Trastuzumab is indicated in patients who overexpress Her-2 neu. The recently developed PD-1/PDL-1 antibodies are showing some promising activity in this setting for patients with metastatic disease who progressed on first-line therapy. Ongoing studies are currently evaluating these agents alone and in combination with chemotherapy and radiation. Supportive care and localized therapy to the primary tumor might be indicated to help with pain, obstruction, bleeding, and other localized symptoms. Nutritional support in this patient population is always challenging and might require parenteral administration of nutrients.

胃肠道癌症

邱维 译　王湘　王晰程 审校　巴一 通审

引言

胃肠道癌症是世界范围内最常见的癌症之一。2018年美国预计约有 300 000 例新发胃肠道癌症病例，同时估计有 150 000 人因此死亡。胃肠道癌症通常具有典型的上皮恶性增生——癌——具有明确的肿瘤转化病理模式。胃肠道恶性肿瘤的发病率正在增加。结肠癌和肝细胞癌已经建立了筛查和早期检测流程。亚裔人群应进行胃癌和食管癌筛查。胃肠道恶性肿瘤的危险因素、临床表现和管理均有部位特异性。管理通常涉及先进的诊断程序和多学科治疗手段，包括先进的内镜检查、化疗、放疗和外科手术干预等。晚期疾病的并发症，包括肠梗阻和胆道梗阻、肝功能衰竭、出血和营养不良，在这些疾病的预后和死亡中扮演重要角色。尽管近期免疫治疗和免疫检查点抑制剂展示了前景，但尚未显著改善这些疾病的整体预后。

食管癌

流行病学

食管癌的发病率因地域而异，其中亚洲和东非发病率最高，而西方国家则最低。美国的食管鳞癌发病率正在减少，而腺癌多见于胃食管交界处，部分缘于肥胖、反流性疾病和巴雷特（Barrett）食管，其发病率不断升高。

病理学

鳞状细胞癌（鳞癌）常见于食管上部，与吸烟、饮酒和饮食摄入有关。在某些地区（如中国、伊朗），热饮被认为是鳞癌高发的原因。另一方面，大多数腺癌发生都有巴雷特食管的背景。有意思的是，只有50%的巴雷特食管患者具有慢性反流病史。在巴雷特食管患者中，罹患食管癌的风险至少增加了30倍，在重度不典型增生的情况下则更高。

临床表现

进行性加重的吞咽困难和体重减轻是食管癌最常见的症状。慢性失血导致的缺铁性贫血也不少见，而长期胃食管反流病史却不如预期常见。早期食管癌通常无症状，常在胃肠道出血检查或巴雷特食管的随诊中被发现。

诊断及分期

上消化道内镜检查仍然是食管癌的首选诊断检查。癌症的诊断需对原发肿瘤或疾病晚期时的转移性病变进行组织学病理明确。内镜超声影像提供食管壁受累深度（T分期）和食管周围淋巴结转移（N分期）的具体分期。内镜超声还可观察肝脏左叶，从而发现远处转移病变（M分期）。支气管镜检查则推荐用于肿瘤位于隆突或隆突上方的患者。增强CT和FDG-PET对于检测隐匿性转移病灶更有帮助。

治疗

淋巴结阴性的早期食管癌（T1a：侵及黏膜）可以通过内镜下黏膜切除术治疗。T1b（肿瘤侵及黏膜下层）可直接手术。局部进展期疾病则推荐多学科综合治疗。至少在美国，新辅助同步放化疗序贯手术切除是标准治疗。而根治性放化疗则是在没有手术条件下的可接受替代方案。紫杉醇联合卡铂的同步放化疗是目前最常用的新辅助（术前化疗）或根治性治疗。食管切除手术可采用经胸（Ivor Lewis）或经膈入路，二者具有相似的临床转归。

晚期（Ⅳ期）食管癌致死率高、预后差。治疗目标是延长生存和改善生活质量。多种化疗药物如5-氟尿嘧啶（5-FU）、铂类、伊立替康和紫杉烷类，以单药或联合治疗的方式给晚期食管癌患者带来获益。

两种分子靶向药物，一种是针对人表皮生长因子受体2（HER2）的单克隆抗体曲妥珠单抗，另一种是针对血管内皮生长因子受体2（VEGFR 2）的单克隆抗体雷莫西尤单抗，与化疗联合使用时对晚期疾病显示出活性效应。曲妥珠单抗适用于Her-2 neu过表达的患者。最近开发的PD-1/PD-L1抗体在晚期一线治疗后病情进展的患者中具有应用前景。目前正在进行的研究正在评估这些药物单用或与放化疗联用的效果。支持治疗和原发肿瘤局部治疗可能有助于缓解疼痛、梗阻、出血以及其他局部症状。这类患者的营养支持一向具有挑战性，可能需要给予肠外营养支持治疗。

GASTRIC CANCER

Epidemiology
Gastric adenocarcinoma is one of the most common malignancies worldwide. The disease has shown a remarkable decline in incidence and mortality worldwide secondary in part to refrigeration and the decreased use of food preservatives as well as the recognition of *Helicobacter pylori* infection as a risk factor. However, this disease remains common in Asian countries (China, Japan, and Korea), in the Middle East, and in Eastern Europe, placing it among the five most common cancers worldwide.

Pathology
There are two main histologic subtypes of gastric adenocarcinoma: diffuse and intestinal. The diffuse type (undifferentiated) is increasing in incidence and is associated with younger age, signet ring cells, early metastasis, and worse prognosis. The intestinal type (differentiated) is seen in older patients, is differentiated with a background of intestinal metaplasia, and has a declining incidence and a somewhat better prognosis. The main carcinogenic event in diffuse carcinomas is loss of expression of E-cadherin, the protein responsible for intercellular connections and the organization of epithelial tissues.

Clinical Presentation
Weight loss, nausea, and epigastric abdominal pain are the most common symptoms of gastric cancer at initial diagnosis. Early satiety (with the linitis plastica subtype), dysphagia (gastroesophageal junction or cardia tumors), and gastrointestinal bleeding are also commonly seen. Symptoms of distant metastatic disease might be seen at diagnosis. The most common metastatic sites are the liver, peritoneal surfaces (causing ascites), distant lymph nodes, and less commonly, the ovaries (Krukenberg tumor) and lungs.

Diagnosis
Upper gastrointestinal endoscopy is the standard diagnostic test to obtain tissue and localize the tumor. Endoscopic ultrasound will help with the TNM staging in combination with CT scans of the chest, abdomen, and pelvis. The role of PET scans is still evolving. The diagnosis of the linitis plastica subtype can be challenging because overt mucosal lesions are often not evident. Radiologic and endoscopic features can guide the diagnosis as well as deep biopsies. Staging laparoscopy can upstage 20% to 30% of patients with gastric cancer with otherwise negative work-up and will spare the patient unnecessary laparotomy. Screening endoscopy is recommended in high-incidence countries as well as high-risk patients.

Treatment
Surgery remains the cornerstone of treatment for nonmetastatic disease. The most controversial areas in the surgical management of gastric cancer are whether to perform total gastrectomy for tumors in the upper third of the stomach versus partial gastrectomy for tumors in the lower two thirds. Also controversial is the extent of lymph node dissection. Extended D2 dissection to remove the stomach, all surrounding lymph nodes, and the spleen is superior and recommended compared to D1 dissection (refers to a limited dissection of only the perigastric lymph nodes), but it is associated with excess morbidity and mortality and should be performed by an experienced surgeon. For locally advanced disease, in addition to surgery, either perioperative chemotherapy with a platinum-based regimen or postoperative chemoradiation with 5-FU is an acceptable approach. For metastatic disease, first- and second-line palliative chemotherapy can improve outcomes, including survival. Similar to esophageal cancer (mentioned previously), trastuzumab and ramucirumab have shown activities in metastatic disease when combined with chemotherapy. The role of immune checkpoint inhibitors in gastric cancer is still evolving as with esophageal cancer.

Prognosis
Clinical outcomes depend on the stage at diagnosis. Five-year survival rates are 65%, 40%, 15%, and 5% for stages I, II, III, and IV, respectively. Survival outcomes in Japan and Korea are better than in most Western countries; this disparity may be attributable to routine screening endoscopies or to differences in disease biology.

PANCREATIC CANCER

Epidemiology
Pancreatic cancer is the eighth leading cause of cancer deaths worldwide and is more common in the Western part of the world. Smoking, obesity and chronic pancreatitis are established clinical risk factors. Pancreatic cancer risk increases with inherited mutations in *BRCA1*, *BRCA2*, and *PALB2* and with familial syndromes. Intraductal papillary mucinous neoplasms of the pancreas (IPMN) are at risk for malignant degeneration and are commonly managed with surveillance.

Pathology
Pancreatic ductal adenocarcinoma is the main histologic type of pancreatic cancer (85% of cases). Adenocarcinoma develops with an accumulation of mutations in the pancreatic duct epithelium. Histologic progression occurs in various stages of pancreatic intraepithelial neoplasia, leading to invasive adenocarcinoma with desmoplastic reaction. Neuroendocrine neoplasms of the pancreas are composed of epithelial neoplastic cells with phenotypic neuroendocrine differentiation. Pancreatic neuroendocrine tumors are uncommon malignancies that originate from the endocrine cells in the pancreas. They may be nonfunctional, or they may secrete hormones such as insulin (insulinoma), gastrin (gastrinoma), glucagon (glucagonoma), or vasoactive intestinal peptide (VIPoma).

Clinical Presentation
Pain, jaundice, and weight loss are the most common presenting symptoms in patients with pancreatic ductal adenocarcinoma. New-onset type 2 diabetes mellitus in an adult older than 50 years of age without overt obesity-related risk factors should raise suspicion for pancreatic cancer. Venous thromboembolism is commonly associated with pancreatic cancer and can rarely be a presenting feature. Pancreatic neuroendocrine tumors are usually diagnosed incidentally or can cause symptoms related to excess hormone production including hypoglycemia (insulinoma), Zollinger-Ellison syndrome (gastrinoma), hyperglycemia (glucagonoma), and diarrhea with electrolyte disturbances (VIPoma).

Diagnosis
Imaging of the abdomen using ultrasound can be utilized as an initial screening test if pancreatic cancer is suspected. CT or magnetic resonance imaging (MRI) can further identify the lesions and their relation to the surrounding vessels as well as metastatic disease. Endoscopic ultrasound and endoscopic retrograde cholangiopancreatography help visualize the lesions better, relieve any obstruction by stent placement, and obtain histologic confirmation by biopsies with fine-needle aspirations or bile duct brushings. Somatostatin-receptor scintigraphy can be helpful in localizing occult neuroendocrine tumors.

胃癌

流行病学

胃腺癌是世界范围内最常见的恶性肿瘤之一。该病在全世界的发病率和死亡率已呈显著下降趋势，这在一定程度上归功于食物冷藏技术的推广以及食品防腐剂的限制应用，同时也因为认识到幽门螺杆菌感染是致病的危险因素。然而，该病在亚洲国家（中国、日本和韩国）、中东和东欧仍然常见，位列全世界最常见的癌种前五位。

病理学

胃腺癌有两种主要的组织学亚型：弥漫型和肠型。弥漫型（未分化型）胃癌发病率正在上升，与年轻、印戒细胞、早期转移及预后更差相关。肠型（分化型）多见于老年患者，具有肠道上皮化生的背景，发病率有下降趋势，预后也相对较好。弥漫型的主要致癌事件是 E-钙黏蛋白的表达缺失，而该蛋白负责细胞间连接和上皮组织的组成。

临床表现

体重减轻、恶心和上腹痛是胃癌首诊时最常见的症状。初期饱腹感（皮革胃亚型）、吞咽困难（胃食管交界处或贲门肿瘤）和胃肠道出血也是常见的症状。远处转移疾病的症状在诊断时也可发现。最常见的远处转移部位是肝、腹膜表面（引起腹水）、远处淋巴结，以及不太常见的卵巢[库肯勃（Krukenberg）瘤]和肺。

诊断

上消化道内镜检查是标准的获取组织和定位肿瘤的诊断检查。内镜超声与胸腹盆 CT 结合有助于 TNM 分期。PET 检测仍在发展中。皮革胃亚型的诊断因为黏膜病变常常不明显而具有挑战性。影像学和内镜下特征可以指导其诊断和深挖活检。腹腔镜分期检查可使 20%～30% 的晚期胃癌患者免于不必要的剖腹手术。建议在高发病率国家和高危患者中开展内镜筛查。

治疗

手术仍然是治疗非转移性胃癌的基石。与针对下 2/3 胃部的肿瘤可行部分胃切除术相比，针对上 1/3 胃部肿瘤是否进行全胃切除术，是胃癌外科治疗中最具争议的领域。同样有争议的是淋巴结的清扫范围。扩大 D2 清扫术包括切除胃、所有周围淋巴结以及推荐切除脾脏。与 D1 清扫术（仅对胃周淋巴结有限度的切除）相比，该术式与过多的并发症和死亡率相关，故应由经验丰富的外科医生进行手术。对于局部进展期疾病，除手术外，以铂类为基础的围术期化疗或术后 5-FU 化疗都是可接受的方法。晚期一线和二线姑息化疗可以改善包括生存期在内的总体预后。与食管癌（如前所述）类似，曲妥珠单抗和雷莫西尤单抗联合化疗对晚期患者显示出疗效。胃癌中免疫检查点抑制剂的作用与食管癌中一样，仍在发展中。

预后

临床转归取决于诊断时的分期。Ⅰ、Ⅱ、Ⅲ、Ⅳ期胃癌的 5 年生存率分别为 65%、40%、15% 和 5%。日本和韩国的生存转归好于大多数西方国家；这种差异可能归结于常规内镜筛查或疾病的生物学差异。

胰腺癌

流行病学

胰腺癌是全球癌症死亡的第八大原因。在西方世界更为常见。吸烟、肥胖和慢性胰腺炎已被明确为临床危险因素。胰腺癌患病风险随具有 *BRCA1*、*BRCA2* 和 *PALB2* 的遗传基因突变及家族性综合征而增加。胰腺导管内乳头状黏液肿瘤（IPMN）有恶变的风险，通常通过定期监测来管理。

病理学

胰腺导管腺癌是胰腺癌的主要组织学类型（85% 的病例）。腺癌随胰管上皮的突变累积而发展。组织学进展发生在胰腺上皮内瘤变的不同阶段，伴随结缔组织增生反应从而导致侵袭性腺癌。胰腺神经内分泌肿瘤由神经内分泌分化表型的恶性上皮细胞组成。胰腺神经内分泌肿瘤来源于胰腺中的内分泌细胞，是不常见的恶性肿瘤。它们可能是无功能的，也可能分泌激素如胰岛素（胰岛素瘤）、胃泌素（胃泌素瘤）、胰高血糖素（胰高血糖素瘤）或血管活性肠肽（血管活性肠肽瘤）等。

临床表现

疼痛、黄疸和体重减轻是最常见的症状。50 岁以上新发的 2 型糖尿病患者，如缺乏明显的肥胖相关危险因素，就应怀疑胰腺癌的可能。静脉血栓栓塞通常与胰腺癌相关，但很少成为显性症状。胰腺神经内分泌肿瘤通常是偶然诊断的，或通过与过量激素分泌相关的症状表现出来，包括低血糖（胰岛素瘤）、卓-艾综合征（胃泌素瘤）、高血糖（胰高血糖素瘤）和伴有电解质紊乱的腹泻（血管活性肠肽瘤）。

诊断

腹部超声影像可以作为疑诊胰腺癌的初始筛查。CT 或 MRI 可进一步明确病变范围及其与周围血管的关系。内镜超声与内镜逆行胰胆管造影有助于更好地观察病变，通过置入支架解除梗阻，并通过细针穿刺或胆管刷片活检获得组织学证据。生长抑素受体核素显像有助于定位隐匿性神经内分泌肿瘤。

Treatment

Pancreatic adenocarcinomas are some of the most difficult cancers to treat. Their anatomic locations make them poor candidates for resection. Only 15% to 20% of patients are candidates for surgical resection at the time of diagnosis because the tumor frequently involves the celiac arterial axis and superior mesenteric artery and vein and even the portal vein. Whipple procedure (pancreatoduodenectomy) and distal pancreatectomy are the standard surgeries; however, the 5-year overall survival rate after pancreatic adenocarcinoma resection is less than 20%.

The role of adjuvant therapy following resection is not well established. Recent studies with multiagent regimens such as a combination of 5-FU, irinotecan, and oxaliplatin (FOLFIRINOX) or combined gemcitabine and nab-paclitaxel have demonstrated improved overall survival for metastatic pancreatic cancer and following resection as well. Observation only or somatostatin analogues are both acceptable first-line treatment for unresectable pancreatic neuroendocrine tumors. Recent studies in neuroendocrine tumors have also shown improvement in outcomes with targeted agents such as everolimus and sunitinib. Palliation of symptoms is a large component of care. Early referral to palliative care should be considered, especially in symptomatic patients with adenocarcinoma. Referrals to nutrition consultants, opioids, celiac nerve plexus block, biliary drainage, as well palliative surgeries can help improve patients' quality of life.

Prognosis

Pancreatic adenocarcinoma carries a very poor prognosis; the 5-year overall survival rate remains less than 10%. Survival has not improved significantly over the last few decades, in contrast to several other cancers. Neuroendocrine tumor carries a better prognosis, depending on the stage and the grade of the tumor, with survival measured in years.

CHOLANGIOCARCINOMA (BILE DUCT CANCERS)

Epidemiology

Cholangiocarcinomas (bile duct cancers) arise from the intrahepatic and extrahepatic biliary epithelium of the bile ducts. Cancer of the gallbladder or the ampulla of Vater are sometimes included with cholangiocarcinomas but have different risk factors and clinical behavior. Although uncommon in the United States, the incidence of cholangiocarcinomas has been on the rise for unclear reasons. Established risk factors include sclerosing cholangitis, cholelithiasis, cholecystitis, chronic liver disease, toxin exposure, metabolic syndrome, and infections. Gallbladder cancer is particularly prevalent in South American countries—especially Chile—as well as southeastern Asian countries.

Pathology

The majority of cholangiocarcinomas are adenocarcinoma. Immunohistochemistry staining might appear similar to other malignancies, in particular pancreatic cancer and upper gastrointestinal malignancies. Imaging and clinical correlation might aid in the differential diagnosis.

Clinical Presentation

Painless jaundice, pruritus, dark urine, and light color stool are usually the presenting symptoms of extrahepatic cholangiocarcinoma and are caused by biliary obstruction. Intrahepatic cholangiocarcinoma usually presents with vague right upper quadrant pain or is found incidentally on imaging. Gallbladder cancer can sometimes be an incidental finding during histologic evaluation after cholecystectomy, which is commonly performed for presumed cholelithiasis or cholecystitis.

Diagnosis

Transabdominal ultrasonography can be used to confirm biliary dilation, but to confirm the diagnosis of cholangiocarcinoma, computed tomography scanning or magnetic resonance imaging with magnetic resonance cholangiopancreatography MRCP should be performed. In some patients, an endoscopic retrograde cholangiopancreatography (ERCP) is used as the first test because it allows direct visualization of the suspected area, helps obtain a tissue diagnosis, and allows for therapeutic intervention to alleviate the obstruction. Endoscopic ultrasound can aid in identifying tumor location and extension as well.

Treatment

A negative margin surgical resection is the only curative treatment for intrahepatic and extrahepatic cholangiocarcinoma. Distal cholangiocarcinomas have the highest rate of complete resection (R0), compared to proximal and intrahepatic cholangiocarcinoma. Adjuvant chemotherapy (with or without radiation), following curative resection, is recommended in general, and based upon meta-analysis. Gemcitabine, platinum and 5-fluouracil based treatments are usually recommended in the adjuvant setting.

Surgical resection with lymph node dissection is the standard treatment for gallbladder cancer and ampullary cancer as well. The role of adjuvant therapy is less clear in this setting. Gallbladder cancer is treated in a similar fashion to cholangiocarcinoma, while recommendations following ampullary cancer resection are less clear. Many clinicians recommend surveillance-only, given the more favorable prognosis of ampullary cancer as compared with other biliary tract cancers and the lack of data supporting a survival advantage with further therapy. However, some oncologists tend to treat these patients as they would resected pancreatic cancer, even for those with the intestinal histology. Enrollment in clinical trials in always preferred.

Treatment with gemcitabine and cisplatin is the standard treatment for stage IV cholangiocarcinoma and gallbladder cancer. Stage IV ampullary carcinoma is treated like pancreatic cancer. Tumor profiling and the role of targeted therapy is evolving. The overall prognosis is still poor for all of these stage IV malignancies, with median overall survival less than 12 months.

Prognosis

Even following curative resection, cholangiocarcinoma still carries a poor prognosis. Five-year overall survival rate ranges from 30% in patients with negative lymph nodes to 2% in patients with metastatic disease. Enrollment in clinical trials is always recommended. Several new agents and pathways are being evaluated in this patient population.

HEPATOCELLULAR CARCINOMA

Epidemiology

Hepatocellular carcinoma (HCC), or primary liver cancer, is a common disease around the world. It is the second most common cause of cancer-related death in men worldwide.

Pathology

Most HCCs arise in the setting of underlying cirrhosis, with alcohol use, hepatitis B, and hepatitis C being the most common causes of cirrhosis. Other diseases causing cirrhosis such as hemochromatosis, primary biliary cirrhosis, and α_1-antitrypsin deficiency are also contributory. Cirrhosis involves chronic hepatocyte injury and ensuing cell regeneration, which provides the substrate for cancer development: inflammatory cytokine stress, constant cell cycling, and aberrant cell development and differentiation.

治疗

胰腺癌是最难治疗的癌症之一。其解剖位置使之难以通过手术切除。因为肿瘤经常累及腹腔干和肠系膜上动静脉甚至门静脉,只有15%～20%的患者在诊断时适合手术切除。Whipple手术(胰十二指肠切除术)和胰远端切除术是标准手术;然而,胰腺癌术后的5年生存率低于20%。

术后辅助治疗的作用尚不明确。近期5-FU、伊立替康和奥沙利铂(FOLFIRINOX)或者吉西他滨和白蛋白结合型紫杉醇联合化疗的研究已显示出对转移性胰腺癌总体预后以及术后治疗有一定获益。对于不可切除的胰腺神经内分泌肿瘤,仅作观察或生长抑素类似物均是可接受的一线方案。最近对神经内分泌肿瘤的研究结果,也显示了靶向药物如依维莫司和舒尼替尼可改善预后。缓解症状是治疗的一个重要组成部分。尤其是有症状的腺癌患者,应考虑尽早转诊缓和医疗。及时营养咨询、阿片类药物应用、腹腔神经丛阻滞、胆道引流以及姑息手术可以帮助提高患者的生活质量。

预后

胰腺癌预后极差;5年总生存率仍低于10%。与其他癌症相比,在过去几十年中生存未获显著改善。神经内分泌肿瘤预后较好,取决于肿瘤分期和分级,其生存期以年为单位计算。

胆管细胞癌(胆管癌)

流行病学

胆管细胞癌(胆管癌)起源于肝内和肝外的胆管上皮。胆囊或乏特(Vater)壶腹癌有时被归类在胆管癌中,但具有不同的危险因素和临床特征。尽管并不常见,但在美国胆管癌的发病率一直在上升,其原因不明。已明确的危险因素包括硬化性胆管炎、胆结石、胆囊炎、慢性肝病、毒物暴露、代谢综合征和感染。胆囊癌在南美洲国家特别流行,尤其是智利,在东南亚国家同样如此。

病理学

大多数胆管癌是腺癌。免疫组化染色可能看起来与其他恶性肿瘤相似,特别是胰腺癌和上消化道恶性肿瘤。影像与临床相结合可能有助于鉴别诊断。

临床表现

肝外胆管癌的常见临床表现为无痛性黄疸、瘙痒、尿色加深和粪便颜色变浅,由胆道梗阻引起。肝内胆管癌通常表现为右上腹隐痛或偶然在影像检查中被发现。胆囊癌有时在预期胆石症或胆管炎行胆囊切除术后,于病理组织评价中被偶然发现。

诊断

经腹超声检查可用于确认胆道扩张。但为了确认胆管癌的诊断,应完善CT或磁共振胰胆管成像(MRCP)。内镜下逆行胰胆管造影(ERCP)被作为某些患者的首选检查,因为它可以直接观察可疑区域,有助于获得组织学诊断并可行治疗干预以缓解梗阻。内镜超声也可以帮助显示肿瘤位置和进展情况。

治疗

肝内和肝外胆管癌唯一的根治方案是切缘阴性的手术切除。与近端和肝内胆管癌相比,远端胆管癌的完全切除率(R0)最高。基于荟萃分析的结果,推荐根治性术后的辅助化疗(联合或不联合放疗)。吉西他滨、铂类和5-氟尿嘧啶为基础的治疗通常在辅助方案中推荐。

手术切除加淋巴结清扫对胆囊癌和壶腹癌均是标准的治疗方法;辅助治疗的疗效还不太明确。对于胆囊癌是以对胆管癌相似的方式进行治疗,而壶腹癌术后的推荐治疗尚不明确。许多临床医生建议仅进行定期监测,因为壶腹癌与其他胆道癌症相比,预后更好,同时也缺乏进一步治疗的生存获益证据。然而,一些肿瘤科医生倾向于将其视为胰腺癌术后的患者来对待,即使对组织学提示肠道来源的也是如此。因此参加临床研究始终是优选推荐的。

对于Ⅳ期胆管癌和胆囊癌,吉西他滨和顺铂是标准治疗方案。Ⅳ期壶腹癌的治疗方法与胰腺癌相似。肿瘤分子表达谱和靶向治疗的作用正在发展中。对于Ⅳ期恶性肿瘤,总体预后仍然很差,总体中位生存期小于12个月。

预后

即使经过根治性切除,胆管癌仍然预后不良。5年总生存率从淋巴结阴性患者的30%到晚期患者的2%。因此始终建议参加临床研究。多种新的药物和靶向相关信号传导通路药物,也正在评估中。

肝细胞癌

流行病学

肝细胞癌(HCC),又被称为原发性肝癌,是全球范围内常见病。它是全球男性癌症相关死亡的第二大常见原因。

病理学

大多数HCC发生于肝硬化背景下,酒精、乙型肝炎和丙型肝炎是肝硬化的最常见原因。其他引起肝硬化的疾病还包括血色病、原发性胆汁性肝硬化和α1-抗胰蛋白酶缺乏症等。肝硬化涉及慢性肝细胞损伤和随后的细胞再生的一系列病理过程,包括炎性细胞因子应激、细胞不断循环以及细胞发育和分化异常等,为癌症发生、发展提供了基础。

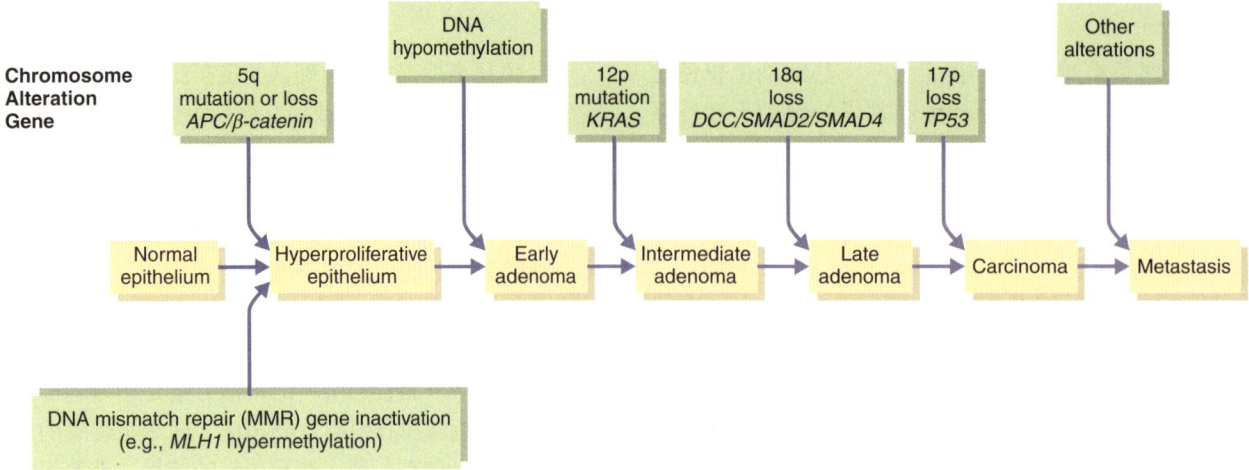

Fig. 5.1 **Model of colorectal carcinogenesis.** Several genes are involved in the stepwise progression from normal colonic epithelium to adenocarcinoma.

Clinical Presentation

HCC is frequently masked by the underlying liver disease. Abdominal distention from ascites, fatigue, muscle wasting, anorexia, and encephalopathy are features of cirrhosis. Acute hepatic decompensation or right upper quadrant pain may herald the development of HCC. HCC can also be an incidental finding during routine surveillance by screening ultrasound for patients with cirrhosis.

Diagnosis

HCC is one of those rare malignancies for which a diagnosis can be made without histologic confirmation. Nonhistologic criteria for diagnosis include underlying cirrhosis, elevated α-fetoprotein level (>400 ng/mL), and a characteristic appearance on contrast-enhanced CT or MRI (arterial enhancement and rapid washout). In the absence of underlying cirrhosis, however, a tissue diagnosis must be obtained. For patients with cirrhosis, a surveillance program incorporating regular measurements of α-fetoprotein and ultrasound imaging can detect early lesions.

Treatment

For small lesions, surgical resection can be curative. Preoperative assessment of liver function to ensure that the patient is an appropriate candidate for partial liver resection is critical. Liver transplantation is an option that will address HCC as well as the underlying cirrhosis. Strict criteria, such as the Milan criteria (i.e., single tumor ≤5 cm, or up to three tumors each <3 cm, and no vascular invasion), are used to determine which patients are eligible for transplantation. For those who are ineligible for surgical approaches, radiofrequency ablation, transarterial chemoembolization, yttrium-90 embolization, and percutaneous ethanol injection can provide local control. Until recently, Sorafenib, a multikinase inhibitor, was the only proven treatment for metastatic HCC. In the last 2 years, two other kinase inhibitors, lenvatinib and cabozantinib, have been approved for the treatment of HCC. Immune check point inhibitors including pembrolizumab and nivolumab are both approved for the second line treatment of HCC after failure of tyrosine kinase inhibitors.

Prognosis

The prognosis in HCC is often determined by the severity of the underlying liver disease. The 5-year survival rate approaches 50% with complete surgical resection or liver transplantation. For advanced HCC, the median overall survival time with therapy is approximately 1 year.

COLORECTAL CANCER

Epidemiology

Colorectal cancer is the third most common cancer as well as the third most common cause of cancer-related death in the United States, with approximately 150,000 new cases diagnosed each year. Worldwide, it is a growing problem and one of the most common cancers. There appears to be an increased association between colon cancer and high dietary fat, red meat consumption, low dietary fiber, obesity, and alcohol use. Conversely, increased physical activity and use of supplemental estrogen, folate, vitamin, aspirin, and nonsteroidal anti-inflammatory drugs appear to be protective. A history of inflammatory bowel disease is a risk factor for colorectal cancer.

Pathology

Adenocarcinoma of the colon progresses from normal epithelium to frank cancer in a stepwise fashion, as illustrated in Fig. 5.1. Most colon cancers arise in polyps. Hamartomatous polyps usually are non-neoplastic but can be part of juvenile polyposis or Peutz-Jeghers polyposis where they can undergo malignant transformation. Serrated polyps 10 mm or greater with dysplasia should be managed as high-risk adenoma. Adenomatous polyps are the most common neoplastic polyps in the colon and can progress to cancer.

Several inherited abnormalities lead to a genetic predisposition to colon cancer. Such syndromes are responsible for 3% to 5% of all colon cancers. They can be divided into syndromes associated with underlying polyps and those without polyps. Classic familial adenomatous polyposis (FAP) is caused by an autosomal dominant mutation in the *APC* gene. The colon is full of polyps—hundreds to thousands—that start forming during adolescence, leading to development of cancer in early adulthood. Patients with attenuated FAP have fewer polyps and later development of malignancy. *MYH*-associated polyposis is caused

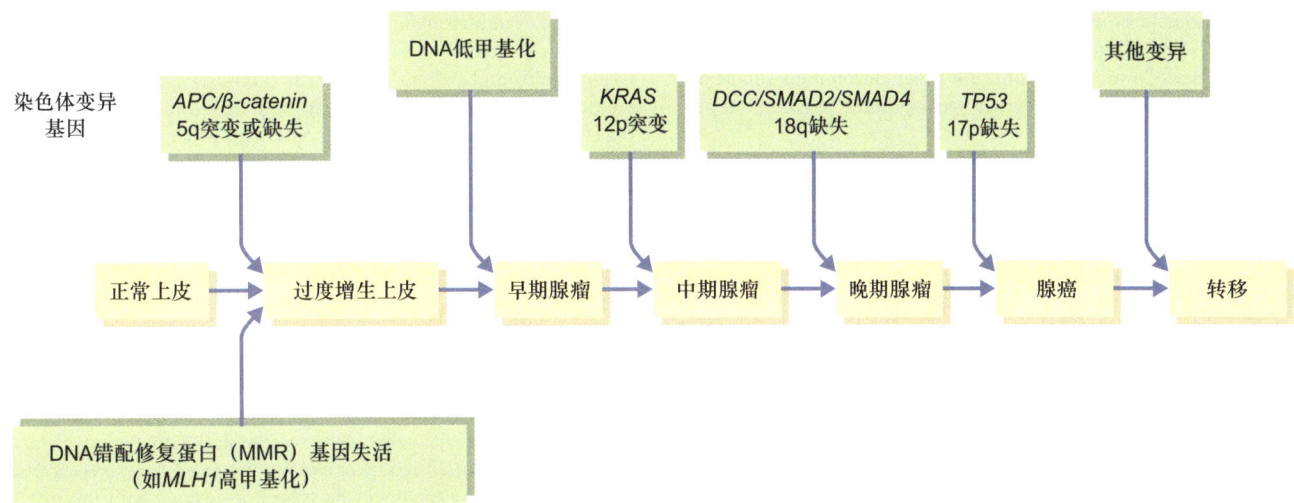

图 5.1 结直肠癌发生的模型。多个基因参与了从正常结肠上皮到腺癌的逐步发展过程

临床表现

HCC 经常被基础肝病掩盖。腹水引起的腹胀、乏力、肌肉萎缩、厌食和肝性脑病是肝硬化的特征。急性肝功能失代偿或右上腹疼痛可能提示 HCC 的发生。HCC 也可在对肝硬化进行常规监测过程中被偶然发现。

诊断

HCC 是少数不需要组织学证实即可诊断的恶性肿瘤之一。非组织学诊断标准包括肝硬化背景、甲胎蛋白水平升高（> 400 ng/ml）以及增强 CT 或 MRI 上的特征性表现（动脉期增强和"快进快出"征象）。然而，在没有肝硬化背景的情况下，必须获得组织学诊断。对于肝硬化患者，定期监测甲胎蛋白水平和肝脏超声可以检测早期病变。

治疗

对于小病灶，手术切除可治愈。术前评估肝功能以确保患者是部分肝切除术的合适对象至关重要。肝移植是一种治疗 HCC 和其基础肝硬化的选择。通常采用严格的标准，如米兰标准（即单个肿瘤 ≤ 5 cm，或直径 < 3 cm 的肿瘤 ≤ 3 个，无血管侵犯）来确定哪些患者适合移植。对于不适合手术的患者，射频消融、经动脉化疗栓塞、钇 90 栓塞和经皮乙醇注射可用于局部治疗。以往，索拉非尼（一种多激酶抑制剂）一直是唯一被证实的转移性 HCC 的治疗方法。在过去 2 年中，另外两种激酶抑制剂——仑伐替尼和卡博替尼已被批准用于治疗 HCC。免疫检查点抑制剂（如帕博利珠单抗和纳武利尤单抗）被获批用于酪氨酸激酶抑制剂治疗失败后的 HCC 二线治疗。

预后

HCC 的预后通常取决于基础肝病的严重程度。完全手术切除或肝移植后 HCC 的 5 年生存率接近 50%。对于晚期 HCC，经过治疗后的中位总生存时间约为 1 年。

结直肠癌

流行病学

在美国，结直肠癌是第三大常见癌症，也是癌症相关死亡的第三大常见原因，每年约有 15 万新诊断病例。在全球范围内，结直肠癌是一个日益严重的问题，也是最常见的癌症之一。结肠癌与高脂肪饮食、食用红肉、低膳食纤维、肥胖和饮酒之间的关系密切。相反，增加体育活动和补充雌激素、叶酸、维生素、阿司匹林和非甾体抗炎药似乎具有保护作用。炎症性肠病是结直肠癌的危险因素之一。

病理学

如图 5.1 所示，结肠腺癌从正常上皮逐步演变为明确的腺癌。大多数结肠癌起源于息肉。错构瘤性息肉通常是非肿瘤性的，但可能是幼年性息肉病或 Peutz-Jeghers 息肉病的一部分，后者可以发生恶变。对于伴有异型增生的锯齿状息肉（直径 ≥ 10 mm）应作为高危腺瘤进行管理。腺瘤样息肉是结肠最常见的肿瘤性息肉，可发展为癌症。

数种遗传异常可导致遗传易感性结肠癌。这类综合征占所有结肠癌的 3%～5%。它们可分为与息肉病相关的综合征和无息肉的综合征。经典的家族性腺瘤样息肉病（FAP）是由 *APC* 基因的常染色体显性突变引起的，结肠中长满了成百上千枚息肉，在青春期开始形成，导致成年早期发生癌症。衰减型 FAP 患者息肉较少，发展为癌症的时间更晚。*MYH* 相关性息肉病

by an autosomal recessive mutation in the *MYH* gene, and the phenotype mimics that of attenuated FAP. Peutz-Jeghers syndrome, juvenile polyposis, and Cowden syndrome are other uncommon conditions that are associated with an inherited predisposition to colorectal polyps leading to cancer.

The classic nonpolyposis syndrome is hereditary nonpolyposis colorectal cancer, also called Lynch syndrome. Germline recessive mutations in genes involved in the mismatch repair pathway *(MSH2, MSH3, MSH6, MLH1, MLH3, PMS1, PMS2)* lead to adenocarcinoma. These cases are indistinguishable from sporadic cases associated with defective mismatch repair, except for the family history of colon and other associated cancers in the inherited syndrome (e.g., endometrial, ovarian, gastric, and small bowel cancer).

Clinical Presentation

Hematochezia and altered bowel habits are the classic symptoms of colon cancer. Early cases are essentially asymptomatic and are typically identified by screening. Advanced cases can manifest with bowel obstruction or perforation, frank rectal bleeding, weight loss, abdominal pain, and ascites due to hepatic or peritoneal metastases. Cancers associated with the mismatch repair pathway have certain typical features: They are right-sided, more common in women, and occur in younger patients. They are usually poorly differentiated and locally advanced without significant lymph node involvement.

Diagnosis

Screening for colorectal cancer is an important public health tool. Screening methods include fecal occult blood testing, imaging (barium enema, CT-guided colonography), and endoscopy (flexible sigmoidoscopy, colonoscopy). Colonoscopy is the "gold standard" for visual confirmation and histologic diagnosis of colon cancer. Once a cancer diagnosis is established, CT scans of the chest, abdomen, and pelvis are indicated to evaluate for distant disease. MRI of the pelvis or endoscopic ultrasound are used in rectal cancer to determine the exact tumor location and its extent prior to neoadjuvant therapy.

Treatment

For patients with resectable disease, surgical resection is the treatment of choice. Removal of the involved segment of the colon, along with the associated mesentery containing all draining lymph nodes, is recommended. Such procedures are being increasingly performed with the use of laparoscopic techniques, resulting in decreased perioperative morbidity. Decisions regarding chemotherapy after surgery (i.e., adjuvant chemotherapy) are based on the pathologic findings. For stage I disease (T1 or T2, N0), no chemotherapy is recommended. For stage III disease (any T, N+), chemotherapy is strongly recommended. A combination of a fluoropyrimidine (5-FU, capecitabine) with oxaliplatin, administered for 6 months, is the standard of care. For stage II disease (T3 or T4, N0), data are controversial. A careful risk-benefit evaluation for each patient is recommended to determine whether adjuvant chemotherapy is appropriate. Rectal cancer is associated with a high rate of local recurrence that can lead to significant morbidity. To improve outcomes, preoperative chemotherapy and radiation therapy are used, and surgery should include total mesorectal excision.

For metastatic colorectal cancer, treatment options include chemotherapy agents such as fluoropyrimidines, oxaliplatin, and irinotecan. The advent of targeted therapies has improved clinical outcomes. These therapies include anti-angiogenic agents (bevacizumab, ziv-aflibercept, ramucirumab), anti–epidermal growth factor receptor antibodies (cetuximab, panitumumab). The multikinase inhibitors (regorafenib) and trifluridine-tipiracil (Lonsurf) are both approved for patients who progress after first- and second-line chemotherapy but efficacy is only modest. Another option for patients with metastatic colorectal cancer who have MSI-H/dMMR tumors is immunotherapy. The immune checkpoint inhibitor nivolumab, both as a single agent or in combination with ipilimumab, are approved by the FDA for patients who progressed after standard of therapy. Colon cancer is one of the few malignancies in which some cases of metastatic disease can also be cured with aggressive systemic therapy and surgery. Therefore, close surveillance after treatment of the initial cancer is recommended to detect early recurrences. Surveillance should include regular physical evaluation, CT scanning, and measurement of serum levels of carcinoembryonic antigen (CEA), a protein synthesized disproportionately by malignant epithelial cells. Increased physical activity and dietary modifications (reduced red meat and fat; increased fruits, vegetables, and fiber) following treatment have been associated with improved outcomes. Another important component of colorectal cancer care is family risk assessment, because this is a common disease, with up to 7500 cases each year in the United States being attributable to heritable syndromes. Referral for genetic counseling should be made if such a syndrome is suspected.

Prognosis

Among gastrointestinal cancers, colorectal cancer has the best overall prognosis. For nonmetastatic disease, the 5-year survival rate ranges from 50% to 95%, depending on the extent of lymph node involvement. For metastatic disease, newer therapies, given in succession, can achieve a median overall survival time of more than 2 years. The key remains early detection by screening, which can improve outcomes.

ANAL CANCER

Epidemiology

Anal cancer is an uncommon malignancy, with about 7000 cases reported annually in the United States. It is strongly associated with human papillomavirus (HPV) infection. It is also more common in patients with human immunodeficiency virus (HIV) infection and in those who engage in anal-receptive sexual intercourse, most likely because of poor host immunity and increased transmission of HPV, respectively. Condyloma acuminata are precursor lesions for this cancer.

Pathology

The histology is typical of a squamous cell carcinoma, with sheets of hyperproliferative keratinized cells. HPV, especially types 16 and 18, causes inactivation of the tumor suppressor genes *TP53* and *RB1* via the viral proteins E6 and E7, predisposing to eventual development of carcinoma. Chronic local inflammation due to inflammatory bowel disease or recurrent anal fissures and fistulas can also lead to anal cancer.

Clinical Presentation

Local symptoms, such as perianal pruritus or pain, bleeding, discharge, and a masslike sensation, are common presentations. In cases of chronic underlying disease such as Crohn's disease, the presence of a nonhealing anal or perianal lesion despite good disease control elsewhere should raise suspicion for malignancy.

是由 MYH 基因的常染色体隐性突变引起的，表型酷似衰减型 FAP。Peutz-Jeghers 综合征、幼年性息肉病和 Cowden 综合征是其他不常见的遗传病，与结直肠息肉恶变导致癌症相关。

经典的非息肉病综合征是遗传性非息肉病性结直肠癌，也称为林奇（Lynch）综合征。参与错配修复途径的基因（MSH2、MSH3、MSH6、MLH1、MLH3、PMS1、PMS2）出现胚系隐性突变（译者注：原文有误，应为显性突变）导致腺癌。除了其他遗传性综合征（如，子宫内膜癌、卵巢癌、胃癌和小肠癌）的结肠和肿瘤家族史，这些病例与散发的错配修复缺陷相关的结直肠癌难以区分。

临床表现

便血和排便习惯改变是结肠癌的典型症状。早期病例基本无症状，通常通过筛查才能发现。晚期病例可表现为肠梗阻或穿孔、明显的直肠出血、体重减轻、腹痛和肝或腹膜转移所致的腹水。与错配修复途径相关的癌症具有一定的典型特征：位于右侧结肠，更常见于女性，好发于年轻患者。通常分化差，局部分期晚，无明显淋巴结受累。

诊断

结直肠癌筛查是一项重要的公共卫生工具。筛查方法包括粪便潜血试验、影像学（钡灌肠、CT 结肠成像）和内镜检查（软式乙状结肠镜、结肠镜）。结肠镜检查是结肠癌可视化和组织学诊断的"金标准"。结肠癌一旦确诊，应行胸部、腹部和盆腔的 CT 扫描，以评估有无远处转移。在直肠癌中，盆腔 MRI 或内镜超声用于确定肿瘤的确切位置和范围，以便进行新辅助治疗。

治疗

对于可切除的患者，手术切除是首选的治疗方法。建议切除受累的肠段，以及包含所有引流淋巴结的相关系膜。随着腹腔镜技术的普及，此类手术越来越多地使用腹腔镜，从而降低了围术期并发症的发生率。术后化疗（即辅助化疗）的决策基于病理分期。对于 I 期病变（T1 或 T2，N0），不建议化疗。对于 III 期病变（任何 T、N＋），强烈建议化疗。为期 6 个月的氟尿嘧啶类药物（5-FU、卡培他滨）联合奥沙利铂化疗是标准治疗。对于 II 期病变（T3 或 T4，N0），结论存在争议。建议对每例患者进行仔细的风险-获益评估，以确定是否需要辅助化疗。直肠癌的局部复发率高，可导致严重后果。为改善结局，需采用术前化疗和放疗，手术应包括全直肠系膜切除。

对于转移性结直肠癌，治疗选择包括氟尿嘧啶、奥沙利铂和伊立替康等化疗药物。靶向治疗的出现改善了临床结局。这些治疗包括抗血管生成药物（贝伐珠单抗、阿柏西普、雷莫西尤单抗）、抗表皮生长因子受体抗体（西妥昔单抗、帕尼单抗）。多激酶抑制剂（瑞戈非尼）和曲氟尿苷-替匹嘧啶（朗斯弗）均获批用于一线和二线化疗后进展的患者，但疗效相对有限。MSI-H/dMMR 转移性结直肠癌患者的另一种选择是免疫治疗。免疫检查点抑制剂纳武利尤单抗（nivolumab）作为单一药物或与伊匹单抗联合使用，已获得 FDA 批准用于标准治疗后进展的患者。结肠癌是为数不多的，即使转移后，也能通过积极全身治疗和手术治愈的恶性肿瘤之一。因此，建议在初始治疗后进行密切监测，以发现早期复发。检测手段应包括定期体检、CT 检查和血清癌胚抗原（CEA）监测，CEA 是在有恶性上皮细胞时会不成比例地合成增加的蛋白。治疗后增加体力活动和调整饮食结构（减少红肉和脂肪；增加水果、蔬菜和纤维）与改善结局相关。结直肠癌护理的另一个重要内容是家庭风险评估，因为这是一种常见疾病，在美国每年高达 7500 例病例归因于遗传综合征。如果怀疑存在此类综合征，应转诊进行遗传咨询。

预后

在消化道肿瘤中，结直肠癌的总体预后最好。对于非转移性病变，5 年生存率约为 50%～95%，具体取决于淋巴结受累的程度。对于转移性病变，新的疗法相继应用可以实现超过 2 年的中位总生存时间。关键仍在于通过筛查实现早期发现，这可以改善结局。

肛门癌

流行病学

肛门癌是一种少见的恶性肿瘤，美国每年约报告 7000 例。它与人乳头瘤病毒（HPV）感染密切相关。同时，它也常见于人类免疫缺陷病毒（HIV）感染者以及进行肛交的人群，这可能是因为宿主免疫力差和 HPV 传播增加所致。尖锐湿疣是肛门癌的前驱病变。

病理学

组织学表现是典型的鳞状细胞癌，伴有成片过度增生的角化细胞。HPV，尤其是 16 型和 18 型，通过病毒蛋白 E6 和 E7 的作用，导致抑癌基因 TP53 和 RB1 失活，最终导致肿瘤发生。炎症性肠病或复发性肛裂、肛瘘所致的慢性局部炎症也可导致肛门癌。

临床表现

局部症状，如肛周瘙痒或疼痛、出血、肛周分泌物和肿块样感觉是常见表现。在有克罗恩病等慢性基础疾病的患者中，如果其他病变控制满意，而肛门或肛周病变迟迟不愈合，应怀疑恶性肿瘤。

Diagnosis

Physical examination is adequate to identify suspicious lesions. A biopsy should be obtained to confirm the diagnosis. Evaluation for distant spread should include CT scans of the chest, abdomen, and pelvis. Special attention should be paid to examination of inguinal lymph nodes, because they are common sites of early spread.

Treatment

Anal cancer is one of the few solid tumor malignancies that are curable without surgical resection. For very small, early lesions, complete excision may suffice. However, for most cases, combined chemotherapy with 5-FU and mitomycin, together with radiation therapy, is the standard curative modality. This regimen has significant short-term toxicities that should be managed aggressively. This treatment can obviate the need for a large operation that would result in a permanent colostomy.

Prognosis

More than 70% of cases can be cured with chemoradiation. Relapsed disease is usually treated with surgical excision (if local) or systemic chemotherapy (if distant). Widespread vaccination against HPV, anal Pap smears in high-risk populations, and better prevention and treatment of HIV infection should lower the incidence of anal cancer.

SUGGESTED READINGS

Bang YJ, Van Cutsem E, Feyereislova A, et al: Trastuzumab in combination with chemotherapy versus chemotherapy alone for treatment of HER2-positive advanced gastric or gastro-oesophageal junction cancer (ToGA): a phase 3, open-label, randomised controlled trial, Lancet 376:687–697, 2010.

Conroy T, Desseigne F, Ychou M, et al: FOLFIRINOX versus gemcitabine for metastatic pancreatic cancer, N Engl J Med 364:1817–1825, 2011.

Grothey A, Van Cutsem E, Sobrero A, et al: Regorafenib monotherapy for previously treated metastatic colorectal cancer (CORRECT): an international, multicentre, randomised, placebo-controlled, phase 3 trial, Lancet 381:303–312, 2013.

Hvid-Jensen F, Pedersen L, Drewes AM, et al: Incidence of adenocarcinoma among patients with Barrett's esophagus, N Engl J Med 365:1375–1383, 2011.

Valle J, Wasan H, Palmer DH, et al: Cisplatin plus gemcitabine versus gemcitabine for biliary tract cancer, N Engl J Med 362:1273–1281, 2010.

van Hagen P, Hulshof MC, van Lanschot JJ, et al: Preoperative chemoradiotherapy for esophageal or junctional cancer, N Engl J Med 366:2074–2084, 2012.

Von Hoff DD, Ervin T, Arena FP, Chiorean EG, et al: Increased survival in pancreatic cancer with nab-paclitaxel plus gemcitabine, N Engl J Med 369(18):1691–1703, 2013.

Yao JC, Shah MH, Ito T, et al: Everolimus for advanced pancreatic neuroendocrine tumors, N Engl J Med 364:514–523, 2011.

诊断

体格检查足以发现可疑病变。确诊的手段为组织活检。同时，应进行胸部、腹部和盆腔 CT 检查以明确有无远处转移。另外，应特别注意腹股沟淋巴结的检查，因为该处是早期转移的常见部位。

治疗

肛门癌是为数不多的无需手术切除即可治愈的恶性肿瘤之一。对于非常小的早期病变，完全切除可能就足够。然而，对于大多数病例，联合化疗（5-FU 和丝裂霉素）和放疗是标准的治疗方法。该方案短期毒性明显，应积极管理。但这种治疗方法可以避免需进行永久性结肠造口的大手术。

预后

超过 70% 的病例可通过放化疗治愈。复发性疾病通常采用手术切除（如果是局部的）或全身化疗（如果是远处的）治疗。HPV 疫苗的广泛接种、在高危人群中进行肛门巴氏涂片检查，以及更好地预防和治疗 HIV 感染，有助于降低肛门癌的发病率。

推荐阅读

Bang YJ, Van Cutsem E, Feyereislova A, et al: Trastuzumab in combination with chemotherapy versus chemotherapy alone for treatment of HER2-positive advanced gastric or gastro-oesophageal junction cancer (ToGA): a phase 3, open-label, randomised controlled trial, Lancet 376:687–697, 2010.

Conroy T, Desseigne F, Ychou M, et al: FOLFIRINOX versus gemcitabine for metastatic pancreatic cancer, N Engl J Med 364:1817–1825, 2011.

Grothey A, Van Cutsem E, Sobrero A, et al: Regorafenib monotherapy for previously treated metastatic colorectal cancer (CORRECT): an international, multicentre, randomised, placebo-controlled, phase 3 trial, Lancet 381:303–312, 2013.

Hvid-Jensen F, Pedersen L, Drewes AM, et al: Incidence of adenocarcinoma among patients with Barrett's esophagus, N Engl J Med 365:1375–1383, 2011.

Valle J, Wasan H, Palmer DH, et al: Cisplatin plus gemcitabine versus gemcitabine for biliary tract cancer, N Engl J Med 362:1273–1281, 2010.

van Hagen P, Hulshof MC, van Lanschot JJ, et al: Preoperative chemoradiotherapy for esophageal or junctional cancer, N Engl J Med 366:2074–2084, 2012.

Von Hoff DD, Ervin T, Arena FP, Chiorean EG, et al: Increased survival in pancreatic cancer with nab-paclitaxel plus gemcitabine, N Engl J Med 369(18):1691–1703, 2013.

Yao JC, Shah MH, Ito T, et al: Everolimus for advanced pancreatic neuroendocrine tumors, N Engl J Med 364:514–523, 2011.

Genitourinary Cancers

Andre De Souza, Benedito A. Carneiro, Anthony Mega, Timothy Gilligan

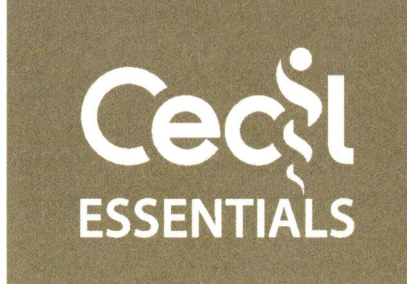

RENAL CELL CARCINOMA

Definition and Epidemiology

Renal cell carcinoma (RCC) represents approximately 3% to 5% of all malignancies and 85% of kidney tumors. It is the sixth most common cancer in men and the eighth most common cancer in women, with approximately 74,000 new cases diagnosed in the United States in 2019 that will contribute to 14,770 deaths. Aside from age and male sex, most patients do not have an identifiable risk factor. The median age of diagnosis is about 65 years and the incidence is twice as high in men as in women. Smoking, obesity, and hypertension are well-established risk factors for RCC. Smokers have a relative risk 2-fold greater than that of nonsmokers whereas hypertension is associated with a 70% increased risk. RCC is also more common in patients with end-stage renal failure. A small number (3%) of cases of RCC are inherited. Approximately 65% of cases of RCC are diagnosed as localized disease with an estimated 5-year survival of 92%. The 5-year survival for advanced disease is 12%.

The most recognized inherited RCC is Von Hippel–Lindau (VHL) syndrome, an autosomal dominant disorder that is characterized by the development of multiple vascular tumors including clear cell RCC. The genetic events underlying VHL syndrome (loss of function truncating mutations or deletions of the *VHL* gene) also occur in sporadic (noninherited) clear cell tumors, leading to the remarkable RCC reliance on blood vessels for growth. Research into this syndrome has led to modified treatment options for advanced disease (see later discussion).

Pathology

The histologic subtypes of RCC are characterized by distinct genetic characteristics, histologic features, and clinical phenotypes. Clear cell RCC (75% of all RCCs) is the most common subtype and is characterized by *VHL* gene inactivation. Less common are the papillary, chromophobe, unclassified subtypes, and medullary RCC, which occurs almost exclusively in patients with sickle cell trait. Although these RCC subtypes are biologically distinct, the current surgical approaches are most frequently uninfluenced by subtype. However, the histologic subtype impacts the medical treatment of advanced disease.

Diagnosis and Differential Diagnosis

Masses in the kidney may be benign or malignant, with an increasing likelihood of malignancy with increasing size. Most clear cell RCC tumors are distinguishable based on their contrast enhancement. Other considerations for renal masses include benign tumors (e.g., oncocytoma), metastatic disease from another primary site (rare), angiomyolipoma, a lipid-containing benign tumor (most commonly occurring in young females), and infectious processes. The diagnosis is made on the basis of a biopsy or at the time of nephrectomy, although the radiographic appearance of each of the differential diagnoses is often characteristic.

Clinical Presentation

RCC is more common in males (2:1), and the median age at presentation is approximately 65 years. Patients diagnosed with RCC below 46 years of age and those presenting with multifocal or bilateral renal masses should be considered for genetic counseling because these features can be associated with hereditary RCC. In the United States, most RCCs are diagnosed as incidental findings on imaging studies (70% of the cases). Classic signs and symptoms include hematuria, flank pain, and a palpable abdominal mass. Systemic symptoms can include pain caused by bone metastases or adenopathy, respiratory symptoms related to involvement of lung parenchyma, or neurologic symptoms when presenting with brain metastases. Symptoms also occur with paraneoplastic syndromes. A renal mass is discovered, usually on computed tomography (CT) scanning, and has an appearance that is characteristic of RCC (i.e., highly vascular). Subsequently, a full staging work-up is performed, including CT scanning of the chest; CT or MRI of the brain is performed if signs or symptoms suggest brain metastases; bone scan is recommended in the presence of bone pain or elevation of alkaline phosphatase. Diagnosis is usually made at the time of nephrectomy, although a biopsy of the renal mass may be indicated, such as in a patient with distant metastases in whom nephrectomy is not pursued or in a patient with a small renal mass that may be initially observed.

Treatment

Renal Masses

Some renal masses (approximately 20%) are not cancerous, and the likelihood of malignancy increases with size, so a diagnostic biopsy should be considered for lesions smaller than 4 cm to confirm diagnosis and guide local treatment or surveillance strategies. If the mass has a radiographic appearance suggestive of RCC, biopsy is often not necessary before surgery, and larger masses are more likely to have such features. The differential diagnosis for enhancing renal masses includes non-RCC malignancies (e.g., upper tract urothelial carcinoma), metastases, and benign tumors. One option for small renal masses, even if proven to be RCC, is initial observation. Retrospective series have defined this approach for renal masses smaller than 4 cm in a select group of patients with significant comorbidities or limited life expectancy. The growth rate is approximately 3 mm/year, and the reported incidence of development of metastases is very low. If surgery is pursued, then removal of either part of the kidney (partial nephrectomy or nephron-sparing surgery) or the entire kidney (radical nephrectomy) is the standard of care, depending on factors such as the extent and anatomy of the tumor, native renal function, and surgical skill. Cancer outcomes are equivalent, although renal

泌尿生殖系统肿瘤

张智旸 译　李孝远　周建凤 审校　巴一 通审

肾细胞癌

定义和流行病学

肾细胞癌（RCC）约占所有恶性肿瘤的 3%～5%，占肾脏肿瘤的 85%。它是男性第六、女性第八常见的癌症，2019 年美国约有 74 000 例新发病例，导致 14 770 人死亡。除年龄和男性性别外，大多数患者没有明确的危险因素。RCC 中位诊断年龄约为 65 岁，男性发病率是女性的 2 倍。吸烟、肥胖和高血压是已明确的 RCC 危险因素。吸烟者患 RCC 的相对风险比非吸烟者高 2 倍，而高血压与 70% 的风险增加相关。慢性肾衰竭患者中 RCC 的发病率也更高。仅有少数（3%）RCC 病例是遗传性的。约 65% 的 RCC 病例确诊时为局部疾病，5 年生存率为 92%；进展期疾病的 5 年生存率为 12%。

最常见的遗传性肾细胞癌是冯·希波·林道（VHL）综合征。这是一种常染色体显性遗传疾病，特征是发生多发性血管肿瘤，包括肾透明细胞瘤。引起 VHL 综合征的遗传事件（导致 VHL 基因功能丧失的截短突变或序列删失）也可发生在散发性（非遗传性）肾透明细胞癌中，导致 RCC 生长非常依赖于血管。对这种综合征的研究已为晚期疾病提供了改进治疗的选择（见下文）。

病理学

RCC 的组织学亚型具有独特的遗传学特征、组织学特点和临床表型。透明细胞 RCC（占所有 RCC 的 75%）是最常见的亚型，以 *VHL* 基因失活为特征。较少见的是乳头状、嫌色细胞癌、未分类亚型以及肾髓质 RCC，后者几乎仅发生在镰刀细胞特征的患者中。尽管这些 RCC 亚型在生物学上各不相同，但目前的手术方法通常不受亚型的影响。然而，组织学亚型会影响晚期疾病的治疗。

诊断和鉴别诊断

肾脏肿物可能是良性或恶性，随着肿物大小的增加，恶性的可能性增加。大多数透明细胞 RCC 可以根据其对比增强而区分出来。肾脏肿块的其他鉴别诊断包括良性肿瘤（如嗜酸细胞瘤）、来自其他原发部位的转移性疾病（罕见）、血管平滑肌脂肪瘤（一种含脂良性肿瘤，最常见于年轻女性）以及感染性疾病等。虽然每种不同诊断的影像学表现通常具有特征性，但确诊需要根据活检病理或肾切除术后病理。

临床表现

RCC 在男性中更常见（2:1），中位发病年龄约为 65 岁。46 岁以下诊断为 RCC 的患者，或呈多发性或双侧肾肿块的患者应考虑遗传咨询，因为这些特征可能与遗传性 RCC 有关。在美国，大多数 RCC 在影像学检查中偶然被发现（70% 的病例）而诊断出来。典型的症状和体征包括血尿、侧腹痛和可触及的腹部肿块。全身症状包括由骨转移或肿瘤压迫引起的疼痛、与肺实质受累相关的呼吸系统症状，或者合并脑转移时的神经系统症状。还可能出现副肿瘤综合征的表现。肾脏肿物通常在计算机断层成像（CT）中被发现，具有 RCC 特点（即高度血管化）。需进行完整分期，包括胸部 CT 扫描；如有迹象或症状提示脑转移，则应行脑部 CT 或 MRI 扫描；如存在骨痛或碱性磷酸酶升高，则建议进行骨扫描。RCC 通常在进行肾切除术后可明确诊断，但对于存在远处转移而不准备行肾切除术的患者，或对于较小的肾肿物开始时选择随诊观察的患者，可考虑肾脏肿物活检。

治疗

肾肿物

一些肾肿物（约 20%）并非癌性，但恶性的可能性随着肿物大小增加而增加，因此对于直径小于 4 cm 的病变，应考虑进行诊断性活检以确认诊断，并指导局部治疗或监测策略。如肿块的影像学表现提示为 RCC，则通常无需术前活检，而较大肿块更有可能具有这些特征。有强化的肾肿块的鉴别诊断包括：非 RCC 的恶性肿瘤（如上尿路上皮癌）、转移性癌和良性肿瘤等。即使被证实为 RCC，处理小病灶的选择之一是先进行观察。有回顾性研究结果表明，在有显著合并症或预期寿命有限的患者中，对小于 4 cm 的肾肿块可选择观察。肿瘤的生长速度约为每年 3 mm，远处转移发生率非常低。如进行手术，则应根据肿瘤范围和解剖部位、基础肾功能和手术技巧等因素，选择切除肾脏的一部分（部分肾切除术或保留肾单位手术）或整个肾脏（根治性肾切除术）。两者预后相当，但部分肾切除

TABLE 6.1 Therapeutic Approaches in Metastatic RCC

Agent	Objective Response Rate	PFS (mo)	Comments
Hormonal therapy	2%	N/A	Limited, palliative role in the treatment of metastatic RCC
Chemotherapy	5-6%	N/A	Not generally used
Interleukin-2	≈20-25% (high dose)	3.1	Durable complete response rate of 7-8%
Interferon-α	10-15%	4.7	Modest improvement in overall survival compared with inactive therapy
VEGF inhibitors[a]	≈30%	9-11	Common toxicity includes fatigue, mucositis, hand-foot syndrome, diarrhea, hypertension, and hypothyroidism
Checkpoint inhibitors[b]	25-42%	4.6-11	Adverse effects include fatigue, pruritus and immune-related hypothyroidism, colitis, adrenal insufficiency. Complete response rates of 9% were observed with the combination of nivolumab (anti-PD-1) and ipilimumab (anti-CTLA4).
mTOR inhibitors[c]	2% (treatment refractory) to 9% (treatment naive)	4	Increased overall survival of temsirolimus monotherapy vs. IFN monotherapy in poor-risk patients. Toxicity includes fatigue, mucositis, rash, and hypertriglyceridemia/hyperglycemia/hypercholesterolemia
mTOR inhibitor (everolimus) + lenvatinib	41%	14.6	Combination of everolimus with lenvatinib improved the outcomes compared to everolimus monotherapy

IFN, Interferon; *mTOR*, mammalian target of rapamycin; *N/A*, not applicable; *PFS*, progression-free survival; *RCC*, renal cell carcinoma; *VEGF*, vascular endothelial growth factor.
[a]VEGF inhibitors: sorafenib, sunitinib, pazopanib, axitinib.
[b]Anti-PD-1 agents such as pembrolizumab and avelumab have also been combined with axitinib.
[c]mTOR inhibitors: temsirolimus, everolimus.

function is better preserved with partial nephrectomy. Another management option for renal masses is exposure to temperature extremes: freezing (cryotherapy) or burning (radiofrequency ablation). This approach is usually pursued in patients with contraindications to surgery, significant comorbidities, and/or small tumors (<3 cm). Although metastasis-free survival and cancer-specific survival rates for partial nephrectomy and ablation techniques are comparable, local recurrence rates can be higher with ablation. Biopsy of kidney mass is recommended prior to ablation to confirm diagnosis and guide subsequent surveillance strategies.

Surgery in Metastatic RCC

Removal of the primary renal tumor in the face of metastatic disease (i.e., debulking or cytoreductive nephrectomy) has been pursued in patients with good performance status, limited extrarenal disease, and low comorbidities based on results from patients receiving systemic treatment with interferon-α (INF-α) in the 1990s. However, results of a randomized clinical trial showed that systemic treatment alone with contemporary tyrosine kinase inhibitor (TKI) sunitinib had comparable overall survival to nephrectomy followed by sunitinib in patients with intermediate- or poor-risk disease, but the study did not address cytoreductive nephrectomy in patients with good-risk disease. In addition, surgical removal of solitary metastatic sites is associated with disease control in up to 30% of highly selected patients.

One randomized clinical trial demonstrated that 1 year of treatment with sunitinib administered following nephrectomy (i.e., adjuvant treatment) improved the disease-free survival of patients at high risk for recurrence, but no difference in overall survival or quality of life was reported. Patient selection and shared decision making are critical in light of treatment toxicities, lack of demonstrated overall survival benefit, and negative results of other clinical trials. To date, no clinical trial evidence has demonstrated improvement in patient outcome with systemic therapy administered before nephrectomy (i.e., neoadjuvant treatment).

Systemic Therapy for Metastatic RCC

The initial treatments for metastatic RCC—hormone therapy and chemotherapy—produced only minimal benefits (Table 6.1). Immunotherapy with cytokines interleukin-2 (IL-2) and INF-α has yielded modest benefits, the majority of benefit realized in highly selected patients who have a durable complete response to high-dose IL-2. The discovery of clear cell RCC reliance on stimulation of the vascular endothelial growth factor (VEGF) pathway, which results from *VHL* gene inactivation, led to the clinical development of several VEGF pathway inhibitors that include TKIs and monoclonal antibodies against VEGF (see Table 59.1). In general, 70% to 75% of patients who receive these drugs have some reduction or stabilization of tumor burden. Periods of disease control typically last for months, although they can extend to several years in a small minority of patients. The incorporation of immune checkpoint inhibitors, such as antibodies against cytotoxic T lymphocyte–associated protein 4 (CTLA-4) and programmed death receptor-1 (PD-1) or its ligand (PD-L1), represents another relevant advancement in the treatment of metastatic RCC. These agents promote antitumor immune response by blocking stimulation of PD-1 or CTLA-4 receptors that suppress T cell immune function. These agents have significant antitumor activity both as anti-PD-1 monotherapy (e.g., nivolumab) or in combination with ipilimumab (anti-CTLA4). Anti-PD-1 and PD-L1 antibodies (pembrolizumab and avelumab, respectively) have also shown strong antitumor activity in combination with the multikinase inhibitor axitinib. Inhibitors of mammalian target of rapamycin (mTOR) represent treatment alternatives as monotherapy or in combination with the multikinase inhibitor lenvatinib. The data supporting the use of TKIs and checkpoint inhibitors for RCC are strongest for clear cell RCC; the optimal treatment of non–clear cell RCC is much less well defined. In the context of growing treatment options, advances in biomarkers of treatment response as well as molecular drivers of prognosis will guide optimal sequencing of agents.

表 6.1 转移性肾细胞癌的治疗方法

药物	客观缓解率	PFS（月）	注释
激素治疗	2%	N/A	有限，转移性肾细胞癌的姑息治疗
化疗	5%~6%	N/A	通常情况下不适用
白介素-2	约20%~25%（高剂量）	3.1	持久的完全缓解率为7%~8%
干扰素-α	10%~15%	4.7	相比安慰剂，整体生存率略有改善
血管内皮生长因子抑制剂（即 VEGF 抑制剂）[a]	约30%	9~11	常见的毒性包括疲劳、口腔炎、手足综合征、腹泻、高血压和甲状腺功能减退
免疫检查点抑制剂[b]	25%~42%	4.6~11	副作用包括疲劳、皮肤瘙痒和免疫相关的甲状腺功能减退、结肠炎、肾上腺功能不全。纳武利尤单抗（抗PD-1单抗）和伊匹木单抗（抗CTLA4单抗）的联合疗法可观察到9%的完全缓解率
mTOR 抑制剂[c]	2%（难治性）至9%（初始治疗）	4	替西罗莫司对比干扰素单药治疗在预后差的患者中延长总生存期。毒性包括疲劳、口腔炎、皮疹和高甘油三酯/高血糖/高胆固醇血症
mTOR 抑制剂（依维莫司）+仑伐替尼	41%	14.6	依维莫司联合仑伐替尼对比依维莫司单药治疗，可改善预后

mTOR，哺乳动物雷帕霉素靶蛋白；N/A，不适用；PFS，无进展生存期；VEGF，血管内皮生长因子。
[a] VEGF 抑制剂：索拉非尼、舒尼替尼、培唑帕尼、阿昔替尼。
[b] 抗 PD-1 药物如帕博利珠单抗和阿维鲁单抗也已与阿昔替尼联合使用。
[c] mTOR 抑制剂：替西罗莫司、依维莫司。

术对肾功能保留更好。肾脏肿瘤的另一种治疗选择是暴露于极端温度：冷冻（冷冻治疗）或烧灼（射频消融）。这种方法通常适用于有手术禁忌证、重要合并症和（或）小肿瘤（<3 cm）的患者。尽管部分肾切除术与消融术的无转移生存率和癌症特异性生存率相当，但消融术的局部复发率可能更高。建议在消融前进行肾脏肿块活检以明确诊断并指导后续监测策略。

转移性 RCC 的手术治疗

对存在转移性疾病的患者，基于 20 世纪 90 年代在接受干扰素-α（INF-α）系统治疗患者中的研究结果，在体力评分好、肾脏以外病灶有限和合并症少的患者中，推荐去除原发性肾脏肿瘤（即减瘤性或细胞减灭性肾切除术）。然而，一项在中危和高危患者中开展的随机临床试验结果显示，单纯接受酪氨酸激酶抑制剂（TKI）舒尼替尼系统治疗与肾切除术后服用舒尼替尼相比，总生存率相似，但这项研究并未涉及低危患者是否应该进行细胞减灭性肾切除术。此外，在高度选择的患者中，孤立性转移灶手术切除的疾病控制率可达 30%。

一项随机临床试验结果证实，肾切除术后口服舒尼替尼治疗 1 年（即辅助治疗）改善了高复发风险患者的无病生存率，但未报告总生存率或生活质量存在差异。鉴于治疗毒性、缺乏总生存获益的证据以及其他临床试验阴性结果，患者选择和医患共同决策至关重要。迄今，尚无临床试验证据表明在肾切除术之前进行全身治疗（即新辅助治疗）可以改善预后。

转移性 RCC 的系统治疗

转移性肾细胞癌的初始治疗——激素治疗和化疗——只有微弱的益处（表6.1）。细胞因子白细胞介素-2（IL-2）和干扰素-α（INF-α）的免疫疗法已体现出适中的益处，其中大部分获益见于高度选择的患者中，他们对高剂量 IL-2 具有持久的完全反应。肾透明细胞癌依赖于 VHL 基因失活导致的血管内皮生长因子（VEGF）通路激活，因此包括 TKI 和 VEGF 单克隆抗体在内的几种 VEGF 通路抑制剂得以临床研发（见表59.1）。一般来说，在接受这些药物治疗的患者中，有 70%~75% 的患者肿瘤负荷有所减轻或稳定。尽管在少数患者中疾病控制期可延长至数年，但一般持续几个月。免疫检查点抑制剂如针对细胞毒性 T 淋巴细胞相关蛋白4（CTLA-4）和程序性死亡受体 1（PD-1）或其配体（PD-L1）的抗体应用，是转移性 RCC 治疗的另一项重要进展。这些药物通过阻断 PD-1 或 CTLA-4 受体，解除 T 细胞免疫功能抑制而促进抗肿瘤免疫反应。抗 PD-1 单抗单药（如纳武利尤单抗）或与抗 CTLA-4 单抗（如伊匹木单抗）联合应用都显示了显著的抗肿瘤活性。抗 PD-1 和 PD-L1 抗体（分别是帕博利珠单抗和阿维鲁单抗）与多靶点激酶抑制剂阿昔替尼联用，也表现出强大的抗肿瘤活性。哺乳动物雷帕霉素靶蛋白（mTOR）抑制剂单药或与多靶点激酶抑制剂仑伐替尼联合应用是替代治疗方案。对肾透明细胞癌，支持使用 TKI 和免疫检查点抑制剂的研究数据最为强大；非透明细胞型 RCC 的最佳治疗方案则远远逊色。伴随不断增加的治疗选择，治疗应答的生物标志物和预后相关分子驱动因素的研究进展，将指导上述药物的最佳用药顺序。

Prognosis

The prognosis of localized kidney cancer is determined largely by the stage and grade of the primary tumor. In metastatic disease, established schemas divide patients into prognostic groups based on performance status, time from diagnosis to metastatic disease, and laboratory values (lactate dehydrogenase [LDH], hemoglobin, calcium, neutrophils, and platelets). Good-, intermediate- and poor-risk groups have median survivals of about 43, 22, and 8 months, respectively.

BLADDER CANCER

Definition and Epidemiology

Urothelial carcinoma of the bladder (UCB) represents 4% of all malignancies and about 3% of cancer-related deaths in the United States. It is more common in developed countries and is the fourth most common cancer among men and ninth among women in the Western world. Smoking is an established risk factor for bladder cancer; the incidence rate is four times higher for smokers than for nonsmokers. Occupational exposures from a range of agents that contain aromatic amines, as chlorinated hydrocarbons and polycyclic aromatic hydrocarbons are believed to account for up to 20% of all bladder cancers. Genetic susceptibility is increasingly recognized as an important risk factor. The risk of bladder cancer is doubled in first-degree relatives of patients with bladder cancer. Inherited genetic factors, such as the slow acetylator *N*-acetyltransferase 2 (NAT2) variants and the glutathione *S*-transferase Mu 1 (GSTM1)–null genotypes, are established risk factors.

Pathology

Urothelial carcinoma is the predominant histologic subtype in the United States and Europe, where it accounts for 90% of all bladder cancers. Adenocarcinoma, squamous cell carcinoma, and small cell cancers account for most of the remaining 10%, although there are parts of the world where nonurothelial carcinomas are more common. The bladder wall consists of four layers: urothelium (the innermost epithelial lining), lamina propria, muscularis propria (detrusor muscle), and adventitia (serosa).

Clinical Presentation

UCB is more common in males (3:1), and the median age at presentation is 73 years. Approximately 75% of newly diagnosed cases of UCB are not muscle invasive; the remaining 25% exhibit de novo invasion of the muscle wall of the bladder at presentation.

Patients with bladder cancer typically have painless hematuria at presentation, although irritative voiding symptoms (frequency, urgency, and dysuria) can be the initial manifestation. Patients with more advanced disease may have progressive flank or pelvic pain from direct extension of disease or as a consequence of ureteral obstruction.

Diagnosis and Differential Diagnosis

The initial evaluation typically involves an office-based cystoscopic evaluation, with the collection of urine for cytology. Upper urinary tract evaluation with either a CT urogram or retrograde pyelogram is also important. When a bladder tumor is found, patients undergo a transurethral resection of bladder tumor (TURBT) under anesthesia to obtain tissue for histologic diagnosis. Inclusion of muscle in the pathologic specimen is necessary to exclude muscle invasion. For patients with muscle-invasive disease, CT imaging of the chest is indicated, and bone scintigraphy in patients with bone pain. Most new cases of UCB are staged as Ta (involvement of epithelial lining), T1 (invasion of lamina propria), or carcinoma in situ (CIS) (Fig. 6.1); these are

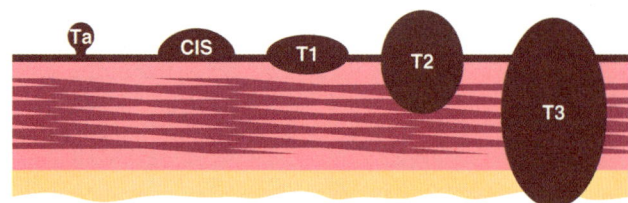

Fig. 6.1 Bladder cancer presentations by depth of invasion.

typically grouped and considered as non–muscle-invasive bladder cancer (NMIBC).

Patients with low-grade, low-stage urothelial carcinoma of the bladder remain at high risk for non–muscle-invasive recurrence but low risk for progression to more advanced stage disease. In contrast, patients with intermediate- or high-grade disease are at increased risk for both recurrence and progression to muscle-invasive and metastatic disease. Secondary involvement of the bladder with other cancers (e.g., lymphoma, sarcoma) is uncommon.

Treatment

Organ-Confined Disease

Low-grade non–muscle-invasive UCBs are typically managed with TURBT and intravesically administered cytotoxic agents. Multifocal, low-grade recurrent disease is managed with intravesically administered bacillus Calmette-Guérin (BCG). High-grade NMIBC (including CIS) is managed with BCG or cystectomy.

Muscle-invasive bladder cancer is optimally managed with radical cystectomy and bilateral pelvic lymphadenectomy. For patients who are deemed poor surgical candidates or who refuse cystectomy, external beam radiotherapy or chemoradiation and TURBT are alternative management options.

Cisplatin-based multiagent chemotherapy administered before cystectomy (i.e., neoadjuvant chemotherapy) has been shown by level I evidence to improve survival. Although it has not been prospectively evaluated in the neoadjuvant setting, the regimen of gemcitabine plus cisplatin (GC) is widely substituted for the older combination of methotrexate, vinblastine, doxorubicin, and cisplatin (M-VAC). Ongoing clinical trials are evaluating the role of perioperative immunotherapy.

Metastatic Disease

Level I evidence from a series of phase III trials provides evidence that cisplatin-based chemotherapy (i.e., M-VAC or GC) in patients with de novo metastatic disease leads to median survival times in the range of 14 to 15 months, with 5% to 15% of patients likely to be cured. The latter group is made up primarily of patients with nodal metastatic disease.

Although there have been no completed randomized phase III trials comparing cisplatin-based chemotherapy with carboplatin-based therapy in patients with advanced UCB, multiple randomized phase II trials have reported superior activity with cisplatin-based regimens. However, between 30% and 50% of patients with advanced UCB are ineligible for cisplatin because of concomitant renal insufficiency, typically as a consequence of age-related renal comorbidity or disease-related extrinsic obstruction. Immunotherapy with checkpoint inhibitors, such as pembrolizumab (anti-PD-1) and atezolizumab (anti-PD-L1), is approved for cisplatin-ineligible patients whose tumors have high expression of PD-L1 (the specific PD-L1 expression cutoff is specific to the immune checkpoint inhibitor used) as well as for patients who have already received or who are ineligible for carboplatin.

预后

局限性肾癌的预后在很大程度上取决于原发肿瘤的分期和分级。在转移性疾病中，已建立根据体能状况、诊断至出现转移性疾病的时间和实验室指标［乳酸脱氢酶（LDH）、血红蛋白、血钙、中性粒细胞和血小板］的预后模型，将患者进行预后分组。低危、中危和高危组的中位生存期分别约为 43 个月、22 个月和 8 个月。

膀胱癌

定义和流行病学

在美国，膀胱尿路上皮细胞癌（UCB）占所有恶性肿瘤的 4%，约占癌症相关死亡的 3%。其在发达国家更为常见，是西方世界男性第四和女性第九常见癌症。吸烟是膀胱癌的已知危险因素；吸烟者的患病率比非吸烟者高 4 倍。职业暴露，比如与含氯化烃和多环芳香烃等芳香胺类的一系列物质接触，被认为与高达 20% 的膀胱癌发生相关。遗传易感性越来越被认为是一个重要的危险因素。患有膀胱癌患者的一级亲属，患膀胱癌的风险增加 1 倍。一些遗传因子，如慢乙酰化酶 N- 乙酰转移酶 2（NAT2）变异和谷胱甘肽 S- 转移酶 Mu 1（GSTM1）缺失基因型，已被确认为危险因素。

病理学

在美国和欧洲，尿路上皮细胞癌是主要的组织学亚型，占所有膀胱癌的 90%。腺癌、鳞状细胞癌和小细胞癌占剩余 10% 的大部分，尽管某些地域的非尿路上皮细胞癌更为常见。膀胱壁包括四层：尿路上皮（最内层上皮内衬）、黏膜固有层、固有肌层（膀胱逼尿肌）和外膜（浆膜）。

临床表现

UCB 在男性中更为常见（3∶1），中位发病年龄 73 岁。约 75% 的新诊断 UCB 病例未侵犯肌层，剩余 25% 在初次发病时已侵犯膀胱肌壁。

膀胱癌患者起病时通常表现为无痛性血尿，但刺激性排尿症状（尿频、尿急和排尿困难）也可能为初始表现。更为晚期的患者可能会因为疾病直接侵犯或输尿管阻塞而出现进行性加重的腰部或骨盆疼痛。

诊断和鉴别诊断

初始评估包括门诊膀胱镜检查、尿液细胞学检查。上尿路评估通常需进行 CT 尿路造影或逆行肾盂造影。当发现膀胱肿瘤时，患者可在麻醉下接受经尿道膀胱肿瘤切除术（TURBT）以获取组织进行组织学诊断。病理标本中必须包含肌层以排除肌肉浸润。对有肌层浸润的患者，需进行胸部 CT 影像学检查，而有骨痛的患者应进行骨扫描。大多数新发 UCB 病例被分为 Ta 期（上皮内侵犯）、T1 期（黏膜固有层侵犯）或原位癌

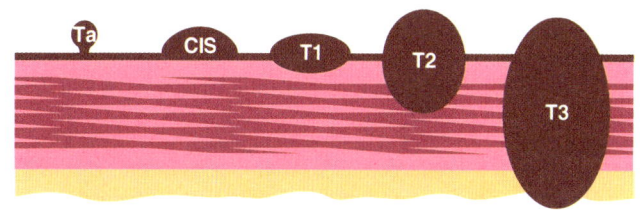

图 6.1　根据浸润深度的膀胱癌分期

（CIS）（图 6.1）；这些通常被归为非肌层浸润性膀胱癌（NMIBC）。

低级别、分期早的 UCB 患者中，非肌层浸润性病变复发风险高，但发展到更为晚期病变的风险较低。相比之下，中级别或高级别病变的患者复发和转变为肌层浸润性和转移性疾病的风险均增高。其他肿瘤（如淋巴瘤、肉瘤）转移到膀胱的情况少见。

治疗

局限于膀胱的疾病

低级别非肌层浸润性 UCB 通常采用 TURBT 和膀胱内给予细胞毒类药物。多灶性、低级别反复复发的疾病，可采用经尿道膀胱内给予卡介苗（BCG）治疗。高级别 NMIBC（包括 CIS）采用 BCG 或膀胱切除术进行治疗。

肌层浸润性膀胱癌的最佳治疗方案是根治性膀胱切除和双侧盆腔淋巴结清扫术。对被认为手术效果不佳或拒绝行膀胱切除术者，外放射治疗或放化疗和 TURBT 是可行的替代治疗方法。

Ⅰ 类证据显示，在膀胱切除术前予以顺铂为基础的多药化疗（即新辅助化疗）可以提高患者的生存率。虽然尚未在新辅助治疗中进行前瞻性评估，但吉西他滨加顺铂（GC）方案被广泛用于代替传统的甲氨蝶呤、长春瑞滨、多柔比星和顺铂（M-VAC）方案。目前正在进行的临床试验正在评估围术期免疫治疗的作用。

转移性疾病

一系列 Ⅲ 期临床试验获得的 Ⅰ 类证据表明，在初诊为转移性疾病的患者中，采用顺铂为基础的化疗（即 M-VAC 或 GC）可使中位生存时间达到 14～15 个月，且有 5%～15% 的患者有可能治愈，后者主要由淋巴结转移的患者组成。

尽管尚缺乏已完成的随机 Ⅲ 期临床试验结果来比较顺铂为基础的化疗与卡铂为基础的治疗在晚期膀胱癌患者中的疗效，但多项随机 Ⅱ 期临床试验报道了顺铂为基础方案的疗效更优。然而，30%～50% 的晚期膀胱癌患者由于并发肾功能不全而不能使用顺铂，肾功能不全通常是由于年龄相关的肾脏并发症或疾病相关的外压性梗阻。免疫检查点抑制剂如帕博利珠单抗（抗 PD-1）和阿替利珠单抗（抗 PD-L1）已被批准用于不能使用顺铂且具有高 PD-L1 表达（不同免疫检查点抑制剂有特定的 PD-L1 表达定义界值）的患者，以及已经接受或不能接受卡铂的患者。

The management of advanced disease after front-line therapy has evolved with various options beyond single-agent chemotherapy. Novel treatments include PD1 and PD-L1 checkpoint inhibitors and the TKI erdafitinib targeting of fibroblast growth factor receptor 3 (FGFR3) in tumors displaying FGFR3 activating mutations or gene fusions. The best sequencing of agents beyond the front-line treatment remains to be defined. Antibodies targeting cell surface protein and delivering cytotoxic payloads (antibody drug conjugates), such as the Nectin-4 antibody enfortumab that delivers the cytotoxic drug vedotin and the trophoblast cell surface 2 antibody sacituzumab with its topoisomerase inhibitor SN-38 payload, have shown promising antitumor activity in advanced bladder cancer, and ongoing trials are comparing these drugs to standard of care treatments. Enfortumab vedotin was granted accelerated approval in the United States for patients previously treated with or ineligible for platinum-based chemotherapy and an immune checkpoint inhibitor.

Prognosis

Patients with low-grade, low-stage NMIBC typically do not progress to muscle-invasive disease. Their disease does not alter life expectancy but is associated with morbidity and use of health care resources and requires long-term follow-up. Patients with muscle-invasive disease who undergo cystectomy are at risk for systemic failure based on the T stage and extent of nodal involvement. Patients with organ-confined disease without nodal involvement have cure rates greater than 50%. Patients with metastatic disease have median survival times in the range of 14 to 16 months with systemic therapy, and only a small subset (5% to 15%) are long-term survivors, although immune checkpoint blockers and new targeted therapies may change these metrics in the near future.

PROSTATE CANCER

Definition, Epidemiology, and Screening

Prostate cancer is the most common malignancy among men in the United States; more than 174,000 cases were expected to be diagnosed in 2019 with 31,000 deaths. The lifetime risk of diagnosis and death is roughly 12% and 2.4%, respectively. The incidence has declined since the United States Preventative Service Task Force (USPSTF) recommended against prostate-specific antigen (PSA)-based screening in 2012 (D recommendation). In 2018, the USPSTF revised the recommendation to shared decision making with men age 55 to 69 years (C Recommendation). Evidence from randomized clinical trials reveals that PSA-based screening programs in men aged 55 to 69 years may prevent 1.3 prostate cancer deaths and three cases of metastatic prostate cancer per 1000 men screened. The USPSTF recommends against PSA-based screening in men 70 years and older (D recommendation).

Multiple risk factors, including age, race, dietary factors, and genetic factors, have been linked to prostate cancer. The median age at diagnosis is 65 years, and younger men (<40 years) rarely develop prostate cancer. African American men have a greater risk of developing prostate cancer compared with white men (16% vs. 11% lifetime risk of diagnosis). Although it is possible that screening may offer greater benefit for African American men, there is no conclusive evidence to support race-based screening recommendations. A man with first-degree relatives affected by prostate cancer has a 5-fold to 10-fold increased risk of prostate cancer. Whereas high animal fat intake has been linked to an increased risk of prostate cancer, no foods, vitamins or dietary supplements have been shown to reduce the likelihood of being diagnosed with the disease.

A large chemoprevention trial (SELECT) demonstrated that intake of selenium and vitamin E does not reduce the risk of prostate cancer. Two studies evaluating the 5α-reductase inhibitors finasteride and dutasteride demonstrated a 23% to 25% reduction in relative risk of prostate cancer. Despite these benefits, the use of these agents remains low. Adverse effects such as erectile dysfunction, loss of libido, and gynecomastia along with concern of a small increase in high-grade tumors have resulted in low acceptance and adoption.

Clinical Presentation

Because prostate cancer can be detected in small subsets even with very low PSA levels (i.e., <1 ng/mL) there is no "normal" PSA value below which there is no risk of prostate cancer. PSA values can be affected by rectal examination, ejaculation, infection, bicycle riding, and urinary obstruction.

Most men with early disease have no symptoms; however, urinary frequency, urgency, nocturia, and hesitancy do occur. The presence of hematuria or hematospermia should prompt consideration of prostate cancer. An abnormal rectal examination result (asymmetric mass/nodule) is also suggestive of cancer.

Men with advanced, metastatic prostate cancer are more frequently symptomatic. Given the proclivity for bone metastasis, skeletal pain is common. Because of the frequency of spine metastases, malignant spinal cord compression and resulting neurologic injury is part of the natural history of prostate cancer. Adenopathy in the abdomen and pelvis is also common, as are deep venous thromboses, and men may thus present with lower extremity edema. Men can also experience urinary obstruction with hydronephrosis due to ureteral obstruction or bladder outlet obstruction. Constitutional symptoms such as weight loss and night sweats have also been described, especially with visceral metastasis.

Diagnosis and Staging

Most patients with prostate cancer are diagnosed with local disease with the use of extended core biopsies (12 cores). Multiparametric magnetic resonance imaging (MRI) is increasingly being utilized in initial assessment of a man with an abnormal PSA. MRI is interpreted using the Prostate Imaging-Reporting and Data System (PI-RADS), a 1-5 scale, with higher numbers indicating a greater likelihood of clinically significant cancer (Gleason score 7-10). In patients with MRI PI-RADS 3 to 5, biopsies can be done with MRI guidance to improve diagnostic accuracy.

After diagnosis, risk stratification based on PSA level, Gleason score, and clinical stage becomes crucial to define management. Bone scans and CT scans are not indicated for men with a new diagnosis of prostate cancer unless they have certain intermediate-risk or high-risk features. In addition to stage, grade, and PSA level, important features determining treatment include age, comorbidities, patient preferences, and life expectancy.

Pathology, Prognosis, and Genetic Mutations

Adenocarcinoma accounts for more than 95% of all prostate cancers. The remaining histologic subtypes include neuroendocrine (small cell carcinoma), squamous, and basal cell neoplasms.

The Gleason scoring system is pivotal in the management of prostate cancer, but its interpretation requires expertise in pathology. The score is based on growth pattern and degree of differentiation and ranges from 3 to 5 (5 being the least differentiated). The composite Gleason score is derived by adding together the numerical values for the two most prevalent differentiation patterns. For instance, if a specimen comprises primarily a grade 3 pattern and secondarily a grade 4 pattern, the score is reported as 7 (3 + 4). In 2016 the World

在一线治疗进展后，晚期疾病的后线治疗已有多种选项，而非仅有单药化疗。新的治疗方法包括 PD-1、PD-L1 的免疫检查点抑制剂以及在成纤维细胞生长因子 3（FGFR3）激活突变或基因融合的肿瘤中应用靶向 FGFR3 的厄达替尼。在一线治疗进展后的药物最佳顺序尚待确定。靶向细胞表面蛋白并释放细胞毒药物的单抗（抗体偶联药物），如 Nectin-4 抗体恩弗妥单抗释放细胞毒药物维汀（vedotin），以及 Trop-2 抗体戈沙妥珠单抗携带拓扑异构酶抑制剂 SN-38，在晚期膀胱癌中显示了有希望的抗肿瘤活性。恩弗妥单抗（EV）用于治疗既往接受过 PD-1/PD-L1 抑制剂和含铂化疗治疗的局部晚期或转移性尿路上皮细胞癌患者，已在美国获得加速批准。

预后

低级别、分期早的非肌层侵袭性膀胱癌患者通常不会进展为肌层侵袭性疾病，疾病不会改变预期寿命，但与发病率和卫生资源配置等因素相关，且需长期随访。接受膀胱切除术的肌层侵袭性疾病患者根据 T 分期和淋巴结受累程度，可能有转移进展的风险。局限于膀胱、没有淋巴结受累的患者治愈率超过 50%。转移性疾病患者在全身治疗后中位生存时间为 14～16 个月，只有一小部分患者（5%～15%）可获长期生存。免疫检查点抑制剂和新型靶向药物的研发，未来有望改变现状。

前列腺癌

定义，流行病学和筛查

前列腺癌是美国男性中最常见的恶性肿瘤，预计 2019 年新增病例超过 17.4 万，3.1 万人死于前列腺癌。诊断和死亡的终生风险分别约为 12% 和 2.4%。自 2012 年美国预防服务工作组（USPSTF）不建议进行前列腺特异性抗原（PSA）筛查（D 级推荐）以来，发病率有所下降。2018 年，USPSTF 修订建议为，与 55～69 岁的男性共同决策（C 级推荐）。来自随机临床试验的证据表明，在 55～69 岁的男性中，基于 PSA 的筛查可预防每 1000 名筛查男性中 1.3 例前列腺癌死亡和 3 例转移性前列腺癌。USPSTF 不建议对 70 岁及以上的男性进行 PSA 筛查（D 级推荐）。

包括年龄、种族、饮食因素和遗传因素在内的多种危险因素与前列腺癌的发生有关。诊断时的中位年龄为 65 岁，年轻男性（< 40 岁）罕患前列腺癌。与白人相比，非裔美国男性患前列腺癌的风险更高（终生诊断风险比：16% 比 11%）。虽然筛查为非裔美国人可能带来更大益处，但没有确凿证据支持基于种族角度筛查的推荐。一级亲属患有前列腺癌的男性患前列腺癌的风险增加了 5～10 倍。高动物脂肪摄入增加前列腺癌的风险，但无证据表明食物、维生素或膳食补充剂等可降低前列腺癌发生风险。

一项大型化学预防试验（SELECT）结果表明，摄入硒和维生素 E 并不能降低罹患前列腺癌风险。两项评估 5α-还原酶抑制剂非那雄胺和度他雄胺的预防研究表明，药物干预后，前列腺癌的相对发生风险降低了 23%～25%。尽管有获益，这些药物因可能导致勃起功能障碍、性欲减退、男性乳房发育等副作用，使得接受和使用率较低。

临床表现

在即使 PSA 水平非常低（即 < 1 ng/ml）的少数患者中仍可检测到前列腺癌，因此并不存在能排除患前列腺癌风险的"正常"PSA 界值。而经直肠检查、射精、感染、骑自行车和尿路梗阻等，都会干扰 PSA 检测值。

大多数早期病变患者没有症状，但也可能有尿频、尿急、夜尿和尿等待。出现血尿或血精应警惕前列腺癌。直肠指检异常发现（不对称的肿块/结节）提示前列腺癌。

晚期转移性前列腺癌常有症状。骨转移多见，因此骨骼疼痛常见。脊柱转移多见，使得脊髓压迫和神经损伤也是前列腺癌自然病程的一部分。腹盆腔淋巴结转移以及深静脉血栓也很常见，可引起下肢水肿。也可因输尿管梗阻或膀胱出口梗阻而导致梗阻性肾积水。体重减轻和夜间盗汗等全身症状也可能出现，常见于内脏转移患者。

诊断及分期

大多数局限期前列腺癌患者通过粗针穿刺活检（共穿刺 12 针）被诊断。多参数磁共振成像（MRI）越来越多地被用于初步评估 PSA 异常患者，通过前列腺成像报告和数据系统（PI-RADS，1～5 分）进行解读，数字越高则表明临床上患前列腺癌可能性越大（Gleason 评分 7～10）。对于 MRI PI-RADS 为 3～5 分的患者，可在 MRI 引导下进行活检，以提高诊断准确性。

确诊后，基于 PSA 水平、Gleason 评分和临床分期的危险分层是临床管理的关键。骨扫描和 CT 扫描不适用于新诊断前列腺癌患者，除非有某些中危或高危特征。除了分期、分级和 PSA 水平，决定治疗方案的重要因素还包括年龄、合并症、患者意愿和预期寿命。

病理学，预后和基因突变

腺癌占所有前列腺癌的 95% 以上。其余的组织学亚型包括神经内分泌（小细胞癌）、鳞状和基底细胞肿瘤。

Gleason 评分系统在前列腺癌管理中很重要，但需要病理学专业解读。基于生长模式和分化程度，评分范围从 3 到 5（5 是分化最差的）。Gleason 综合评分由主要成分分级和次要成分分级相加所得。例如，一个样本主要成分 3 级，次要成分 4 级，则评分为 7（3 + 4）。

TABLE 6.2	WHO/ISUP Prostate Cancer Histologic Grading System
Grade Group 1	Gleason 3 + 3 = 6
Grade Group 2	Gleason 3 + 4 = 7
Grade Group 3	Gleason 4 + 3 = 7
Grade Group 4	Gleason 4 + 4 = 8, 3 + 5 = 8, 5 + 3 = 8
Grade Group 5	Gleason 4 + 5 = 9, 5 + 4 = 9, 5 + 5 = 10

Health Organization (WHO) defined a new prostate grading system to improve prognostic strata. The WHO histologic grading system includes five grade groups as defined in Table 6.2.

Prognosis and primary management of localized prostate cancer depends on tumor (T) stage, PSA level, tumor grade, and number of positive biopsies. Risk stratification includes very low, low, favorable intermediate, unfavorable intermediate, high, and very high risk prostate cancer.

Genes in the DNA repair pathway, such as *BRCA1/2*, *ATM*, and *CHEK2*, have been found to be pathologically mutated in approximately 20% of metastatic castrate-resistant prostate cancer (mCRPC) and 8% to 12% of localized prostate cancer. *BRCA2* mutations have been associated with more aggressive prostate cancers with higher recurrence and mortality. Recommendations for genetic counseling in men with prostate cancer include presenting with de novo metastatic prostate cancer, significant family history of prostate, breast, pancreatic cancer, and Gleason 8 to 10 disease, and Ashkenazi Jewish heritage.

Treatment

Available treatment options for localized prostate cancer include radical prostatectomy, radiation therapy (either external beam radiation or brachytherapy), and active surveillance. Consensus recommendation favors active surveillance over primary treatment for very-low-risk and low-risk prostate cancer (Gleason score 6, PSA <10 ng/mL, low tumor burden). The selection between radical prostatectomy and radiation therapy is based on risk stratification and patient preferences. Surgery carries risks of urinary incontinence and erectile dysfunction. Radiation therapy has lower rates of urinary incontinence but also causes erectile dysfunction. Late complications from radiation therapy include radiation cystitis and proctitis. There is a small increased risk of second malignancies after radiation therapy, especially bladder cancer in smokers. Primary radiation therapy for intermediate- and high-risk patients is often given in combination with androgen deprivation therapy leading to additional adverse effects.

Once patients have developed advanced disease, androgen deprivation therapy (chemical or surgical castration) is widely used. Intermittent androgen deprivation therapy is an effective alternative for patients whose only sign of recurrence is a rising PSA level. In men with metastatic disease, continuous therapy with luteinizing hormone releasing hormone (LHRH) agonist or antagonist is used. Androgen deprivation therapy also has major side effects, including night sweats, hot flashes, erectile dysfunction, weight gain, loss of muscle mass, fatigue, bone loss, and metabolic syndrome. In men with metastatic prostate cancer, randomized controlled trials have reported longer overall survival when androgen deprivation therapy was combined with any of the four following medications: abiraterone (a novel CYP17A1 inhibitor), docetaxel chemotherapy, or the androgen receptor antagonists enzalutamide and apalutamide.

Bone health is a significant problem in men with prostate cancer. Osteoporosis due to androgen deprivation therapy and skeletal-related events from metastases are both common. Two agents are available to prevent these complications: zoledronic acid, a bisphosphonate, and denosumab, a RANK-ligand inhibitor. Their benefit is primarily in men with mCRPC and skeletal metastasis. All men on ADT should be counseled on osteoporosis screening and prevention and lower-dose bisphosphonate or denosumab can be used if significant bone loss develops.

All patients with metastatic prostate cancer eventually develop castrate-resistant prostate cancer (CRPC), defined by serologic, clinical, or objective progression in the setting of a castrate testosterone level. Although the mechanism of CRPC is not well understood, several treatment options are now available. Sipuleucel-T, an autologous antigen-presenting cell product shown to prolong survival in a randomized trial, is sometimes used in the prechemotherapy setting, but its use has been limited by the fact that it is not associated with a reduction in PSA, and there is thus no way to measure whether it is controlling the cancer. If not used in the castrate-sensitive setting, either abiraterone or one of the new androgen receptor antagonists (enzalutamide, apalutamide, or darolutamide) can be prescribed. Radium 223 improves survival outcomes and reduces skeletal events in men with symptomatic skeletal metastasis and without visceral or bulky, soft tissue metastasis. Two chemotherapy agents, docetaxel and cabazitaxel, are therapeutic options. Finally, the poly ADP-ribose polymerase (PARP) inhibitors are beneficial in men with mCRPC and a documented DNA repair defect.

TESTICULAR CANCER

Definition and Epidemiology

It is estimated that 9,610 new cases of testicular cancer will be diagnosed in men in the United States in 2020 and 440 men are predicted to die from the disease. It accounts for 1% of all cancers in men. The incidence of testis cancer varies widely among racial groups and geographic regions. In the United States, it is the most common cancer diagnosed in men aged 20 to 40 years of age, but it is rarely diagnosed before age 15 or after age 55. It is four times more common in white than in Black individuals. The incidence has increased by more than 50% since 1975. Risk factors include cryptorchidism, a personal or family history of testis cancer, gonadal dysgenesis, and Klinefelter's syndrome. Cryptorchidism increases risk in the undescended testicle and the normally descended contralateral testicle. Orchiopexy for cryptorchidism before puberty reduces the risk of testis cancer.

Pathology

Approximately 98% of testis cancers are germ cell tumors; the others are lymphomas, sex-cord stromal tumors, and adenocarcinomas of the rete testis. Germ cell tumors are divided into two broad categories: seminomas and nonseminomas (i.e., nonseminomatous germ cell tumors, or NSGCTs). Seminomas by definition are 100% seminoma, whereas most NSGCTs are a mixture of two or more of the five types of germ cell tumors: seminoma, embryonal carcinoma, teratoma, yolk sac tumor, and choriocarcinoma. A tumor that contains any elements of embryonal carcinoma, teratoma, yolk sac tumor, or choriocarcinoma is considered to be an NSGCT even if most of the tumor is seminoma. Because seminomas do not produce α-fetoprotein (AFP), patients who have a significantly elevated AFP level have an NSGCT regardless of the histopathology.

Diagnosis and Differential Diagnosis

Whenever a testis tumor is suspected, transscrotal ultrasound should be performed; if a mass suspicious for cancer is seen, the standard diagnostic procedure is an inguinal orchiectomy. Transscrotal orchiectomy or biopsy is contraindicated because of the risk of seeding the tumor in the scrotum and altering the pattern of spread. Differential diagnosis

表 6.2　WHO/ 国际泌尿病理协会（ISUP）前列腺癌组织学分级系统	
1 级	Gleason 3 + 3 = 6
2 级	Gleason 3 + 4 = 7
3 组	Gleason 4 + 3 = 7
4 组	Gleason 4 + 4 = 8, 3 + 5 = 8, 5 + 3 = 8
5 组	Gleason 4 + 5 = 9, 5 + 4 = 9, 5 + 5 = 10

2016 年世界卫生组织（WHO）定义了一个新的前列腺癌 5 级分级系统，优化预后分层，见表 6.2。

局限性前列腺癌的预后和初始治疗取决于肿瘤（T）分期、PSA 水平、肿瘤分级和活检阳性数。风险分层包括了极低、低、中危预后良、中危预后差、高和极高危组。

在约 20% 的转移性去势抵抗性前列腺癌（mCRPC）和 8%～12% 的局限期前列腺癌中可检测到 DNA 修复通路相关基因如 *BRCA1/2*、*ATM* 和 *CHEK2* 病理性突变。*BRCA2* 突变前列腺癌更具侵袭性，有更高的复发率和死亡率。起病即为转移性前列腺癌，有前列腺癌，乳腺癌和胰腺癌的显著家族史、Gleason 评分 8～10 分及德裔犹太人血源前列腺癌患者，建议行遗传咨询。

治疗

局限期前列腺癌治疗方案包括根治性前列腺切除术、放射治疗（外照射或近距离放射治疗）和主动监测。对于极低危和低危前列腺癌（Gleason 评分 6，PSA < 10 ng/ml，低肿瘤负荷），一致推荐主动监测。应基于风险分层和患者意愿，选择根治性前列腺切除术或放射治疗。手术有引起尿失禁和勃起功能障碍的风险。放射治疗虽尿失禁发生率减少，但也会引起勃起功能障碍。放射治疗的晚期并发症包括放射性膀胱炎和直肠炎等。放射治疗后第二恶性肿瘤的风险略有增加，特别是在吸烟者中发生膀胱癌。中高危患者的放射治疗常与雄激素剥夺治疗联合使用，需警惕额外不良反应。

一旦进展为晚期，雄激素剥夺治疗（药物或手术去势）被广泛使用。间歇性雄激素剥夺治疗是一种有效的可选方案，用于仅有 PSA 升高考虑复发的患者。转移性前列腺癌，需使用促黄体素释放激素（LHRH）激动剂或拮抗剂进行连续性治疗。雄激素剥夺治疗的常见副作用包括盗汗、潮热、勃起功能障碍、体重增加、肌少症、疲劳、骨质丢失和代谢综合征等。针对转移性前列腺癌的随机对照试验结果发现，雄激素剥夺治疗与以下四种药物之一联合使用时，总生存期更长：阿比特龙（一种新型 CYP17A1 抑制剂），多西紫杉醇化疗药物或雄激素受体拮抗剂恩扎卢胺和阿帕他胺。

需重视前列腺癌患者的骨骼健康。由雄激素剥夺治疗引起的骨质疏松症和转移所致骨相关不良事件一样常见。有两种药物可以预防这些并发症：唑来膦酸（一种双膦酸盐）和地舒单抗（一种 RANK- 配体抑制剂）。主要用于改善转移性去势抵抗前列腺癌骨转移患者。雄激素剥夺治疗中都建议接受骨质疏松筛查和预防咨询，若发生明显骨质丢失，可使用低剂量的双膦酸盐或地舒单抗。

所有转移性前列腺癌患者最终会进展为去势抵抗（CRPC）：睾酮达到去势水平，而生化、临床或影像学检查提示进展。去势抵抗的机制尚未完全阐明，但目前已有多种治疗选择。Sipuleucel-T 是一种自体抗原提呈细胞产物，在随机试验中显示延长患者生存时间，有时用于未经化疗患者，但因其未能降低 PSA，难以评价肿瘤是否被控制，而使这项治疗应用受限。若在激素敏感期未使用过，可处方阿比特龙或新的雄激素受体拮抗剂（恩扎卢胺、阿帕他胺或达罗他胺）之一。镭 223 用于无内脏转移或大的软组织转移的症状性骨转移患者，可减少骨相关不良事件，改善预后。两种化疗药物：多西紫杉醇和卡巴他赛，也是治疗选择。多聚 ADP 核糖聚合酶（PARP）抑制剂也已被用于 DNA 修复缺陷的转移性 CRPC 患者。

睾丸癌

定义和流行病学

据估计，2020 年美国有 9610 名男性被诊断为睾丸癌，预计 440 名男性死于这种疾病。睾丸癌占男性所有癌症的 1%。在不同种族和地理区域之间，睾丸癌发病率差异很大，而在美国，是 20～40 岁男性最常见的肿瘤类型，但在 15 岁以前或 55 岁以后罕见。白人中的发病率是黑人的 4 倍。1975 年以来，其发病率增加了 50% 以上。危险因素包括隐睾症、有睾丸癌个人或家族史、性腺发育不全和克氏综合征。隐睾症增加隐睾和对侧正常下降睾丸的患癌风险。在青春期前行睾丸固定术，可降低睾丸癌的风险。

病理学

睾丸肿瘤大约 98% 是生殖细胞肿瘤，其他包括淋巴瘤、性索间质肿瘤和睾丸网状腺癌。生殖细胞肿瘤分为两大类：精原细胞瘤和非精原细胞瘤［即非精原细胞性生殖细胞肿瘤（NSGCT）］。纯精原细胞瘤的定义是 100% 为精原细胞的肿瘤，而大多数非精原细胞瘤为精原细胞瘤、胚胎性癌、畸胎瘤、卵黄囊瘤和绒毛膜癌五种类型中两种或多种类型的混合。一个包含有胚胎性癌、畸胎瘤、卵黄囊瘤或绒毛膜癌中任何成分的肿瘤，即便大部分是精原细胞瘤，也被认为是非精原细胞瘤。由于精原细胞瘤不产生甲胎蛋白（AFP），如 AFP 水平显著升高，无论组织病理学如何，都诊断为非精原细胞瘤。

诊断和鉴别诊断

怀疑睾丸肿瘤，应行阴囊超声检查；若发现肿块怀疑癌症，则行经腹股沟睾丸切除术。禁用经阴囊睾丸切除术或活检，因可能形成阴囊内种植而改变播散

includes testicular lymphoma, torsion, epididymitis, orchitis, and other benign scrotal lesions.

Clinical Presentation

Testis cancer most often manifests as testicular enlargement, mass, or induration. It may or may not be painful or tender, and the presence of pain does not exclude a diagnosis of cancer. Testicular atrophy, gynecomastia, back pain, and thromboembolic disease can also occur.

Staging the cancer requires measuring postorchiectomy levels of serum AFP, human chorionic gonadotropin (β-HCG), and LDH as well as assessing for nodal and organ metastases, which should be done with a CT scan of the abdomen and pelvis and either chest CT or a chest radiography. The testes drain to the retroperitoneal lymph nodes, and retroperitoneal nodal spread constitutes stage II disease. In practice, testis cancer is divided into three categories: stage I (localized), with no evidence of spread to lymph nodes or beyond; stage II (regional), with enlarged retroperitoneal lymph nodes but no distant metastases; and disseminated disease. Disseminated disease includes stage I or II disease in which serum AFP and/or β-HCG levels are persistently elevated after orchiectomy, bulky stage II disease, and all stage III disease. Metastases to other organs or to pelvic or other non-retroperitoneal lymph nodes represent stage III disease, as does spread to retroperitoneal nodes in the setting of highly elevated serum tumor markers. Disseminated disease is divided into three categories: good-risk, intermediate-risk, and poor-risk disease; treatment differs for the different risk groups.

Treatment

Stage I seminomas and NSGCTs are usually managed with surveillance after surgery. The risk of relapse is about 18% for seminomas and 30% for NSGCTs. For pure seminomas, larger tumor size and lymphovascular invasion are each associated with a higher risk of recurrence. For nonseminomas, lymphovascular invasion has been most strongly associated with risk of relapse and tumors that are pure or predominantly embryonal carcinoma are also at higher risk. Alternatives to surveillance are single-agent carboplatin chemotherapy or radiation therapy for seminomas and bleomycin and etoposide and cisplatin (BEP) chemotherapy or retroperitoneal lymph node dissection (RPLND) for NSGCTs. Long-term disease-specific survival for stage I disease is 99% regardless of which of these approaches is used.

Stage II seminomas are usually treated with radiation therapy or chemotherapy (with BEP or etoposide plus cisplatin [EP]). Chemotherapy is preferred when the disease bulk is greater than 5 cm and sometimes for less bulky tumors. Management of stage II NSGCTs depends on the disease bulk and the levels of serum AFP and β-HCG. If either marker is elevated, then chemotherapy is preferred regardless of disease bulk. If no nodes are bigger than 2 cm and there are fewer than six enlarged nodes, then RPLND or chemotherapy can be considered. For bulkier disease, chemotherapy is preferred.

Treatment of stage III disease depends on the sites of metastases and the levels of serum tumor markers. For good-risk disease, the treatment is three cycles of BEP or four cycles of EP chemotherapy. For intermediate- and poor-risk disease, the treatment is four cycles of BEP chemotherapy (or etoposide, ifosfamide, and cisplatin [VIP] chemotherapy). In NSGCT, all residual masses should be resected after chemotherapy if feasible. In cases of seminoma, residual masses are typically observed unless they grow. Sometimes, post-chemotherapy residual masses greater than 3 cm in patients with pure seminoma are evaluated with an FDG-PET/CT, but the value of that approach is limited by the incidence of false-positive results. Patients with pure seminomas and residual masses after chemotherapy are the only testis cancer patients who should be considered for PET scans.

Relapsed disease after chemotherapy is treated with salvage chemotherapy given either at standard doses or at high doses with hematopoietic stem cell support.

Prognosis

Overall, the long-term disease-specific survival rate for testis cancer is 96%. By stage, the survival rates are 99% for stage I, 96% for stage II, and 73% for stage III. By disseminated disease risk category, survival is about 90% for good-risk disease, about 80% for intermediate-risk disease, and about 50% for poor-risk disease.

SUGGESTED READINGS

Burger M, Oosterlinck W, Konety B, et al: ICUD-EAU international consultation on bladder cancer 2012: non–muscle-invasive urothelial carcinoma of the bladder, Eur Urol 63:36–44, 2012.

Calabrò F, Albers P, Bokemeyer C, et al: The contemporary role of chemotherapy for advanced testis cancer: a systematic review of the literature, Eur Urol 61:1212–1220, 2012.

Capitanio U, Bensalah K, Bex A, et al: Epidemiology of renal cell carcinoma, Eur Urol 75(1):74–84, 2019.

Choueiri TK, Motzer RJ: Systemic therapy for metastatic renal-cell carcinoma, N Engl J Med 376(4):354–366, 2017.

Cooperberg MR, Carroll PR, Klotz L, et al: Active surveillance for prostate cancer: progress and promise, J Clin Oncol 29:3669–3676, 2011.

Eulitt P, Bjurlin M, Milowsky M: Perioperative systemic therapy for bladder cancer, Curr Opin Urol 29(3):220–226, 2019.

Gakis G, Efstathiou J, Lerner S, et al: ICUD-EAU international consultation on bladder cancer 2012: radical cystectomy and bladder preservation for muscle-invasive urothelial carcinoma of the bladder, Eur Urol 63:45–57, 2013.

Gourdin T: Optimization of therapies for men with advanced prostate cancer, Curr Opin Oncol 31(3):188–193, 2019.

Honecker F, Aparicio J, Berney D, et al: ESMO consensus conference on testicular germ cell cancer: diagnosis, treatment and follow-up, Ann Oncol 29(8):1658–1686, 2018.

Inamura K: Prostate cancer: understanding their molecular pathology and the 2016 WHO Classification, Oncotarget 9(18):14723–14737, 2018.

James N, Hussain S, Hall E, et al: Radiotherapy with or without chemotherapy in muscle-invasive bladder cancer, N Engl J Med 366:1477–1478, 2012.

James ND, Sydes MR, Clarke NW, et al: STAMPEDE investigators addition of docetaxel, zoledronic acid, or both to first-line long-term hormone therapy in prostate cancer (STAMPEDE): survival results from an adaptive, multiarm, multistage, platform randomised controlled trial, Lancet 387:1163–1177, 2016.

Kasivisvanathan V, Ranikko A, Borghi M, et al: MRI-Targeted or standard biopsy for prostate cancer diagnosis, N Engl J Med 378:1767–1777, 2018.

Motzer RJ, Escudier B, McDermott DF, et al: Nivolumab versus everolimus in advanced renal-cell Carcinoma, N Engl J Med 373(19):1803–1813, 2015.

Motzer RJ, Penkov K, Haanen J, et al: Avelumab plus axitinib versus sunitinib for advanced renal-cell carcinoma, N Engl J Med 380(12):1103–1115, 2019.

Motzer RJ, Tannir NM, McDermott DF, et al: Nivolumab plus ipilimumab versus sunitinib in advanced renal-cell carcinoma, N Engl J Med 378(14):1277–1290, 2018.

Nadal R, Bellmunt J: Management of metastatic bladder cancer, Cancer Treat Rev 76:10–21, 2019.

Ravaud A, Motzer RJ, Pandha HS, et al: Adjuvant sunitinib in high-risk renal-cell carcinoma after nephrectomy, N Engl J Med 375(23):2246–2254, 2016.

Rini BI, Plimack ER, Stus V, et al: Pembrolizumab plus axitinib versus sunitinib for advanced renal-cell carcinoma, N Engl J Med 380(12):1116–1127, 2019.

Siegel R, Miller K, Ahmedin J: Cancer statistics 2019, CA Cancer J Clin 69:7–34, 2019.

United States Preventative Service Task Force recommendation Statement. JAMA 319(18): 1901–1913, 2018.

模式。鉴别诊断包括睾丸淋巴瘤、睾丸扭转、附睾炎、睾丸炎和其他良性阴囊病变。

临床表现

睾丸癌最常表现为睾丸增大、肿块或硬结。伴有疼痛或无痛性，或有压痛。疼痛症状并不能除外癌症诊断。睾丸萎缩、男性乳房发育、背痛和血栓栓塞性疾病也可能发生。

癌症分期需行术后血清甲胎蛋白（AFP）、人绒毛膜促性腺激素（β-HCG）和乳酸脱氢酶（LDH）测定，也需要行腹盆CT以及胸部CT或胸部X线摄像来评估淋巴结和脏器转移。睾丸淋巴引流至腹膜后淋巴结，腹膜后淋巴结转移即为Ⅱ期。在临床实践中，睾丸癌分为三类：Ⅰ期（局限期）无淋巴结或其他转移证据；Ⅱ期（进展期）有腹膜后淋巴结转移，但没有远处转移；以及播散期。播散期包括在睾丸切除术后血清AFP和（或）β-HCG水平持续升高的Ⅰ期或Ⅱ期，腹膜后淋巴结病变较大的Ⅱ期疾病以及所有Ⅲ期疾病。如有转移到其他脏器或骨盆或其他非腹膜后区域淋巴结，则为Ⅲ期，也包括腹膜后淋巴结转移伴有血清肿瘤标志物明显升高。播散期分为三类：预后良好、中等或预后差；不同分层治疗方法不同。

治疗

Ⅰ期精原细胞瘤和NSGCT通常选择术后监测。精原细胞瘤的复发风险约为18%，非精原细胞瘤的复发风险约为30%。对于纯精原细胞瘤，肿瘤较大和淋巴血管浸润，均与较高的复发风险相关。对于非精原细胞瘤，淋巴管血管浸润与复发的风险密切相关，而纯或以胚胎性癌为主的肿瘤也有较高的复发风险。术后监测的替代方案，如精原细胞瘤可选择卡铂单药化疗或放疗，非精原细胞肿瘤可选择博来霉素、依托泊苷和顺铂（BEP）化疗或腹膜后淋巴结清扫术（RPLND）。无论采用哪种方法，Ⅰ期患者长期疾病特异性生存率为99%。

Ⅱ期精原细胞瘤通常采用放疗或化疗［BEP或依托泊苷加顺铂（EP）］。当腹膜后淋巴结直径大于5 cm时，首选化疗，有时也用于淋巴结稍小的情况。Ⅱ期非精原细胞瘤的治疗取决于腹膜后淋巴结大小和血清AFP、β-HCG水平。任一肿瘤标志物升高，不论腹膜后淋巴结大小如何，均首选化疗。若腹膜后淋巴结肿大，直径不大于2 cm，数量少于6个，则腹膜后淋巴结清扫术或化疗都可考虑。而腹膜后淋巴结超大，则首选化疗。

Ⅲ期治疗取决于转移部位和血清肿瘤标志物的水平。预后良好组予3周期BEP或4周期EP化疗。预后中等组和预后差组，则4周期BEP［或依托泊苷、异环磷酰胺和顺铂（VIP）］化疗。非精原细胞瘤化疗后，若可行，所有的残余病变都应予以切除。而精原细胞瘤治疗后残余病变多选择观察，除非有肿瘤增大。有时，纯精原细胞瘤患者化疗后残留肿块大于3 cm，可用FDG-PET/CT进一步评估，但其价值受一定的假阳性率的限制。在睾丸癌中，只有纯精原细胞瘤化疗后残留肿块推荐考虑PET扫描。

化疗后出现复发，应行标准剂量或需造血干细胞支持的高剂量化疗方案进行挽救性化疗。

预后

总体来说，睾丸癌的长期疾病特异性生存率为96%。Ⅰ期生存率为99%，Ⅱ期为96%，而Ⅲ期为73%。按播散性疾病风险分类，预后良好组生存率约为90%，预后中等组约为80%，预后差组约为50%。

推荐阅读

Burger M, Oosterlinck W, Konety B, et al: ICUD-EAU international consultation on bladder cancer 2012: non–muscle-invasive urothelial carcinoma of the bladder, Eur Urol 63:36–44, 2012.

Calabrò F, Albers P, Bokemeyer C, et al: The contemporary role of chemotherapy for advanced testis cancer: a systematic review of the literature, Eur Urol 61:1212–1220, 2012.

Capitanio U, Bensalah K, Bex A, et al: Epidemiology of renal cell carcinoma, Eur Urol 75(1):74–84, 2019.

Choueiri TK, Motzer RJ: Systemic therapy for metastatic renal-cell carcinoma, N Engl J Med 376(4):354–366, 2017.

Cooperberg MR, Carroll PR, Klotz L, et al: Active surveillance for prostate cancer: progress and promise, J Clin Oncol 29:3669–3676, 2011.

Eulitt P, Bjurlin M, Milowsky M: Perioperative systemic therapy for bladder cancer, Curr Opin Urol 29(3):220–226, 2019.

Gakis G, Efstathiou J, Lerner S, et al: ICUD-EAU international consultation on bladder cancer 2012: radical cystectomy and bladder preservation for muscle-invasive urothelial carcinoma of the bladder, Eur Urol 63:45–57, 2013.

Gourdin T: Optimization of therapies for men with advanced prostate cancer, Curr Opin Oncol 31(3):188–193, 2019.

Honecker F, Aparicio J, Berney D, et al: ESMO consensus conference on testicular germ cell cancer: diagnosis, treatment and follow-up, Ann Oncol 29(8):1658–1686, 2018.

Inamura K: Prostate cancer: understanding their molecular pathology and the 2016 WHO Classification, Oncotarget 9(18):14723–14737, 2018.

James N, Hussain S, Hall E, et al: Radiotherapy with or without chemotherapy in muscle-invasive bladder cancer, N Engl J Med 366:1477–1478, 2012.

James ND, Sydes MR, Clarke NW, et al: STAMPEDE investigators addition of docetaxel, zoledronic acid, or both to first-line long-term hormone therapy in prostate cancer (STAMPEDE): survival results from an adaptive, multiarm, multistage, platform randomised controlled trial, Lancet 387:1163–1177, 2016.

Kasivisvanathan V, Ranikko A, Borghi M, et al: MRI-Targeted or standard biopsy for prostate cancer diagnosis, N Engl J Med 378:1767–1777, 2018.

Motzer RJ, Escudier B, McDermott DF, et al: Nivolumab versus everolimus in advanced renal-cell carcinoma, N Engl J Med 373(19):1803–1813, 2015.

Motzer RJ, Penkov K, Haanen J, et al: Avelumab plus axitinib versus sunitinib for advanced renal-cell carcinoma, N Engl J Med 380(12):1103–1115, 2019.

Motzer RJ, Tannir NM, McDermott DF, et al: Nivolumab plus ipilimumab versus sunitinib in advanced renal-cell carcinoma, N Engl J Med 378(14):1277–1290, 2018.

Nadal R, Bellmunt J: Management of metastatic bladder cancer, Cancer Treat Rev 76:10–21, 2019.

Ravaud A, Motzer RJ, Pandha HS, et al: Adjuvant sunitinib in high-risk renal-cell carcinoma after nephrectomy, N Engl J Med 375(23):2246–2254, 2016.

Rini BI, Plimack ER, Stus V, et al: Pembrolizumab plus axitinib versus sunitinib for advanced renal-cell carcinoma, N Engl J Med 380(12):1116–1127, 2019.

Siegel R, Miller K, Ahmedin J: Cancer statistics 2019, CA Cancer J Clin 69:7–34, 2019.

United States Preventative Service Task Force recommendation Statement. JAMA 319(18): 1901–1913, 2018.

7

Breast Cancer

Mary Anne Fenton, Rochelle Strenger

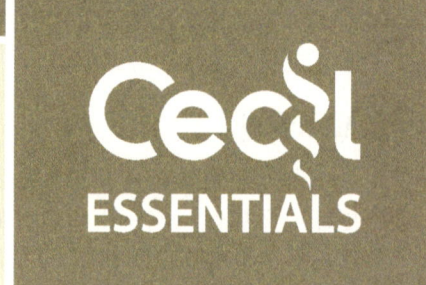

EPIDEMIOLOGY

Worldwide and in the United States, breast cancer is the number one malignancy in women. In 2019 in the United States approximately 271,270 new cases were diagnosed including 268,600 in females and 2670 in males. Breast cancer is the second leading cause of female cancer deaths in the United States. Projected 2019 breast cancer mortality is estimated to be 42,260 (41,760 female, 500 male breast cancer patients). A woman has a 12.4% lifetime risk of breast cancer, and her risk increases with age (Table 7.1). The mortality risk from breast cancer in the United States declined by 39% between 1989 and 2015 due to early detection and more effective treatment; the current 5-year survival rate is 90%. For most solid tumors 5-year survival is predictive of a cure. Unfortunately, however, for the ER+ breast cancer subtype systemic recurrences continue to occur beyond 20 years.

Not all women share equally in improved breast cancer outcomes. Socioeconomic barriers may limit access to early detection and effective therapies. In addition, there are significant ethnic differences in breast cancer incidence and outcome. While breast cancer is less common in African American women, they are more likely to present at a later stage, have a higher incidence of the more aggressive triple-negative subtype and have a higher breast cancer specific mortality rate. The difference in mortality rate is in part related to tumor biology comorbidities, access and adherence to care.

RISK FACTORS

A women's risk of breast cancer increases with age (see Table 60.1) with a lifetime risk of 12%. To put it another way, 1 in 8 women in the United States will develop breast cancer during the course of their lifetime. Reproductive factors such as early onset of menses, late onset of menopause, first live birth after age 35 or nulliparity correlate with a mild increased risk of breast cancer. A positive personal history of dense breasts, findings on a breast biopsy of atypical ductal hyperplasia (ADH) or lobular carcinoma in situ (LCIS) increase breast cancer risk 4-fold.

The risk of breast cancer is increased when there is family history of breast cancer and other cancers such as ovarian, high-risk pancreatic, and prostate. When there is one family member with breast cancer the risk is increased 2-fold. The presence of a familial breast cancer predisposition to gene mutation BRCA1/2 increases breast cancer risk over 4 fold (Table 7.2).

Breast Cancer Genetics

Approximately 10% of breast cancers are associated with inheritable genetic mutations. The first high-penetrance genes, *BRCA1* and *BRCA2*, were identified by screening families with early-onset breast cancer. Mutations in the tumor suppressor genes *BRCA1/2* are also associated with ovarian cancer and other malignancies. Screening recommendations and guidelines for genetic testing and counseling from organizations such as Medicare and the National Comprehensive Cancer Network (NCCN) Guidelines focus on individuals with first-, second-, and third-generation maternal and paternal family histories of cancer, including age of onset.

NCCN guidelines from 2019 recommend referral for genetic counseling for patients diagnosed with breast cancer below the age of 50, or triple-negative (ER/PR, HER2-negative) disease below the age of 60, two breast primaries in an individual, family member with diagnosis of breast cancer below age of 50, family member with ovarian cancer, patient or relative with male breast cancer, and individuals of Eastern European Jewish ancestry who may be at risk for founder mutations. Unfortunately, many individuals are unaware of their family history of cancer including site of cancer and age of onset (Table 7.3).

The identification of a high-penetrant mutation in a family member without breast cancer will afford them the opportunity to consider preventative and early detection strategies. Prior to 2012, breast cancer genetic testing focused on *BRCA1/2* testing and was performed by the Sanger method of sequencing a single DNA fragment at a time, a sequencing technique known to miss large deletions. Next-generation sequencing (NGS) allows for testing of multiple genes, and the number of "clinically actionable mutations" has increased beyond *BRCA1/2*. Patients with *BRCA1/2* testing with negative results prior to 2012 should be referred for genetic counseling and updated testing. In the metastatic setting, patients with germline *BRCA1/2* (g*BRCA1/2*) mutations may be candidates for PARP inhibitor therapy (see metastatic breast cancer section).

CLINICAL PRESENTATION AND DIAGNOSIS

In the United States, over 50% of breast cancers are detected on a screening mammogram, and 33% of cases will present with a self-detected or clinically detected breast mass. In the majority of mammogram and ultrasound detected masses, calcifications and clinically palpable lesions are amenable to core needle biopsy in order to establish a diagnosis, determine breast cancer histology, assess tumor grade, and assess ER, PR, and HER2 expression by immunohistochemistry. The presence or absence of estrogen receptor (ER), progesterone receptor (PR), and human epidermal growth factor receptor 2/neu (HER2) are prognostic for survival and predict response to systemic therapies for breast cancer. Patients presenting with a palpable mass should be referred for diagnostic mammogram and ultrasound and biopsy. If imaging and biopsy are not concordant with the patient's presentation and clinical examination the patient should be referred to a breast surgeon.

乳腺癌

刘媛 译 李宁宁 应红艳 审校 巴一 通审

流行病学

无论在全球还是美国，乳腺癌均是女性最常见的恶性肿瘤。2019年美国的新发病例约271 270例，其中268 600例为女性，2670例为男性。乳腺癌是美国女性癌症死亡的第二大病因。预计2019年因乳腺癌死亡人数约为42 260人（41 760名女性，500名男性乳腺癌患者）。女性一生中患乳腺癌的风险为12.4%，并且随着年龄的增长而增加（表7.1）。得益于早期诊断和更有效的治疗，1989年至2015年间美国乳腺癌的死亡风险下降了39%；目前5年生存率为90%。尽管对于大多数实体肿瘤来说，5年生存率预示着治愈。遗憾的是，对于雌激素受体阳性（Estrogen Receptor+，ER+）亚型的乳腺癌，即便在患病20年后仍会发生肿瘤复发转移。

乳腺癌的诊治不断进步，但并非所有患者均能从中同等获益。社会经济条件的困难可能限制了她们获得早期诊断和有效治疗的机会。此外，乳腺癌的发病率和预后在不同种族之间存在显著差异。虽然非裔美国女性患乳腺癌的概率较低，但她们诊断时分期更晚，更具侵袭性的三阴性亚型发病率更高，且乳腺癌特异性死亡率更高。死亡率的差异与肿瘤生物学特性、医疗资源可及性和依从性部分相关。

危险因素

女性患乳腺癌的风险随年龄增长而增加（见表60.1），终生患病风险为12%。换言之，在美国，每8名女性中就有1人将在其一生中患乳腺癌。如月经初潮早、绝经晚、首次活产年龄超过35岁或未育等生育相关因素可能导致乳腺癌风险的轻度增加。而有致密性乳房的阳性个人病史，不典型导管增生（ADH）或小叶原位癌（LCIS）的乳腺活检结果会使癌症风险增加4倍。

当有乳腺癌及其他癌症（如卵巢癌、高风险胰腺癌和前列腺癌）的家族史时，患乳腺癌的风险增加。如果家庭中有一名成员患有乳腺癌，则患乳腺癌风险增加2倍。家族性乳腺癌易感基因BRCA1/2存在突变则使乳腺癌风险增加超过4倍（表7.2）。

乳腺癌遗传学

大约10%的乳腺癌与遗传的基因突变有关。BRCA1和BRCA2是通过筛查早发性乳腺癌家族发现的第一个高易感风险基因。抑癌基因BRCA1/2的突变也与卵巢癌及其他恶性肿瘤有关。Medicare和美国国家综合癌症网络（NCCN）等组织的关于筛查和基因检测与咨询的指南，均聚焦于有第一、第二和第三代母系或父系癌症家族史的个体，包括其患病亲属的发病年龄。

2019年的NCCN指南建议：50岁以前确诊的乳腺癌患者或60岁以前确诊的三阴性（ER/PR、HER2阴性）乳腺癌患者、有两个乳腺癌原发病灶的患者、家庭成员中有50岁以前确诊乳腺癌患者、家庭成员中有卵巢癌患者、男性乳腺癌患者或亲属以及可能有奠基者突变风险的东欧犹太裔人均应进行遗传咨询。不幸的是，许多人不了解其癌症家族史，包括癌症部位和发病年龄（表7.3）。

识别带有高易感风险突变的未患乳腺癌的家庭成员，这将为他们提供预防和早期筛查的机会。在2012年之前，乳腺癌基因检测集中于BRCA1/2基因，采用的是桑格（Sanger）测序方法，每次测序单个DNA片段，这种测序技术会遗漏大片段缺失。二代测序（next generation sequencing，NGS）可检测多个基因，临床可靶向突变的检出也已远不止于BRCA1/2基因。2012年之前行BRCA1/2基因检测且结果为阴性的患者，推荐进行基因咨询并重新检测。对于转移的患者，携带胚系BRCA1/2（gBRCA1/2）突变者可能从PARP抑制剂治疗中获益（见转移性乳腺癌部分）。

临床表现与诊断

在美国，超过50%的乳腺癌是在进行乳房X线筛查中发现的，33%的病例则是患者自检或临床查体发现乳房肿块而诊断。大多数通过乳房X线片和超声检测出的肿块、钙化病变和临床可扪及的病变，均可通过空芯针活检确诊，明确乳腺癌组织学类型、病理分级，并通过免疫组化评估雌激素受体（ER）、孕激素受体（PR）和人类表皮生长因子受体2/neu（HER2）的表达。ER、PR和HER2的表达情况是患者生存的预后因素，也对肿瘤接受系统性治疗的反应具有预测意义。因此，发现可触及的肿块的患者应推荐进行诊断性乳房X线摄片和超声检查以及穿刺活检。如果影像检查和活检病理的结果与患者的临床表现和体格检查不一致，应推荐患者至乳腺外科就诊。

TABLE 7.1 Age-Specific Probabilities of Developing Invasive Breast Cancer for US Women

Age	10-Year Probability	Or 1 in
20	0.1%	1567
30	0.5%	220
40	1.5%	68
50	2.3%	43
60	3.4%	29
70	3.9%	25
Lifetime	12.4%	8

Note: Probability is among those free of cancer at the beginning of each age interval based on cases diagnosed 2012-2014 American Cancer Society, Inc. Surveillance Report 2017.
From Desantis C, Ma J, Goding Sauer A, et al. Breast Cancer Statistics, 2017, Racial Disparity and Mortality by State, CA Cancer J Clin 67;439-448, 2017.

TABLE 7.2 Risk Factors for Breast Cancer

		Relative Risk
Family history of breast cancer	First-degree relative	2
	More than one first degree relative	3-4
	BRCA1/2 mutation carrier	>4
Age over 65		>4.0
Early menses	age < 12	1.1-2
Nulliparous		1.1-2
First birth	>35 years	1.1-2
Late menopause	>55 years	1.1-2
Never breast fed		1.1-2
Postmenopausal obesity (BMI greater than or equal to 30)		1.1-2
Mammographically dense breasts		4
Proliferative breast lesions	Atypical ductal hyperplasia	4
	Lobular carcinoma in situ	
High-dose radiation to the chest	Hodgkin's lymphoma age 10-30	2.1-4

Data from American Cancer Society. Breast Cancer Facts and Figures 2017-2018 Atlanta, GA; American Cancer Society, 2017.

Traditionally, breast cancer histology and anatomic stage have driven patient stage, prognosis, and decision making for surgery, radiation, and medical oncology care. In current practice, and as delineated in the latest American Joint Commission (AJCC) 8th edition *Staging Manual*, ER, PR, HER2 status, tumor grade, and genomics impact breast cancer prognosis in the prognostic breast cancer stage.

Histology

Breast cancer arises from the epidermal cells of the terminal ductal lobular unit and progresses in a continuum from intraductal hyperplasia, atypia, ductal carcinoma in situ, to invasion through the basement membrane of the duct.

Ductal Carcinoma in Situ

Ductal carcinoma in situ (DCIS) is a clonal disorder of cancer cells contained within the milk duct basement membrane with the potential to

TABLE 7.3 NCCN Guideline on Referral for Genetic Counseling 2019

No history of breast cancer	Personal history of ovarian cancer
	Family history of pancreatic cancer
	Family history of metastatic prostate cancer
	Eastern European Jewish ancestry and personal history of breast cancer or high-grade Gleason 7 or greater prostate cancer in family member
Patient with breast cancer	Age under 50
	Triple-negative breast cancer under the age of 60
	Ovarian cancer
	Two breast primaries
	Male breast cancer
	Pancreatic cancer
	Greater than or equal to two family members with breast cancer
	Family member with ovarian cancer Gleason 7 or greater or metastatic prostate cancer

Data from National Comprehensive Cancer Network Genetic/familial high-risk assessment: breast/ovarian version 3.2019 http://www.nccn.org/professionals/physician_gls/pdf/breast.pdf. Accessed September 25, 2019.

progress to invasive ductal carcinoma (Fig. 7.1). Twenty-five percent of breast cancers diagnosed each year in the United States are classified as DCIS (Tis, Stage 0). Fifteen to fifty percent of DCIS will progress to invasive cancer. Treatment for DCIS is excision to 2-mm negative margins and local breast radiation. Low-grade DCIS less than 2.5 mm considered "low risk" DCIS may be treated with excision alone. The option of "watchful waiting" is being investigated in ongoing studies on molecular features of DCIS. Patients with DCIS are not at risk for systemic spread unless it progresses or recurs as invasive disease.

DCIS treated with mastectomy has a local regional recurrence rate less than 1%. Lumpectomy and radiation recurrence rate is 6% to 16%, of which 50% of recurrences are invasive. There is no difference in survival for mastectomy versus lumpectomy/radiation therapy. For ER-positive DCIS, tamoxifen or anastrozole (reserved for postmenopausal patients) reduces local recurrence by 32% and contralateral breast cancer by 50%.

Lobular Carcinoma in Situ

LCIS is a spectrum of lobular cells with varying potential for invasion. A patient with LCIS and/or atypical ductal hyperplasia has an increased risk of bilateral breast cancer. Patients with DCIS, LCIS, and atypical hyperplasia are candidates for risk reduction with selective estrogen receptor modulators (SERMS) such as tamoxifen and raloxifene or aromatase inhibitors.

Invasive Breast Cancer

Breast cancer is classified histologically by morphology and grade based on nuclear pleomorphism, gland formation, and mitotic index. The most commonly used grading system is Bloom Richardson or Nottingham, with grade 1 less aggressive and grade 3 more aggressive and with higher invasion potential.

Infiltrating ductal carcinoma (IDC) (49% to 75%), is the most common histology, seen as a density on mammography and gross pathology assessment. The clinical behavior of IDC is dependent on grade and ER, PR and HER2 expression. **Invasive lobular carcinoma (ILC)** comprises 5% to 15% of invasive breast cancer, has a slight increased risk of bilateral

表 7.1 美国女性各年龄段罹患浸润性乳腺癌的概率

年龄段	10 年内罹患浸润性乳腺癌的概率	或 1/
20	0.1%	1567
30	0.5%	220
40	1.5%	68
50	2.3%	43
60	3.4%	29
70	3.9%	25
终生	12.4%	8

注：患癌概率是基于美国癌症协会 2017 年监测报告（American Cancer Society, Inc. Surveillance Report 2017），针对每个年龄段启始时未患癌症的人群中，于 2012—2014 年确诊癌症病例。
引自 Desantis C, Ma J, Goding Sauer A, et al. Breast Cancer Statistics, 2017, Racial Disparity and Mortality by State, CA Cancer J Clin 67；439-448，2017.

表 7.2 乳腺癌的危险因素

		相对风险
乳腺癌家族史	一级亲属	2
	多个一级亲属	3~4
	BRCA1/2 基因突变携带者	>4
年龄超过 65 岁		>4.0
初潮早	年龄 < 12 岁	1.1~2
未生育		1.1~2
首次生育年龄	> 35 岁	1.1~2
晚绝经	> 55 岁	1.1~2
从未哺乳		1.1~2
绝经后肥胖（BMI ≥ 30 kg/m²）		1.1~2
X 线片示致密乳房		4
增生性乳腺病变	不典型导管增生	4
	小叶原位癌	
高剂量胸部放射治疗	10~30 岁间患霍奇金淋巴瘤	2.1~4

引自 American Cancer Society. Breast Cancer Facts and Figures 2017—2018 Atlanta, GA; American Cancer Society, 2017.

表 7.3 2019 年 NCCN 遗传咨询转诊指南

无乳腺癌病史	个人有卵巢癌病史 有胰腺癌家族史 有转移性前列腺癌家族史 东欧犹太裔者，个人有乳腺癌病史或家族成员有高级别（Gleason 评分 ≥ 7 分）前列腺癌病史
有乳腺癌病史	年龄 < 50 岁 三阴性乳腺癌 < 60 岁 卵巢癌 双原发乳腺癌 男性乳腺癌 胰腺癌 家族中有 ≥ 2 名乳腺癌患者 家族中有卵巢癌患者，或 Gleason 评分 ≥ 7 分或转移性前列腺癌患者

引自 National Comprehensive Cancer Network Genetic/familial high-risk assessment: breast/ovarian version 3.2019 http://www.nccn.org/professionals/physician_gls/pdf/breast.pdf. Accessed September 25, 2019.

乳腺癌传统上通过组织学和解剖分期来决定患者的分期、预后及手术、放疗和抗肿瘤药物治疗的决策。在当前的临床实践中，以及如最新的美国癌症联合委员会（AJCC）第 8 版分期手册中所述的乳腺癌预后分期，ER、PR、HER2 状态，肿瘤的组织学分级和基因组学均会影响乳腺癌的预后。

组织学

乳腺癌起源于终末导管小叶单位的上皮细胞，可表现为从导管内增生、不典型增生、导管原位癌到突破导管基底膜的浸润癌的连续谱系。

导管原位癌

导管原位癌（DCIS）是一种局限于乳腺导管基底膜内的癌细胞克隆性病变，有进展为浸润性导管癌的潜力（图 7.1）。在美国，每年诊断的乳腺癌中有 25% 被分类为 DCIS（Tis，0 期）。15%~50% 的 DCIS 将进展为浸润性癌。DCIS 的治疗应行肿物切除，保证至少 2 mm 阴性切缘，之后行乳腺局部放疗。小于 2.5 mm 的低级别 DCIS 被认为是"低风险"DCIS，可只行手术切除。目前有针对 DCIS 的分子特征的临床研究正在进行，探索是否可对其采取"观察等待"的策略。除非 DCIS 进展或复发为浸润性疾病，患者不会面临肿瘤全身扩散的风险。

接受乳房切除术治疗的 DCIS 局部复发率不到 1%。肿瘤广泛切除术和放疗患者的复发率为 6%~16%，其中 50% 的患者复发时为浸润性疾病。乳房切除术与肿瘤广泛切除术/放射治疗的生存无差异。对于 ER 阳性 DCIS，使用他莫昔芬或阿那曲唑（仅限于绝经后患者）可减少 32% 的局部复发和 50% 的对侧乳腺癌的发生。

小叶原位癌

小叶原位癌（LCIS）是一系列具有不同侵袭潜力的小叶细胞病变谱系。患有 LCIS 和（或）不典型导管增生的患者发生双侧乳腺癌的风险增加。患有 DCIS、LCIS 和不典型增生的患者可考虑通过选择性雌激素受体调节剂（SERMS）如他莫昔芬和雷洛昔芬或芳香化酶抑制剂进行治疗以降低风险。

浸润性乳腺癌

乳腺癌根据形态学和组织学分级进行组织学分类，组织学分级基于细胞核多形性、腺体形成和有丝分裂指数。最常用的分级系统是 Bloom Richardson 或 Nottingham 系统，一级表示侵袭性较低，三级表示侵袭性较高，具有更高的侵袭潜力。

浸润性导管癌（IDC）（占 49%~75%）是最常见的组织类型，在乳腺 X 线片和大体病理中表现为致密病变。IDC 的临床行为取决于组织学分级和 ER、PR 及 HER2 的表达情况。**浸润性小叶癌（ILC）** 占浸润性乳腺癌的 5%~15%，其双侧乳腺癌的风险略增加，并且

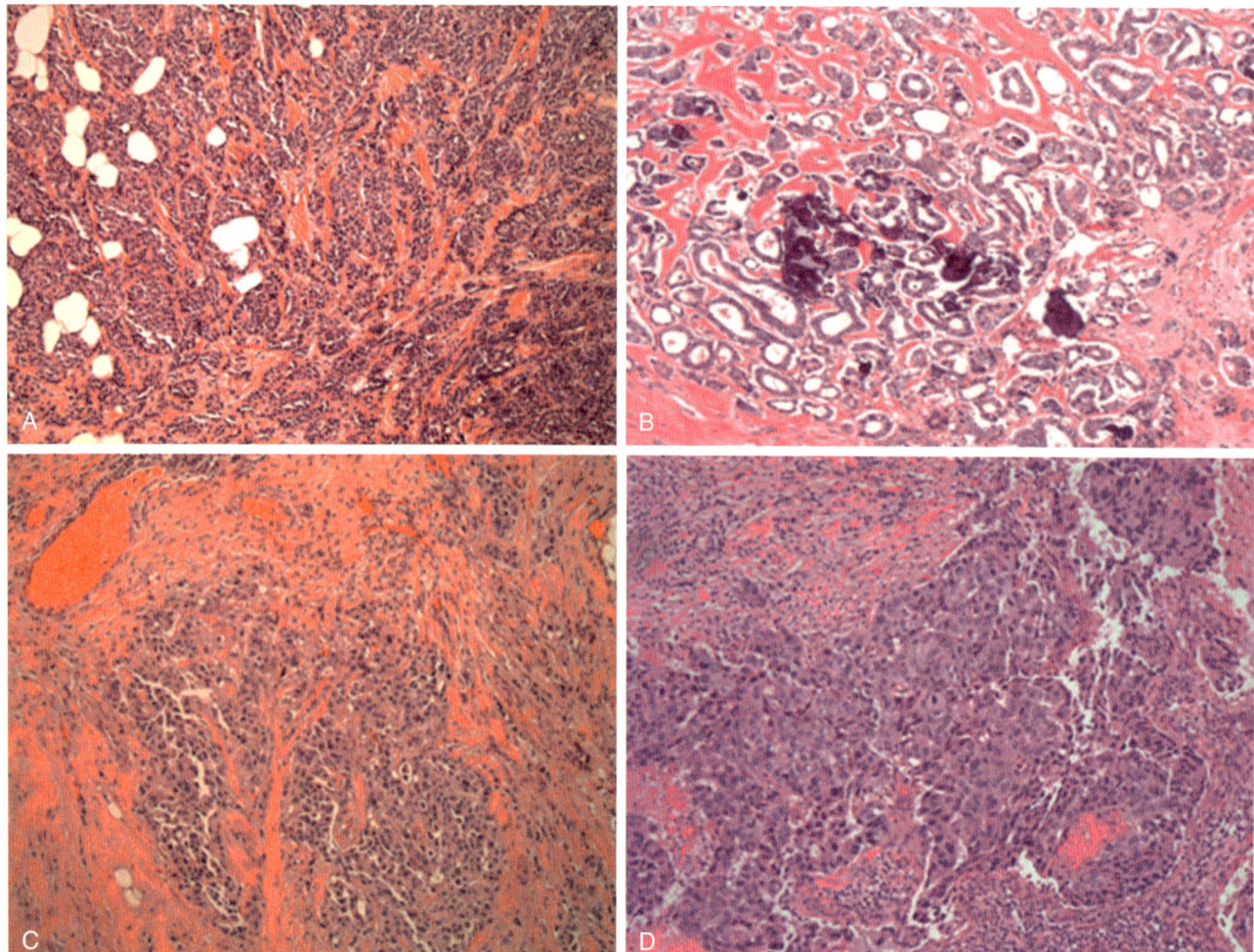

Fig. 7.1 (A-D) Four cases of invasive ductal carcinoma. (Korourian S: Infiltrating carcinomas of the breast: not one disease. In: Bland K, editor. The Breast: Comprehensive Management of Benign and Malignant Diseases, 145-155.e4, 64, 2018, Elsevier Press.).

breast cancer and slight propensity for abdominal mesenteric dissemination. ILC is characterized by single cell tissue infiltration, loss of heterozygosity or 16q chromosome, and absence of epithelial e-cadherin. **Medullary carcinoma** (3% to 9%) is associated with *BRCA1* germline mutations and higher grade. The histologic appearance is described as "pushing borders" rather than single cell invasion. **Mucinous and tubular breast cancer** subtypes, 1% to 2% and 1% to 3% respectively, are less common and present a lower risk for systemic metastasis.

BREAST CANCER STAGING

Approximately 90% of breast cancer at presentation is confined to the breast and axilla. Clinical evaluation includes history, including careful review of systems; screening for signs or symptoms of metastasis such as headache, weight loss, and bone pain; clinical examination; and laboratory evaluation including CBC, liver tests, and alkaline phosphatase. Clinical breast cancer staging is based on clinical breast exam including breast inspection for nipple discharge or retraction, skin dimpling, ulceration, erythema, edema, and palpable masses, and palpation of supraclavicular, axillary, and cervical lymph nodes.

Inflammatory breast cancer (Fig. 7.2) is an aggressive subtype of breast cancer with tumor invasion of the dermal lymphatics presenting with rapid skin changes of edema, erythema, and *peau d'orange* change, involving greater than one third of the breast. Patients with breast cancer considered clinical stage III or signs or symptoms concerning for distant metastasis should be referred for systemic staging with bone scan and CT scan and in select cases PET scan. If a suspicious site is noted on staging, biopsy should be performed to confirm distant spread of breast cancer.

Breast cancer staging is based on the AJCC of anatomic cancer staging using tumor size (T in centimeters), regional node metastasis (N), and distant metastasis (M). The TNM system has prognostic significance. In the AJCC 8th edition *Staging Manual*, released in 2019, clinical stage (c) and pathologic stage (p) are supplemented with an additional pathologic prognostic stage incorporating grade and ER, PR, and HER2 gene overexpression. As an example, patients with T2 (2 to 5 cm) node-negative (N0) ER-positive HER2-negative tumors with gene expression profiles such as an Oncotype® Recurrence Score less than 11 have an excellent 5-year prognosis. This is reflected in the patient's AJCC 8th edition pathological prognostic stage of 1A (previously, by the AJCC 7th edition system, the patient would have been staged as IIA).

TREATMENT

Breast cancer is a story of the old and the new. Tamoxifen, the first cancer targeted therapy, was approved for ER-positive metastatic breast

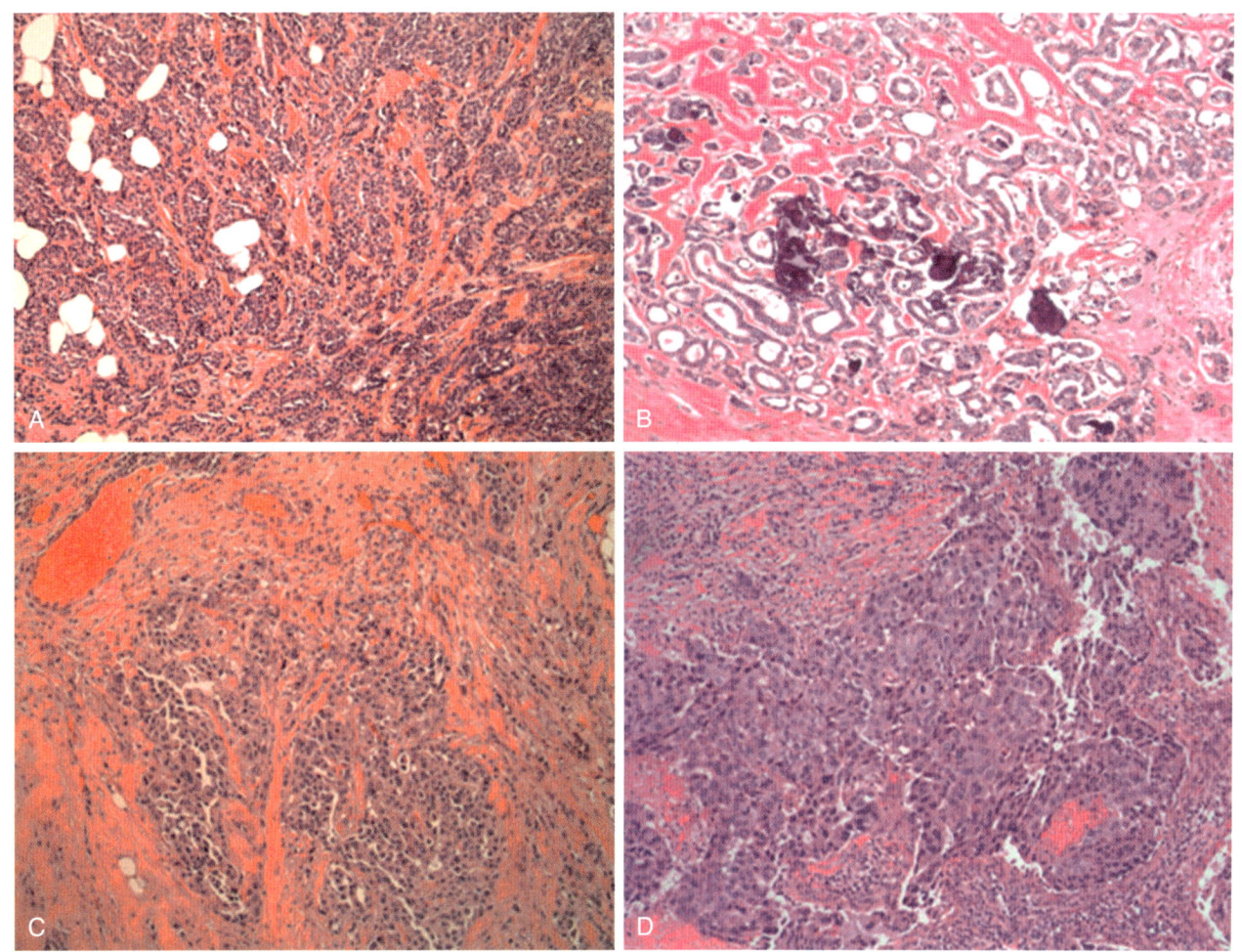

图7.1 （A-D）浸润性导管癌的4个病例（Korourian S：Infiltrating carcinomas of the breast：not one disease. In：Bland K，editor. The Breast：Comprehensive Management of Benign and Malignant Diseases，145-155.e4，64，2018，Elsevier Press.）

具有轻微向腹腔肠系膜播散的倾向。ILC的特征是单细胞组织浸润，16q染色体杂合性缺失，以及上皮e-钙黏蛋白缺失。髓样癌（占3%～9%）与 *BRCA1* 胚系突变相关，具有较高的组织学分级。其组织学外观被描述为"推挤性边界"而不是单细胞浸润。黏液性和管状乳腺癌亚型分别占1%～2%和1%～3%，较少见，全身转移风险较低。

乳腺癌分期

大约90%的乳腺癌在确诊时局限于乳房和腋窝。临床评估包括病史，详细的系统回顾；筛查有无转移的症状体征，如头痛、体重减轻和骨痛；临床体格检查；以及全血细胞计数、肝功能检测和碱性磷酸酶等实验室检查。乳腺癌的临床分期基于乳房查体，应包括是否有乳头溢液或回缩、皮肤凹陷、溃疡、红斑、水肿和可触及的肿块，以及对锁骨上、腋窝和颈部淋巴结的触诊。

炎性乳腺癌（图7.2）是一种侵袭性乳腺癌亚型，肿瘤侵入真皮淋巴管，皮肤迅速出现水肿、红斑和橘皮样改变，累及超过1/3的乳房。临床Ⅲ期或有远处转移症状/体征的乳腺癌患者应进行系统的分期检查，包括骨扫描和CT检查，部分患者在特定情况下进行PET扫描。如果在分期过程中发现可疑的转移部位，应进行活检以确认。

乳腺癌分期基于AJCC的解剖学癌症分期，使用肿瘤大小（T，以厘米为单位）、区域淋巴结转移（N）和远处转移（M）。TNM系统对预后具有指导意义。在2019年发布的AJCC第8版分期手册中，在临床分期（c）和病理分期（p）的基础上，增加了一个结合了组织学分级和ER、PR及HER2基因过表达的病理预后分期。例如，具有T2（肿瘤大小2～5 cm）N0（淋巴结阴性）ER阳性HER2阴性且基因表达谱如Oncotype®复发评分小于11的患者有很好的5年预后。这个患者按AJCC第8版病理预后分期，分为1A期（在之前的AJCC第7版系统中，该患者将被分为ⅡA期）。

治疗

乳腺癌的治疗是一个新旧交替的"故事"。他莫昔芬，是首个癌症靶向治疗药物，1977年被批准用于ER阳性的转移性乳腺癌。在这最常见类型的乳腺癌的

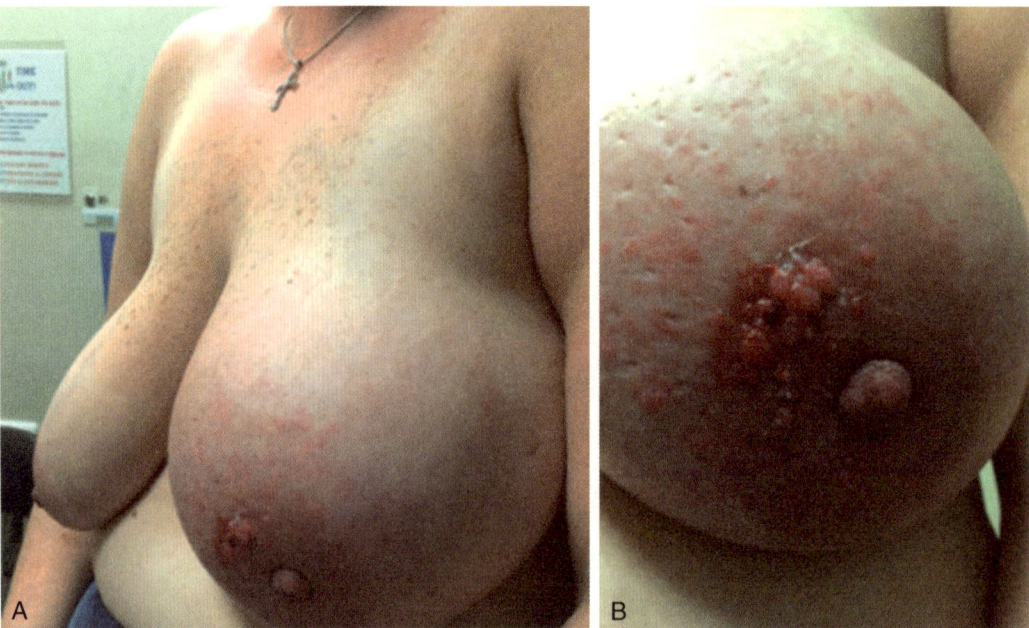

Fig. 7.2 (A and B) Inflammatory breast cancer with erythema and edema occupying the majority of the breast. (Somlo G, Jones V: Inflammatory breast cancer. In: Bland K, editor. The Breast: Comprehensive Management of Benign and Malignant Diseases, 2018, Elsevier Press.).

cancer in 1977. In the adjuvant setting for the most common type of breast cancer, tamoxifen has proven to reduce systemic recurrence by 50%. Scientific discoveries of pathways of tamoxifen resistance have led to additional therapeutic strategies for ER-positive breast cancer including aromatase inhibition to decrease estrogen production in postmenopausal patients, ovarian suppression of estrogen production in the premenopausal setting, and estrogen receptor downregulation with fulvestrant. Recent discoveries have led to FDA approval of cell cycle inhibitors of cyclin D 4/6 in combination with endocrine therapy with improved overall survival of ER-positive metastatic breast cancer.

By gene expression profiling, ER-positive breast cancer is further subdivided into luminal A, with a low cell proliferation signature and high endocrine therapy response, and luminal B, with a high cell proliferation signature and higher recurrence rate indicating relative endocrine insensitivity and relatively higher chemotherapy sensitivity. In the current era of personalized medicine, gene expression profiles such as Oncotype Recurrence Score testing of ER-positive node-negative breast cancer can identify patients who can forgo chemotherapy.

Other applications of personalized medicine for metastatic breast cancer include screening tumor samples with genomic sequencing for actionable mutations with specific targeted agents. PIK3CA-mutant ER-positive stage IV breast cancer patients have improved progression-free survival (PFS) with the PIK3CA inhibitor alpelisib. Approximately 10% of patients with breast cancer harbor somatic mutations in specific tumor suppressor genes such as *BRCA1* and *BRCA2*. These patients are at higher risk of breast cancer and other malignancies with early age of onset. Some patients who harbor these genes are candidates for more intense screening and prevention strategies. Patients with stage IV disease who are *BRCA1/2* mutation carriers may benefit from PARP inhibitor therapy.

Early-Stage Breast Cancer
Local Therapy
Stage I and II breast cancer clinical trials demonstrate equivalent outcomes of overall survival with breast preservation surgery with lumpectomy or segmental mastectomy to achieve negative surgical margins and breast external beam radiation compared to modified radical mastectomy and axillary dissection. Patients age 70 and older with ER+ stage 1 disease willing to take 5 years of endocrine therapy have an equivalent overall survival with or without radiation and can safely omit radiation.

Unfortunately, not all breast cancer patients are candidates for breast preservation. Patients with multicentric disease (more than one breast quadrant), extensive malignant appearing calcifications, surgical inability to achieve negative margins, prior breast radiation, connective tissue disorder or who are unable to access a radiation facility treatment center are candidates for mastectomy. Patients with inflammatory breast cancer need neoadjuvant chemotherapy, prior to surgery, to eradicate dermal lymphatic cancer metastasis from the skin. In addition, patients with large unresectable tumors or large tumor-to-breast ratio may be candidates for neoadjuvant chemotherapy or endocrine therapy to downstage the tumor and allow for breast preservation.

For patients with no palpable lymph nodes on clinical exam, sentinel lymph node staging with removal and examination of the first draining lymph node accurately reflects the status of axillary metastases. Based on the ACOSZ-0011 trial of patients with clinically negative axillary lymph nodes staged with sentinel lymph nodes (with up to two positive lymph nodes), radiation and systemic therapy provide adequate local control.

Systemic Therapy
Prognosis estimation of systemic recurrence. The indication for breast cancer staging is to estimate the risk of systemic metastasis and help direct therapy. Historically, the most accurate indicators are tumor size, axillary metastasis, tumor grade, and ER, PR, and HER2 neu expression. ER, PR, and HER2 gene expression are detected by immunohistochemistry (IHC). Equivocal HER2 IHC testing is further evaluated by *HER2* gene duplication detected by invitro hybridization (ISH).

Another chapter in breast cancer care is systemic therapy to reduce the risk of recurrence by elimination of micro-metastatic disease. Effective systemic therapy for breast cancer is the result of patient participation in well-designed randomized sequential clinical trials and identification of effective systemic therapies to decrease recurrence. The use of genomic signatures for personalized medicine allows us to

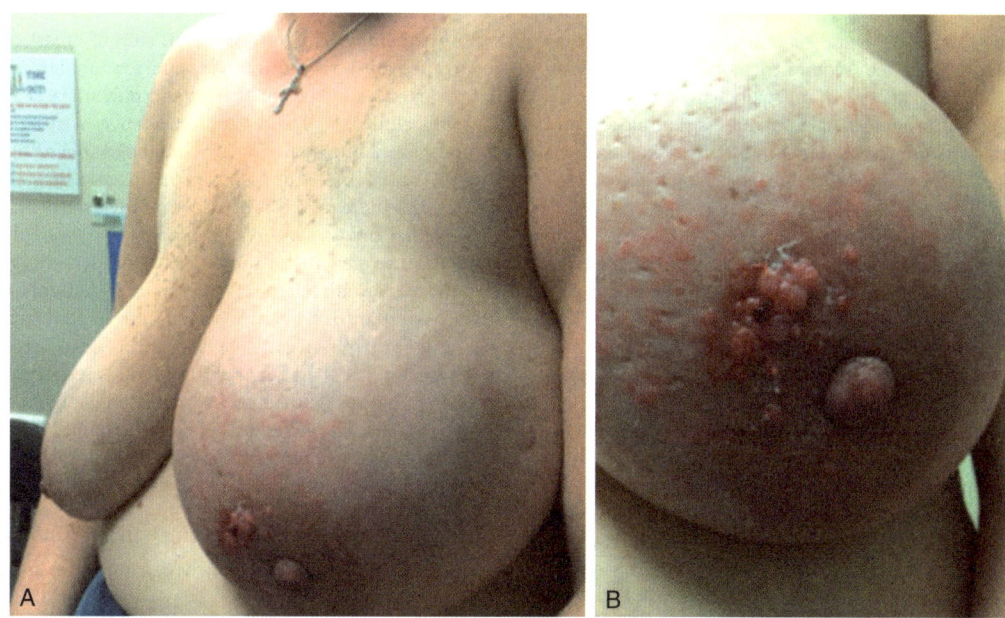

图 7.2 （**A** 和 **B**）炎性乳腺癌，大部分乳房出现红斑和水肿（Somlo G，Jones V：Inflammatory breast cancer. In：Bland K，editor. The Breast：Comprehensive Management of Benign and Malignant Diseases，2018，Elsevier Press.）

辅助治疗中，他莫昔芬已被证明可将全身复发率降低50%。对他莫昔芬耐药途径的科研探索为 ER 阳性的乳腺癌提供了新的治疗策略，包括在绝经后患者中抑制芳香化酶以减少雌激素的产生，在绝经前抑制卵巢产生雌激素，以及用氟维司群下调雌激素受体。最近的发现促使美国食品药物管理局批准了细胞周期蛋白 D（cyclin D）4/6 抑制剂与内分泌治疗联合使用，改善了 ER 阳性转移性乳腺癌患者的总生存。

通过基因表达谱分析，ER 阳性乳腺癌进一步细分为管腔 A 型（luminal A），具有低细胞增殖特征及内分泌治疗高反应性；管腔 B 型（luminal B）具有高细胞增殖特征和较高的复发率，表明其对内分泌治疗相对不敏感和但有相对较高的化疗敏感性。在当前的个体化医疗时代，基因表达谱如肿瘤复发风险评分（Oncotype Recurrence Score）可对 ER 阳性、淋巴结阴性乳腺癌患者进行检测，识别出哪些患者可以豁免化疗。

个体化医疗在转移性乳腺癌中的其他应用包括通过基因组测序筛查肿瘤样本，以发现可靶向的突变。PIK3CA 突变的 ER 阳性的Ⅳ期乳腺癌患者应用 PIK3CA 抑制剂阿培利司可改善无进展生存期。约有 10% 的乳腺癌患者存在特定肿瘤抑制基因（如 *BRCA1* 和 *BRCA2*）的胚系突变（译者注：原文体细胞突变有误）。这些患者患乳腺癌和其他恶性肿瘤的风险较高，而且发病年龄较早。对有这些基因突变的患者可遵循更严格的筛查和预防策略。Ⅳ期的 *BRCA1/2* 突变携带的患者可能从 PARP 抑制剂治疗中获益。

早期乳腺癌
局部治疗

Ⅰ期和Ⅱ期乳腺癌的临床研究表明，与改良根治术和腋窝淋巴结清扫术相比，采用乳房肿块切除或节段性乳房切除的方式进行保乳手术以达到阴性切缘，并联合乳腺外照射，两者总生存期相当。愿意接受 5 年内分泌治疗的 70 岁及 70 岁以上 ER 阳性的Ⅰ期患者，接受与不接受放疗的总生存期相当，可以安全地免于放疗。

遗憾的是，并非所有乳腺癌患者都适合保乳手术。患有多中心疾病（≥1 个乳腺象限）、广泛的恶性钙化、手术无法达到阴性切缘、既往乳腺放疗史、结缔组织病或无法在有放射设施的中心治疗等，都应选择乳房切除术。炎性乳腺癌患者需要在手术前进行新辅助化疗，以根除皮肤内淋巴转移癌。此外，肿瘤较大无法切除，或肿瘤大小/乳房体积比例大的患者，可能更适合新辅助化疗或内分泌治疗，使肿瘤降期从而适合保留乳房。

对于临床查体未触及淋巴结的患者，可进行前哨淋巴结分期，切除并检查第一个引流淋巴结能准确反映腋窝淋巴结转移的情况。根据 ACOSZ-0011 研究，对临床腋窝淋巴结阴性患者进行了前哨淋巴结分期（最多有两个阳性淋巴结），放射治疗和全身治疗可提供充分的局部控制。

全身治疗

全身复发的预后评估 乳腺癌的分期是为了估计全身转移的风险并协助指导治疗。传统来说，最准确的指标是肿瘤大小、腋窝转移、肿瘤分级以及 ER、PR 和 HER2 表达。ER、PR 和 HER2 表达应用免疫组织化学的方法检测。如果 HER2 免疫组织化学检测结果不明确，则通过体外杂交（ISH）检测 *HER2* 基因重复的方法进一步评估。

乳腺癌治疗的另一个篇章是全身治疗，全身治疗通过消除微转移以降低疾病复发风险。乳腺癌有效的全身治疗是通过患者参与精心设计的随机序列临床研究，并找到有效的可降低复发率的全身治疗方法来实现的。将基因组特征应用于个体化治疗使我们可超越"化疗万能论"，真正去了解是哪些乳腺癌对化疗敏感或需要化疗。PREDICT.NHS.UK 等工具可根据患者的

move beyond "chemo for all" to an understanding of which breast cancers are chemotherapy sensitive or require chemotherapy. Tools such as PREDICT.NHS.UK calculate risk of mortality based on a patient's age, anatomic stage, and prognostic factors and assist clinicians and patients in estimating risk of recurrence and mortality reduction from chemotherapy, endocrine therapy, and validated genomic assays.

Therapy for HR+ Breast Cancer

Hormone receptor positive (HR+) breast cancer is the most common form of breast cancer and HR positivity is prognostic for a better 5-year disease-free survival compared to HR-negative breast tumors. HR+ also predicts those who will respond to antiestrogen directed therapies, although the risk of local and systemic recurrence extends past 10 years and is estimated to occur at a rate of 2% per year.

Tamoxifen was the first "targeted therapy" and ER expression the first biomarker for response to therapy. The Early Breast Cancer Trialists Group (EBCTCG) published series of breast cancer trial meta-analyses. EBCTCG trials of tamoxifen for HR+ breast cancer showed decreases in systemic recurrence by 50% and mortality by 25%; reduction in recurrence continues after 5 years. Further incremental improvement for subsets of patients include ovarian suppression for high-risk HR+ premenopausal patients and addition of aromatase inhibitors for postmenopausal patients. Based on the persistent risk of late recurrences in HR+ disease, trials of extended endocrine therapy with tamoxifen or aromatase inhibitors have shown further decrease in disease recurrence. Extended therapies and ovarian suppression come at a cost of increase in side effects and symptoms including hot flashes, decreased bone density, and for tamoxifen, increase in vaginal bleeding and risk of endometrial cancer.

A subset of HR+ patients is less responsive to endocrine therapy. In the current era of personalized medicine, gene expression profiles such as Oncotype Recurrence Score for HR+ node-negative breast cancer evaluates 16 genes including ER, proliferation, and invasion genes and predicts for risk of recurrence with endocrine therapy as well as a response to chemotherapy. Luminal A patients have low Oncotype Recurrence Scores and can forgo chemotherapy, and luminal B patients may derive benefit from addition of chemotherapy to endocrine therapy. Results of these assays can be used by clinicians for risk-benefit discussions with patients.

Approximately 20% of breast cancers are HER2 positive. *HER2* gene overexpression is a marker of a more aggressive phenotype. Targeted therapy with trastuzumab, a humanized monoclonal antibody to HER2 in combination with chemotherapy reduces systemic recurrence by 40%. Since the identification of trastuzumab, additional HER2-directed monoclonal antibodies have been developed and documented to have clinical utility. Pertuzumab, a monoclonal antibody directed to HER2 that prevents HER2 heterodimerization and cell activation added to trastuzumab and chemotherapy clinically improves the pathologic response rate. Future directions with HER2-directed therapies may be the ability to tailor therapy based on response and potentially to deescalate chemotherapy for HER2-positive patients.

Triple-negative breast cancer, defined as the absence of ER, PR and HER2 expression, is an aggressive breast cancer phenotype and comprises 10% to 15% of all breast cancers. Gene array analysis has identified six subtypes. Triple-negative breast cancer has a high systemic recurrence rate that typically occurs within the first 5 years of diagnosis. Due to high recurrence rates and shortened life expectancy after triple-negative breast cancer recurrence, systemic chemotherapy should be considered for a triple-negative breast cancer greater than 0.5 cm. Neoadjuvant chemotherapy may be considered if tumor size is over 2 centimeters.

Metastatic Breast Cancer

Metastatic breast cancer is "treatable not curable," and while the goal of therapy is palliative, many patients will live months to years on systemic therapy. The most frequent sites of breast cancer systemic recurrence are bone, lung, liver, and for lobular cancer, abdominal recurrences including ovaries and mesentery. Patients presenting with clinical or radiographic evidence of systemic recurrence should have a biopsy to confirm diagnosis including evaluation of ER, PR, and HER2 expression of metastatic cells. Results from a small series indicate receptor status on metastasis may change from the original breast cancer approximately 10% of the time. Next-generation sequencing of tumor metastasis screening for actionable mutations may direct cancer therapies in patients demonstrating PIK3CA-mutant ER-positive stage IV, to include alpelisib and fulvestrant. For triple-negative breast cancers, testing for programmed death ligand 1 (PD-L1) expression predicts response to checkpoint inhibitor therapy with atezolizumab. Single-agent chemotherapy for stage IV breast cancer is as effective as combination chemotherapy. Combination chemotherapy is reserved for patients at risk for a visceral crisis.

ER-Positive HER2-Negative Metastatic Breast Cancer

Bone only metastatic disease may have a long disease-free interval and patients may live many months to years with treatment as a chronic disease. Recurrence of ER-positive breast cancer within 6 months of initiation of antiestrogen therapy may indicate primary endocrine therapy resistance. Although chemotherapy response rate is more rapid, in the absence of impending visceral crisis there is no advantage in survival to chemotherapy over initial endocrine therapy.

Triple-Negative Breast Cancer

Unfortunately, systemic recurrence of triple-negative breast cancer (TNBC) frequently occurs in first 2 years after diagnosis. Chemotherapy options for stage IV ER-positive breast cancer resistant to endocrine therapy or TNBC include anthracyclines, taxanes, eribulin, carboplatin, and other single agents.

Targeted therapies for TNBC subtypes have expanded therapeutic options for selected patients. Patients with *BRCA1/2* germline mutations may benefit from disease control with an oral polyadenosine diphosphate-ribose polymerase (PARP) inhibitor. Olaparib and talazoparib are FDA approved for *BRCA*-associated *HER2*-negative breast cancer based on improved progression free survival. Immune checkpoint inhibition is one of many pathways for cancer to evade the immune system. Tumors expressing PD-L1 may activate PD-1 on tumor infiltrating immune cells resulting in immune cell apoptosis. In the Impassion130 trial of checkpoint inhibitor therapy, tumor-infiltrating immune cells with expression of 1% or greater PD-L1 expression derive increase in progression free survival with nab-paclitaxel and atezolizumab.

Special Circumstances
Bone Metastasis

Osteoclast inhibitors zoledronic acid bisphosphonates or denosumab, a RANK ligand inhibitor, prolong the time to skeletal related events such as pathologic fractures or need for surgery or radiation for bone metastases. Risks include renal dysfunction, hypocalcemia, and osteonecrosis.

Survivorship

A cancer patient becomes a cancer survivor on the day of diagnosis, regardless of whether they are currently without evidence of disease or are living with advanced or metastatic breast cancer. There are 15 million cancer survivors in the United States. Forty-four percent are breast cancer survivors. The Institute of Medicine report on cancer survivorship notes the transition of patients from active treatment to cancer survivor. The concern for patients "lost in transition" led the American College of Surgeons Commission on Cancer and the American Society

年龄、解剖分期、预后因素计算死亡风险，并协助临床医生和患者估计复发风险以及化疗、内分泌治疗和有效基因组检测降低死亡率的情况。

激素受体阳性乳腺癌的治疗

激素受体（HR）阳性乳腺癌是最常见的乳腺癌类型，与 HR 阴性的乳腺肿瘤相比，HR 阳性预示着较高的 5 年无病生存率。HR 阳性也可预测出对抗雌激素治疗有反应的患者，然而局部和全身复发的风险会持续 10 年以上，估计每年复发率为 2%。

他莫昔芬是首个"靶向疗法"，ER 表达是首个提示治疗反应的生物标志物。早期乳腺癌试验协作组（EBCTCG）发表了一系列乳腺癌研究荟萃分析。EBCTCG 研究显示，应用他莫昔芬治疗 HR 阳性乳腺癌，全身复发率降低了 50%，死亡率降低了 25%，5 年后全身复发率继续降低。对一部分患者的进一步改善方法包括，对于高危 HR 阳性绝经前患者进行卵巢功能抑制，及对绝经后患者加用芳香化酶抑制剂。基于 HR 阳性疾病持续长期复发风险，应用他莫昔芬或芳香化酶抑制剂的延长内分泌治疗研究已显示出疾病复发率的进一步降低。延长治疗和应用卵巢功能抑制剂的代价是副作用和症状的增加，包括潮热、骨密度降低，而他莫昔芬增加了阴道出血和患子宫内膜癌的风险。

一部分 HR 阳性患者对内分泌治疗反应较差。在当前的个体化医疗时代，基因表达谱如 Oncotype 复发风险评分，对 HR 阳性淋巴结阴性乳腺癌评估包括 ER、增殖和侵袭基因在内的 16 个基因，预测内分泌治疗的复发风险和化疗反应。luminal A 型患者肿瘤复发风险评分较低，可以避免化疗，luminal B 型患者可能从内分泌治疗基础上加用化疗中获益。临床医生可利用这些检测结果与患者进行风险-获益讨论。

大约 20% 的乳腺癌患者 HER2 呈阳性。*HER2* 基因过表达是更具侵袭性表型的标志。使用曲妥珠单抗（一种针对 HER2 的人源化单克隆抗体）进行靶向治疗并联合化疗，可降低 40% 全身复发率。自曲妥珠单抗问世以来，有更多的针对 HER2 靶向单克隆抗体已经被开发出来，并被证实具有临床效用。帕妥珠单抗，是一种针对 HER2 的单克隆抗体，可阻止 HER2 异源二聚化和细胞活化，与曲妥珠单抗和化疗一起使用，可提高病理缓解率。HER2 靶向疗法的未来发展方向可能是根据治疗反应定制治疗方案，以及 HER2 阳性患者的化疗可能降级。

三阴性乳腺癌，是指无 ER、PR 和 HER2 表达的一种侵袭性乳腺癌表型，占所有乳腺癌的 10%～15%。基因阵列分析确定了六种亚型。三阴性乳腺癌的全身复发率高，复发通常发生于确诊的前 5 年内。由于三阴性乳腺癌的高复发率和复发后预期寿命缩短，肿瘤大小超过 0.5 cm 的三阴性乳腺癌应考虑接受全身化疗。如果肿瘤直径超过 2 cm，可以考虑进行新辅助化疗。

转移性乳腺癌

转移性乳腺癌是"可治疗而不可治愈"的，虽然治疗目标是姑息治疗，很多患者在接受全身治疗后可存活数月至数年。乳腺癌最常见的全身复发部位是骨、肺、肝，对于小叶癌，常见腹部复发，包括卵巢和肠系膜。有临床或影像学证据的全身复发患者应进行活检以确诊，包括评估转移细胞的 ER、PR 和 HER2 表达。小规模系列研究结果提示，约 10% 的转移病灶的受体状态较原发乳腺癌有所改变。对肿瘤转移病灶进行二代测序，筛查可靶向的突变，可指导 PIK3CA 突变 ER 阳性Ⅳ期患者的抗肿瘤治疗，包括阿培利司和氟维司群。对于三阴性乳腺癌，检测 PD-L1 表达可预测对检查点抑制剂阿替利珠单抗治疗的反应。Ⅳ期乳腺癌的单药化疗与联合化疗同样有效。联合化疗适用于有内脏危象风险的患者。

ER 阳性 HER2 阴性转移性乳腺癌

仅骨转移的疾病可能有很长的无病间隔期，作为一种慢性疾病，患者在接受治疗后可存活数月至数年。ER 阳性乳腺癌在开始抗雌激素治疗的 6 个月内复发，可能表明其原发性内分泌耐药。尽管化疗的反应速度更快，在无内脏危象的情况下，化疗对比初始内分泌治疗并无生存优势。

三阴性乳腺癌

遗憾的是，三阴性乳腺癌（TNBC）的全身复发经常发生在确诊后的前 2 年。Ⅳ期的内分泌耐药的 ER 阳性乳腺癌或 TNBC 的化疗选择包括蒽环类、紫杉类、艾立布林、卡铂和其他单药。

针对 TNBC 亚型的靶向治疗扩大了特定患者的治疗选择。*BRCA1/2* 胚系突变的患者口服聚腺苷二磷酸核糖聚合酶（PARP）抑制剂可控制病情。为延长无进展生存期，奥拉帕利和他拉唑帕利被 FDA 批准用于治疗 *BRCA* 相关的 HER2 阴性乳腺癌。免疫检查点抑制是肿瘤逃避免疫系统的众多途径之一。肿瘤表达 PD-L1 可激活肿瘤浸润免疫细胞上的 PD-1 导致免疫细胞凋亡。在免疫检查点抑制剂疗法的 Impassion130 研究中，肿瘤浸润免疫细胞的 PD-L1 表达≥1% 的人群应用白蛋白紫杉醇（nab-paclitaxel）和阿替利珠单抗的无进展生存期延长。

特殊情况

骨转移

破骨细胞抑制剂唑来膦酸（双膦酸盐）或地舒单抗（一种 RANK 配体抑制剂）可延长如病理骨折或骨转移需要手术或放射治疗等骨相关事件的发生时间。治疗风险包括肾功能损害、低钙血症和骨坏死。

幸存者

癌症患者自确诊之日起即成为癌症幸存者，无论他们目前是没有疾病迹象还是进展期或转移性乳腺癌患者。美国有 1500 万癌症幸存者。其中 44% 是乳腺癌幸存者。医学研究所关于癌症幸存者的报告关注到患者从积极治疗到癌症幸存者的过渡。对"在过渡中迷失"的患者的关注促使美国外科学院癌症委员会和美

of Clinical Oncology (ASCO) to recommend the creation of a survivorship plan for patient and primary care practitioner and follow-up care as quality standards.

Endocrine Therapy Compliance

It is estimated that 50% of ER-positive breast cancer patients do not complete adjuvant endocrine therapy due to side effects or barriers such as cost. Side effects that may affect quality of life and compliance include hot flashes from chemotherapy-induced menopause, tamoxifen or aromatase inhibitors. A recent study showed improvement in hot flashes and sleep quality with the use of cognitive behavioral therapy. Arthralgias from aromatase inhibitors may be attenuated by rotation through drug regimens and/or acupuncture, duloxetine or yoga.

Sexual Dysfunction

Unfortunately, sexual dysfunction is a common side effect following a breast cancer diagnosis secondary to surgery, radiation, chemotherapy, and adjuvant endocrine therapy. Practitioners should use open-ended questions about intimacy issues to normalize patients' concerns. Patients note change in self-image, decrease in sexual drive, vaginal dryness, and dyspareunia. Effective interventions can include use of vaginal moisturizers and lubricants, gabapentin and venlafaxine for hot flashes, topical lidocaine for tender vestibule, and referral to a sexual health expert.

Fertility Preservation

Pregnancy following a breast cancer diagnosis does not appear to increase risk for breast cancer recurrence, based on case control studies. Fertility may be compromised by chemotherapy, and fertility preservation options include egg retrieval and invitro fertilization. A general rule is to avoid pregnancy for 2 years after diagnosis, because this time period is a high-risk time for cancer recurrence. The PROMISE trial will follow a cohort of women following breast cancer diagnosis and treatment for breast cancer outcomes who chose to stop adjuvant endocrine therapy for pregnancy.

Lymphedema

Breast and arm lymphedema can be a complication from surgery and may be exacerbated by radiation. Physical therapy, manual massage, and compression bras and sleeves may attenuate this side effect.

Male Breast Cancer

Male breast cancer represents 1% of all breast cancers in the United States. Approximately 2500 men are diagnosed with breast cancer yearly and 500 men will die each year from male breast cancer. Risk factors for male breast cancer include *gBRCA2* mutations, Klinefelter's syndrome, undescended testes or testicular injury, and environmental radiation exposure, as documented in atomic bomb survivors. Male breast cancer patients are not represented in clinical trials. Available data on male breast cancer are primarily from small cohort studies. Mirroring women, incidence increases with age, but unlike women it is slightly higher in black men than in non-Hispanic white men. Presentation is with a palpable breast mass. Initial evaluation includes diagnostic mammogram, ultrasound, and core needle biopsy. On histologic diagnosis, 90% are ER-positive, HER2-positive. Surgical options and systemic therapy are similar to those of female counterparts. Tamoxifen reduces the risk of systemic disease in male breast cancer, with similar side effects as seen in women. The utility of aromatase inhibitor therapy is unknown in the adjuvant or metastatic setting.

Breast Cancer in Older Women

Breast cancer risk increases with age (see Table 60.1). In the United States a woman has a 1 in 8 risk of breast cancer diagnosis. The majority of patients diagnosed with breast cancer are ER-positive and over 65 years old. Patients age 70 and older with ER-positive stage 1 disease willing to take 5 years of endocrine therapy have an equivalent overall survival with or without radiation therapy and can therefore safely omit radiation. For women over 70 years of age with more aggressive or higher stage breast cancer, estimation of risk of recurrence, life expectancy, comorbidities, and toxicities of therapies are necessary to tailor therapy. Tools such as "ePrognosis" can be used for life-expectancy estimates based on comorbidities and PREDICT.NHS.UK for estimation of mortality based on tumor stage and prognostic features.

SCREENING

One outcome of advances in breast imaging techniques has been earlier detection of invasive and noninvasive breast cancers. Multiple guidelines have attempted to address screening of women without symptoms of breast cancer. In 2019, The American College of Physicians issued an updated guidance statement that addresses the use of screening mammography in women aged 50 to 74.

These guidelines do not address high-risk patients such as those with a personal history of breast cancer, prior abnormal mammogram or who carry a genetic mutation known to predispose to an increased risk of breast cancer.

CONCLUSION AND FUTURE DIRECTIONS

Breast cancer 5-year survival overall is 90% due to early detection and effective therapies such as chemotherapy and endocrine therapy. Unfortunately, chemotherapy and endocrine therapy have short- and long-term side effects of fatigue, cardiac toxicity, neuropathy, hot flashes, and sexual dysfunction. In an era of personalized medicine, ER-positive, node-negative breast cancer gene expression profile has identified a large proportion of patients who do not benefit from chemotherapy. Ongoing prospective trials will aid in decision making for ER-positive node-positive patients. For stage IV ER-positive patients, CDK 4/6 inhibitors and PIK3CA inhibitors appear to prolong time to progression. Triple-negative breast cancer continues to have a high proportion of patients who relapse and die within a few years of diagnosis; novel therapies are currently in phase 3 trials.

SUGGESTED READINGS

Bland KI, Copeland III EM, Klimberg VS, Gradishar WJ: The breast: comprehensive management of benign and malignant diseases, ed 5, Elsevier Inc, 2018.

DeSantis CE, etal: Breast cancer statistics, 2017, racial disparity in mortality by state, CA Cancer J Clin 67:439–448, 2017.

Giordano S: Breast cancer in men, N Engl J Med 378:2311–2320, 2018.

National Comprehensive Cancer Network Breast Cancer Version 3.2019. http://www.nccn.org/professionals/physician_gls/pdf/breast.pdf. Accessed September 25, 2019.

National Comprehensive Cancer Network Genetic/Familial High-Risk Assessment: Breast/Ovarian Version 3.2019. http://www.nccn.org/professionals/physician_gls/pdf/breast.pdf. Accessed September 25, 2019.

Runowicz C, Leach CR, Henry NL, et al: ACS/ASCO breast cancer survivorship guidelines, J Clin Oncol 34:611–635, 2015.

Screening for Breast Cancer in Average-risk Women: A guidance statement from the American College of Physicians, Ann Intern Med 170(8):547–560, 2019. https://doi.org/10.7326/M18-2147.

Siegel R, Miller KD, Jemal A: Cancer statistics, 2019 CA Cancer J Clin 69:7–34, 2019.

国临床肿瘤学会（ASCO）建议为患者和初级保健医生制定幸存者计划，并将随访管理作为质量标准。

内分泌治疗的依从性

据估计，50% 的 ER 阳性乳腺癌患者由于副作用或费用等障碍没有完成辅助内分泌治疗。可能影响生活质量和依从性的副作用包括化疗诱发的停经、他莫昔芬或芳香化酶抑制剂导致的潮热。最近的一项研究显示使用认知行为疗法可改善潮热和睡眠质量。通过换用药物和（或）针灸、度洛西汀或瑜伽可以减轻芳香化酶抑制剂引起的关节痛。

性功能障碍

不幸的是，乳腺癌患者的性功能障碍是继手术、放疗、化疗和辅助内分泌治疗后常见的副作用。医生应就亲密关系提出开放式问题，使患者的担忧正常化。患者会注意到自我形象改变、性欲减退、阴道干涩和性交困难。有效的干预措施包括使用阴道保湿剂和润滑剂、应用加巴喷丁和文拉法辛治疗潮热、外用利多卡因治疗前庭触痛，以及转诊至性健康专家处。

保留生育能力

根据病例对照研究，确诊乳腺癌后妊娠似乎不会增加乳腺癌的复发风险。化疗可能会影响生育能力，保留生育能力的方法包括取卵和体外受精。一般原则是确诊后 2 年内避免怀孕，因为这段时间是乳腺癌复发的高危期。PROMISE 研究将对诊断乳腺癌并接受治疗后选择停止辅助内分泌治疗以备孕的妇女进行队列跟踪，了解乳腺癌治疗效果。

淋巴水肿

乳房和手臂淋巴水肿可能是手术的并发症，也可能因放射治疗而加重。物理治疗、人工按摩以及佩戴压力胸罩和袖子可减轻这种副作用。

男性乳腺癌

男性乳腺癌占美国所有乳腺癌的 1%。每年约有 2500 名男性被诊断，每年将有 500 名男性死于男性乳腺癌。男性乳腺癌的风险因素包括 gBRCA2 基因突变、Klinefelter 综合征、隐睾或睾丸损伤，以及环境辐射（如原子弹爆炸中的幸存者）。临床研究不包括男性乳腺癌患者。现有的有关男性乳腺癌的数据主要来自小型队列研究。与女性相同，男性乳腺癌的发病率随年龄的增长而增加，但与女性不同的是，黑人男性的发病率略高于非西班牙裔白人男性。临床表现为可触及的乳房肿块。初步评估包括诊断性乳房 X 线、超声和空芯针活检。组织学检查发现，90% 男性乳腺癌为 ER 阳性、HER2 阴性（译者注：原文有误）。手术选择和系统治疗与女性患者相似。他莫昔芬可降低男性乳腺癌患者全身性疾病的风险，副作用与女性类似。芳香化酶抑制剂疗法在辅助治疗或转移性疾病中的作用尚不清楚。

老年女性乳腺癌

乳腺癌风险随年龄增长而增加（见表 60.1）。在美国，妇女被诊断出乳腺癌的风险为 1/8。大多数确诊为乳腺癌的患者都是 ER 阳性且年龄在 65 岁以上。愿意接受 5 年内分泌治疗的 70 岁及以上 ER 阳性的 1 期患者，接受或不接受放疗的总生存率相当，因此可以安全地免于放疗。对于 70 岁以上患有侵袭性更强或分期更高的乳腺癌女性来说，需要对复发风险、预期寿命、合并症和疗法毒性进行评估，以便为其量身定制治疗方案。如 "ePrognosis" 等工具可用于根据合并症估计预期寿命，PREDICT.NHS.UK 可根据肿瘤分期和预后特征估算死亡率。

筛查

乳腺影像技术的进步带来的一个成果就是可以更早地发现浸润性和非浸润性乳腺癌。多项指南都试图解决无乳腺癌症状女性的筛查问题。2019 年，美国内科医师学会针对 50～74 岁女性应用乳腺 X 线筛查发布了指南更新说明。

这些指南并未涉及高风险患者，如有乳腺癌病史、既往乳房 X 线检查结果异常的患者或携带已知易导致乳腺癌风险增加的基因突变的患者。

结论和未来方向

由于早期发现和化疗、内分泌治疗等有效疗法，乳腺癌的 5 年生存率达到 90%。不幸的是，化疗和内分泌治疗有疲劳、心脏毒性、神经病变、潮热和性功能障碍等短期和长期副作用。在个体化医疗时代，ER 阳性、淋巴结阴性乳腺癌基因表达谱已识别出很大一部分无法从化疗中获益患者。正在进行的前瞻性试验将有助于 ER 阳性、淋巴结阳性患者的治疗决策。对于 ER 阳性的 Ⅳ 期患者，CDK 4/6 抑制剂和 PIK3CA 抑制剂似乎可延长疾病进展时间。三阴性乳腺癌患者在确诊后几年内复发和死亡的比例仍然很高；新型疗法目前正在进行三期试验。

推荐阅读

Bland KI, Copeland III EM, Klimberg VS, Gradishar WJ: The breast: comprehensive management of benign and malignant diseases, ed 5, Elsevier Inc, 2018.

DeSantis CE, etal: Breast cancer statistics, 2017, racial disparity in mortality by state, CA Cancer J Clin 67:439–448, 2017.

Giordano S: Breast cancer in men, N Engl J Med 378:2311–2320, 2018.

National Comprehensive Cancer Network Breast Cancer Version 3.2019. http://www.nccn.org/professionals/physician_gls/pdf/breast.pdf. Accessed September 25, 2019.

National Comprehensive Cancer Network Genetic/Familial High-Risk Assessment: Breast/Ovarian Version 3.2019. http://www.nccn.org/professionals/physician_gls/pdf/breast.pdf. Accessed September 25, 2019.

Runowicz C, Leach CR, Henry NL, et al: ACS/ASCO breast cancer survivorship guidelines, J Clin Oncol 34:611–635, 2015.

Screening for Breast Cancer in Average-risk Women: A guidance statement from the American College of Physicians, Ann Intern Med 170(8):547–560, 2019. https://doi.org/10.7326/M18-2147.

Siegel R, Miller KD, Jemal A: Cancer statistics, 2019 CA Cancer J Clin 69:7–34, 2019.

8. Gynecological Cancer

Christina Bandera, Tarra B. Evans, Don Dizon

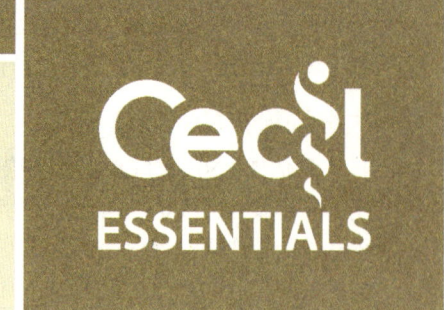

OVARIAN CANCER

Epidemiology

Ovarian cancer is the most difficult gynecologic cancer to cure, because over 70% of cases present with metastatic disease, and over 80% of cases will recur despite treatment. Ovarian cancer is the seventh most common cancer affecting women worldwide. In North America, Europe, Australia, and New Zealand it is the most common cause of death from a gynecologic malignancy.

A woman's lifetime risk of developing ovarian cancer is 1.4%. Most ovarian cancers are sporadic; however, a family history of ovarian cancer is the strongest risk factor for developing disease due to inherited genetic mutations. For example, inherited BRCA1 and BRCA2 mutations carry a 40% to 60% and a 15% to 20% risk of developing ovarian cancer, respectively. Lynch syndrome, the result of inherited mutations in mismatch repair genes, portends a 12% risk of ovarian cancer.

Currently, guidelines recommend that all women with ovarian carcinoma receive genetic counseling. Multigene panel testing is available to detect mutations that may confer a greater risk of developing the disease and can help guide targeted treatment recommendations. Furthermore, genetic screening enables identification of family members at risk who may benefit from prophylactic removal of the ovaries and fallopian tubes, as well as specialized screening programs for other cancers. (Please see Chapter 2.)

Other significant risk factors for ovarian cancer include reproductive factors associated with increased ovulation such as early menarche, late menopause, and nulliparity. Protective factors against ovarian cancer include pregnancy, breast-feeding, and use of oral contraceptives. Talcum powder has been associated with asbestos contamination, and its use on the perineum has been studied for a potential link to ovarian cancer, with conflicting results.

Pathology

Ovarian carcinoma refers to a family of tumors arising from the epithelial lining of the ovary, fallopian tube, and peritoneum. More recently, it is thought that the majority of ovarian cancers originate in the fallopian tube due to the frequent concurrent finding of premalignant serous tubal intraepithelial carcinoma (STIC). The most common cell type is serous carcinoma. Other histologies include endometrioid, mucinous, and clear cell patterns.

Borderline ovarian neoplasms are an unusual category of ovarian neoplasm with a favorable prognosis that can spread and recur but do not exhibit invasion of tissue. Treatment is surgical because these tumors do not respond to chemotherapy.

Nonepithelial ovarian cancers account for less than 5% of ovarian cancers and originate from sex-cord cells, stromal cells, and germ cells of the ovary. These rare tumors often occur in adolescent females, and pathologic classification determines treatment and prognosis.

Clinical Presentation

Ovarian cancer is often called the cancer that "whispers" because symptoms are subtle and nonspecific. Bloating, abdominal pain, gastrointestinal disturbance, and bladder symptoms may present once diffuse carcinomatosis develops with nodules of cancer and ascites throughout the abdomen and pelvis. Cancer is often detected during imaging for work-up of sudden GI or GU symptoms. Common sites of metastasis include the omentum, peritoneal surfaces, lymph nodes in the pelvis and abdomen, and pleural effusions. Distant metastases to the lungs, liver, bone and brain are less common. Over 70% of patients are diagnosed with disease beyond the pelvis considered stage IIIC or IV.

Diagnosis and Staging

Ovarian cancer is diagnosed with histologic confirmation of a pelvic mass or abnormal tissue typically identified on ultrasound, computed tomography (CT), or magnetic resonance imaging (MRI). Advanced ovarian cancer is suspected on imaging with the presence of an adnexal mass accompanied by ascites, peritoneal carcinomatosis or enlarged pelvic and para-aortic lymph nodes. Patients with an enlarged complex ovarian mass and no evidence of metastatic disease should have surgery for resection of the mass with effort made to avoid disrupting the integrity of the neoplasm, because rupture may spread cancer if present. If widespread disease is seen on imaging, a clinician may recommend an image-guided biopsy of solid tumor, drainage of ascites or surgical resection to obtain tumor for tissue diagnosis.

The tumor biomarker carbohydrate antigen 125 (CA 125) is a mucin-type glycoprotein secreted into the bloodstream by cancer cells and can be useful in the initial work-up and for monitoring response to treatment, but the test should not be used for diagnostic purposes alone as the marker is nonspecific. CA 125 may be elevated in noncancer conditions such as menstruation, benign ovarian tumors, endometriosis, fibroids, pelvic infection, congestive heart failure, and pleural effusions.

Ovarian cancer stage is assigned by review of clinical, pathologic, and radiologic evaluation. Early disease is isolated to the ovaries or fallopian tubes (FIGO [International Federation of Gynecology and Obstetrics] stage I) or to the true pelvis (stage II). Diffuse carcinomatosis or abdominal/pelvic adenopathy (FIGO stage III) and distant metastases to sites including liver parenchyma, lungs, bone and brain (FIGO stage IV) comprise advanced stage disease.

Treatment

The treatment for presumed early stage ovarian carcinoma is surgical resection and staging to evaluate for metastatic disease. Because

妇科癌症

周娜 译 程月鹃 邵亚娟 审校 巴一 通审

卵巢癌

流行病学

卵巢癌是最难治愈的妇科癌症，因为超过70%的病例会出现转移性疾病，超过80%的病例虽经治疗仍会复发。卵巢癌是全球女性第七大常见癌症。在北美、欧洲、澳大利亚和新西兰，它是最常见的妇科恶性肿瘤致死原因。

女性一生中患卵巢癌的风险为1.4%。大多数卵巢癌是散发性的，然而，对于由遗传基因突变所导致的卵巢癌而言，卵巢癌家族史是最大的风险因素。例如，携带遗传性BRCA1和BRCA2基因突变的女性患卵巢癌的风险分别为40%～60%和15%～20%。而林奇综合征，即遗传性的错配修复基因突变，预示患卵巢癌的风险为12%。

目前，指南推荐对于所有罹患卵巢癌的女性进行遗传咨询。多基因检测可用于发现可能会增加患病风险的基因突变并帮助指导靶向治疗。此外，基因筛查还可以确定哪些高危家庭成员可受益于卵巢和输卵管的预防性切除，以及针对其他肿瘤的筛查（请见第2章）。

卵巢癌的其他重要风险因素包括与排卵增加有关的生殖因素，如月经初潮早、绝经晚和未生育。卵巢癌的保护因素包括怀孕、母乳喂养和使用口服避孕药。滑石粉被指与石棉污染相关，曾有研究尝试分析会阴部使用滑石粉与卵巢癌的潜在联系，但结果尚不一致。

病理学

卵巢癌是指来源于卵巢、输卵管和腹膜上皮内膜的一系列肿瘤。最近，由于经常同时发现癌前病变，即浆液性输卵管上皮内癌（STIC），人们认为大多数卵巢癌起源于输卵管。最常见的细胞类型是浆液性癌。其他组织形态包括子宫内膜样癌、黏液腺癌和透明细胞癌。

交界性卵巢肿瘤是一种不常见的卵巢肿瘤，预后良好，可以发生扩散和复发，但不会出现组织浸润。由于这些肿瘤对化疗没有应答，因此治疗方法是手术切除。

非上皮性卵巢癌在卵巢癌中占比不到5%，起源于卵巢性索细胞、基质细胞和生殖细胞。这些罕见肿瘤通常发生于青春期女性，病理分类决定了治疗和预后。

临床表现

卵巢癌症状隐匿且缺乏特异性。腹部和盆腔出现弥漫性癌结节和腹水时可能出现腹胀、腹痛、胃肠道不适和膀胱相关症状。卵巢癌也可能因突发消化道或膀胱症状而进行影像学检查时发现。常见的卵巢癌转移部位包括网膜、腹膜表面、腹盆腔淋巴结以及胸腔积液。累及肺、肝、骨和脑的远处转移较少见。超过盆腔的疾病属于ⅢC期或Ⅳ期，占全部卵巢癌患者的70%以上。

诊断和分期

卵巢癌通常是由超声波、计算机断层成像（CT）或磁共振成像（MRI）发现典型的盆腔肿块或异常组织，并由组织学证实。如果影像学检查发现附件肿块并伴有腹水、腹膜转移癌，或盆腔和腹主动脉旁淋巴结肿大，则应怀疑进展期卵巢癌。患者如果仅有卵巢肿物且无转移性疾病证据，应首先寻求手术切除肿物且术中尽量避免破坏肿瘤的完整性，因为如果是癌则肿物破裂会导致癌症扩散。如果影像学检查已确定疾病广泛转移，临床医生可能的建议包括影像引导下的肿瘤活检、腹水引流或手术切除肿瘤以获取组织学诊断。

肿瘤生物标志物糖类抗原125（CA 125）是一种由癌细胞分泌到血液中的黏蛋白型糖蛋白，可用于初步检查和监测治疗反应。但由于不具有特异性，该标志物不能单独用来诊断卵巢癌。此外，CA 125也可能在月经期、良性卵巢肿瘤、子宫内膜异位症、子宫肌瘤、盆腔感染、充血性心力衰竭和胸腔积液等非癌症情况下升高。

卵巢癌的分期可根据临床、病理和放射评估结果确定。早期病变局限于卵巢或输卵管[FIGO（国际妇产科联盟）Ⅰ期]或真骨盆（Ⅱ期）。进展期卵巢癌包括：肿瘤腹/盆腔播散或腹/盆腔淋巴结转移（FIGO Ⅲ期）和远处转移至肝、肺、骨和脑等部位（FIGO Ⅳ期）。

治疗

如推定为早期卵巢癌，其治疗方法是手术切除，同时做分期手术以评估转移病灶。由于卵巢癌可能通过癌细胞脱落于腹腔种植、淋巴道或血行扩散，所以

TABLE 8.1	Addition of Maintenance Bevacizumab to Front-Line Therapy for Ovarian Cancer Shows Improved Progression-Free Survival (PFS) in Two Studies					
Study	Randomization	N	Median PFS	Hazard Ratio	P-value	Survival Advantage
GOG-218	C/P + placebo	625	10.3 mo	0.91	0.16	No
	C/P + bev	625	11.2 mo	0.72	<0.001	
	C/P + bev →7 bev-M	623	14.1 mo			
ICON7	C/P	764	17.3	0.81	0.004	Yes (for those at high risk for PD)
	C/P + bev →7 bev-M	764	19.0			

Data from Burger RA, et al. NEJM 2011; 365:2473-83; Perren TJ, et al. NEJM 2011; 365:2484-96; Tewari, et al. J Clin Oncol. 2019;37:2317-2328.
bev, Bevacizumab; bev-M, bev maintenance; C/P, cisplatin + paclitaxel; PD, progression of disease.

ovarian cancer may spread through peritoneal shedding of cells, lymphatically or through the bloodstream, staging includes removing the ovaries, fallopian tubes, uterus, omentum, lymph nodes, and peritoneal biopsies. High-grade cancers isolated to the ovary, or cancer with any sign of spread beyond the ovary, is treated with adjuvant chemotherapy. The standard of care calls for the administration of intravenous carboplatin and paclitaxel every 3 weeks. For early stage ovarian carcinoma, there is no consensus on whether three or six cycles should be administered; one study that looked at the impact of histology on outcomes following chemotherapy suggested that compared to three cycles, six cycles was associated with a significantly lower risk of recurrence for women with serous cancers (HR 0.33, 95% CI 0.14-0.77) but not for those with nonserous cancers (HR 0.94, 95% CI 0.60-1.49). We continue to recommend six cycles for women with early stage ovarian cancer, though have a lower threshold to discontinue treatment after three cycles for women with nonserous cancers, if they opt to stop or if side effects intervene.

In advanced stage disease, the care team must decide whether to begin treatment with a primary "debulking" surgery or neoadjuvant chemotherapy (NACT). Debulking is favored when imaging suggests all visible tumor may be resected at the time of surgery. NACT is favored with a low likelihood of achieving cytoreduction to no visible disease or in patients with major perioperative risk factors related to comorbidities and frailty, which is consistent with the ASCO/SGO Clinical Guidelines in this population. After three to four cycles of NACT, patients are assessed for an interval debulking surgery (IDS) followed by additional chemotherapy. One randomized trial showed a survival advantage in favor of heated intraperitoneal chemotherapy for patients undergoing an IDS; confirmatory trials are underway. In either case, adjuvant therapy is indicated, and we suggest patients receive up to three cycles following surgery to complete at least six cycles total of chemotherapy. Finally, data show that bevacizumab confers a progression-free survival advantage, though this did not translate into an overall survival benefit in the American trial, GOG 218 (Table 8.1).

Following first-line chemotherapy, women with newly diagnosed ovarian cancer should be offered maintenance treatment using a poly-ADP-ribose polymerase (PARP) inhibitor. Multiple trials have shown that treatment is associated with significant improvement in disease-free survival, particularly in those with a mutation in BRCA (mBRCA, germline or somatic), with one trial also supporting its use in combination with bevacizumab in those without a mutation but with evidence of homologous recombination deficiency (HRD). While niraparib was associated with a survival advantage in women without mBRCA or HRD, the benefit was much smaller than in other groups. As such, while we offer PARP inhibition as maintenance treatment to all patients after completion of adjuvant therapy, we strongly recommend it for women with mBRCA or evidence of HRD.

Recurrent ovarian cancer can be treated with additional chemotherapy and surgery can be considered if there are resectable sites of limited disease. If the recurrence occurs more than 6 months after completing primary platinum-based treatment, the tumor is considered "platinum sensitive" and retreatment with a platinum combination is preferred. In these patients, evidence supports the use of PARP inhibitors in the maintenance setting, regardless of whether patients have mBRCA or HRD. When recurrence occurs in less than 6 months, the cancer is considered "platinum resistant," and an alternative agent is chosen. Patients with recurrent ovarian cancer do not have curable disease; therefore, clinical trials should be offered whenever possible.

Prognosis

Early ovarian cancer is often curable with surgery and chemotherapy. Stage I disease has an 80% to 90% 5-year survival, and stage II disease portends a 60% to 70% 5-year survival. Unfortunately, patients with advanced stage disease usually recur and develop treatment resistance. Eventually treatment turns to best supportive care. Bowel obstruction from massive carcinomatosis is a common terminal event for women with ovarian cancer. Five-year survival for women with stage III to IV disease ranges from 18% to 50% depending on the pattern of disease.

UTERINE CANCER

Epidemiology

Endometrial cancer is the most common gynecologic cancer in North America and in Northern and Eastern Europe. Worldwide, it is the sixth most common malignancy affecting women, and it ranks as the fourteenth cause of cancer death.

Increased circulating estrogen without progesterone to balance stimulation of the endometrial lining is associated with endometrial cancer development. Obesity is a strong risk factor due to high levels of circulating estrogen via conversion of androgens to estrogen by aromatase within adipose cells. Other increased estrogen-related risk factors include anovulatory menstrual cycles, nulliparity, early menarche, late menopause, estrogen producing ovarian neoplasms (benign thecomas and malignant dysgerminomas), and estrogen replacement without the use of protective progesterone. Breast cancer treatment with tamoxifen blocks estrogen action in the breast but has pro-estrogen effects on the endometrium resulting in a 2- to 5-fold increased risk of endometrial cancer after 5 years of use.

Women with hereditary Lynch syndrome (see section on epidemiology of ovarian cancer) have a 60% lifetime risk of developing endometrial cancer and require screening with annual endometrial biopsy, and when childbearing is complete, a hysterectomy with bilateral salpingo-oophorectomy is recommended. Diabetes and hypertension are associated with increased risk of endometrial cancer. Smoking is

表8.1 卵巢癌一线治疗加入贝伐珠单抗维持治疗在两项研究中显示改善无进展生存（PFS）

研究	随机	n	中位PFS	风险比	P值	生存获益
GOG-218	C/P＋安慰剂	625	10.3个月	0.91	0.16	无
	C/P＋贝伐珠单抗	625	11.2个月	0.72	<0.001	
	C/P＋贝伐珠单抗→7贝伐珠单抗-M	623	14.1个月			
ICON7	C/P	764	17.3个月	0.81	0.004	有（对于有高进展风险的患者）
	C/P贝伐珠单抗→7贝伐珠单抗-M	764	19.0个月			

引自 Burger RA，et al. NEJM 2011；365：2473-83；Perren TJ，et al. NEJM 2011；365：2484-96；Tewari，et al. J Clin Oncol. 2019；37：2317-2328.
贝伐珠单抗-M：贝伐珠单抗维持治疗；C/P，顺铂＋紫杉醇。

分期手术应包括切除卵巢、输卵管、子宫、网膜、淋巴结并行腹膜活检。对于仅限于卵巢的高级别肿瘤，或存在任何卵巢外扩散迹象的肿瘤，术后应进行辅助化疗。标准治疗方法为每3周一次的卡铂联合紫杉醇静脉化疗。对于早期卵巢癌术后进行3周期还是6周期的辅助化疗尚无共识；一项研究探讨了组织学类型对化疗疗效的影响，结果显示，与3周期化疗相比，6周期化疗与浆液性癌患者的复发风险显著降低相关（HR 0.33，95% CI 0.14～0.77），但与非浆液性癌女性的复发风险无关（HR 0.94，95% CI 0.60～1.49）。我们继续推荐针对早期卵巢癌患者术后进行6周期的辅助化疗，而针对非浆液性癌患者，如患者选择停止治疗或出现副作用，则更建议3周期后停止治疗。

对于进展期卵巢癌，治疗团队必须决定初始治疗是"细胞减灭"手术，还是新辅助化疗（NACT）。如影像学检查提示手术可能切除所有可见肿瘤，则倾向于"细胞减灭"手术。如细胞减灭至无可见疾病的可能性较低，或患者具有合并症及衰弱等严重围术期危险因素，则倾向于首选新辅助化疗，这与ASCO/SGO临床指南对这一人群的推荐一致。在接受了3～4周期的NACT后，需对患者进行评估能否行化疗间期肿瘤细胞减灭手术（IDS），术后继续化疗。一项随机试验显示腹腔内热灌注化疗使接受了IDS的卵巢癌患者获得生存增益；目前，确证性研究正在进行中。无论初始治疗方式选择哪一种，术后辅助治疗均有必要，我们建议术后进行3周期的化疗，以完成总体至少6周期的化疗。最后，有研究结果显示贝伐珠单抗可带来无进展生存期获益，但在美国开展的GOG 218研究中并没有转化为总生存获益（表8.1）。

新确诊的卵巢癌患者一线治疗后应接受聚ADP核糖聚合酶（PARP）抑制剂的维持治疗。多项研究显示PARP抑制剂可显著提高无疾病生存，尤其是携带BRCA基因突变（mBRCA，胚系或体细胞突变）的卵巢癌患者。一项试验还支持PARP抑制剂与贝伐珠单抗联合用于无mBRCA但携带同源重组缺陷（HRD）特征的患者。虽然尼拉帕利在无mBRCA或HRD的患者中均显示生存获益，但其获益远小于其他患者组别。因此，尽管我们为所有完成辅助化疗的卵巢癌患者提供PARP抑制剂维持治疗，但我们更强烈建议携带mBRCA或HRD特征的卵巢癌患者使用该药物。

复发性卵巢癌可考虑再次化疗，如存在可切除的局限性病变，可手术治疗。如果疾病复发发生在完成以铂类为基础的初始治疗后6个月及以上，则该肿瘤被认为是"铂敏感型"肿瘤，应首选再次应用以铂类为基础的联合化疗。对于这些患者，无论是否携带mBRCA或HRD，临床证据均支持在维持治疗中使用PARP抑制剂。如疾病复发时间少于6个月，则被视为"铂耐药"，应选择其他药物。复发性卵巢癌患者无法治愈，应尽可能提供临床研究选择。

预后

早期卵巢癌通常可以通过手术和化疗治愈。Ⅰ期患者的5年生存率为80%～90%，Ⅱ期患者的5年生存率为60%～70%。不幸的是，晚期患者通常会复发并产生耐药。最终将转为最佳支持治疗。腹盆腔播散导致的肠梗阻是晚期卵巢癌患者的常见症状。Ⅲ～Ⅳ期患者的5年生存率为18%～50%，取决于疾病类型。

子宫癌

流行病学

子宫内膜癌是北美、北欧和东欧最常见的妇科癌症。在全球范围内，子宫内膜癌是影响妇女的第六大常见恶性肿瘤，也是第十四大癌症死因。

循环雌激素增加且缺乏孕激素来平衡雌激素对子宫内膜的刺激，这与子宫内膜癌的发生密切相关。肥胖是导致循环雌激素高水平的一个很强的风险因素，在脂肪细胞内芳香化酶将雄激素转化为雌激素。其他与雌激素增加的风险因素包括：无排卵月经周期、未生育、月经初潮早、绝经晚、产雌激素卵巢肿瘤（良性泡膜细胞瘤和恶性无性细胞瘤），以及未同时使用保护性孕激素的雌激素替代治疗。使用他莫昔芬治疗乳腺癌会阻断雌激素在乳腺中的作用，但会对子宫内膜产生促雌激素作用，导致使用他莫昔芬5年后患子宫内膜癌的风险增加2～5倍。

患有遗传性林奇综合征（见卵巢癌流行病学部分）的女性一生中罹患子宫内膜癌的风险为60%，需要每年进行子宫内膜活检筛查，并推荐其在完成生育后进行子宫切除术和双侧输卵管卵巢切除术。糖尿病和高血压与子宫内膜癌风险增加有关。吸烟则会降低子

associated with a decreased rate of endometrial cancer, likely due to the association with low circulating estrogen.

Pathology

Endometrial cancer traditionally has been divided into two categories: type 1 and type 2. Type 1 endometrial cancers are hormone-induced, arising from the hyperplastic precursor endometrioid intraepithelial neoplasia (EIN). These low-grade endometrioid type cancers are usually limited to the uterus and have a good prognosis. Type 2 endometrial cancer is the more aggressive form of cancer, more likely to metastasize, and carries a worse prognosis. Type 2 histologies include high-grade endometrioid, serous, clear cell, and carcinosarcoma. More recently, genomic analysis has been used to stratify endometrial cancer into four groups: (1) *POLE* gene ultramutated; (2) tumors with microsatellite instability hypermutated; (3) copy number low; and (4) copy number high (serous tumors and one quarter of high-grade endometrioid tumors). Data suggest that the groups confer prognostic information in terms of progression-free survival with POLE-type tumors having the best prognosis and those with high copy number having the worst prognosis.

Mesenchymal cancers of the uterus are rare and include cancers, such as sarcoma, arising from the myometrial wall of the uterus and cancers arising from the endometrial stromal cells.

Clinical Presentation

Studies show that 70% to 90% of women with endometrial cancer present with postmenopausal bleeding. In premenopausal women, irregular or heavy vaginal bleeding is the most common symptom. An abnormal Papanicolaou (Pap) smear, or abnormal imaging of the uterus, may also lead to a diagnosis of endometrial cancer. Mesenchymal cancers may present with abnormal uterine bleeding or pain.

Diagnosis and Staging

Postmenopausal women with any uterine bleeding, even spotting, should be evaluated for endometrial cancer. The work-up includes a full gynecologic exam with endometrial sampling and imaging to evaluate the appearance of the endometrium (normal endometrial thickness measures ≤4 mm after menopause). Endometrial biopsy may be performed as an office procedure and has a high sensitivity when the endometrial lining measures 11 mm or less. A thicker lining may require further evaluation with a dilatation and curettage of the uterus to definitively rule out malignancy. Premenopausal women with persistent bleeding between menses should also be evaluated with endometrial sampling and radiographic imaging, especially those presenting with known risk factors for endometrial cancer.

If a high-grade cancer is identified on endometrial sampling, then CT of the abdomen and pelvis is recommended to assess for the presence of metastatic disease.

Staging of endometrial cancer is surgical. FIGO stage I disease is cancer limited to the uterus, whereas stage II involves the cervical stroma. Stage III includes disease involving the ovaries, tubes, and regional lymph nodes. Stage IV is defined as peritoneal carcinomatosis, liver metastases, or other metastases beyond the abdomen and pelvis.

Treatment

Unless widespread metastatic disease is identified on preoperative imaging, standard treatment for endometrial cancer is a simple hysterectomy (Fig. 8.1) with bilateral salpingo-oophorectomy and assessment for lymph node metastases. If the uterus is small, this procedure may be performed with a laparoscopic or robot-assisted laparoscopic technique. Laparotomy may be indicated for a large uterus that cannot be extracted vaginally. Sentinel nodal evaluation has largely replaced complete pelvic and para-aortic lymphadenectomy. This procedure

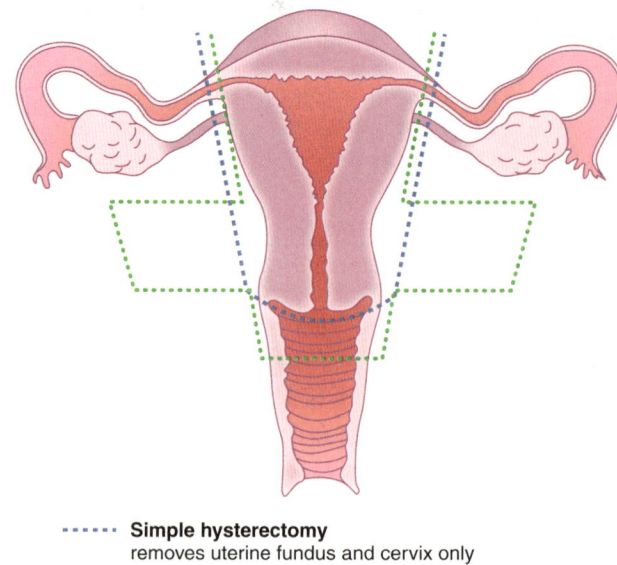

- - - - - **Simple hysterectomy**
removes uterine fundus and cervix only

- - - - - **Radical hysterectomy**
includes parametrial tissue surrounding cervix and upper vagina

Fig. 8.1 Simple hysterectomy involves removal of uterus including fundus and cervix. Radical hysterectomy extends the surgical margin with removal of surrounding parametrial tissue and upper vagina.

involves injecting the cervix with dye and removing lymph nodes that collect the dye. The advantages of sentinel node dissection include a limited, more targeted surgery, with less risk of surgical complications including lower extremity lymphedema.

Early stage endometrial cancer with low grade histology that invades less than 50% of the myometrium has an excellent prognosis for cure with surgery alone. The protocols for administering adjuvant therapy for endometrial cancer after surgical staging are complex. A careful review of pathologic risk factors by a multidisciplinary team that considers the patient's comorbidites is important in the treatment planning process. Recommendations may include vaginal cuff brachytherapy, pelvic radiation, and/or chemotherapy. Stage 1 tumors that invade more than 50% of the myometrium are typically treated with vaginal radiation to prevent local recurrence of cancer. Tumors with cervical stromal involvement are treated with additional whole pelvic radiation. If lymph node metastases or other disease beyond the uterus is identified, then chemotherapy with intravenous carboplatin and paclitaxel with or without radiation is typically recommended. Some patients with high grade cancer such as the serous subtype may also benefit from chemotherapy even if cancer is isolated to the uterus.

Treatment for recurrent endometrial cancer is tailored to the site of recurrence. A vaginal recurrence is typically treated with localized radiation. Distant recurrences often require platinum-based chemotherapy; however, a low-grade metastatic endometrial cancer may respond to antiestrogen hormonal therapy alone. For those who progress on first-line chemotherapy, clinical trials should be pursued. To date, there are no FDA-approved agents in the second- or later-line setting for these patients.

A subset of women with early endometrial cancer may opt to forego standard hysterectomy. This includes young women wishing to preserve fertility and elderly, or frail women, who have a high surgical risk. These women may be treated with high-dose progesterone therapy using a progesterone secreting intrauterine device or oral tablets. Success rates greater than 80% are reported for women with low-grade cancers without evidence of myometrial invasion on pretreatment

内膜癌的发病率，这可能与循环雌激素水平较低有关。

病理学

子宫内膜癌传统上分为 1 型和 2 型。1 型子宫内膜癌是由激素诱发的，产生于增生的前体子宫内膜样上皮内瘤变（EIN）。这些低级别子宫内膜样癌通常局限于子宫，预后良好。2 型子宫内膜癌是侵袭性更强的癌症，更容易转移，预后较差。2 型组织学包括高级别子宫内膜样癌、浆液性癌、透明细胞癌和癌肉瘤。最近，基因组分析将子宫内膜癌分为四个分子亚型：① POLE 基因超突变型；②微卫星不稳定高突变型；③低拷贝数型；④高拷贝数型（浆液性肿瘤和 1/4 高级别子宫内膜样肿瘤）。数据表明这些不同亚型在无进展生存期方面预后不同，其中 POLE 基因超突变型预后最佳，而高拷贝数型肿瘤的预后最差。

子宫间质癌非常罕见，包括子宫肌壁产生的癌（如肉瘤）和源自子宫内膜基质细胞的癌。

临床表现

研究表明，70%～90% 的子宫内膜癌妇女存在绝经后出血。绝经前妇女最常见的症状是不规则的或大量的阴道出血。巴氏涂片异常或子宫影像异常也可能提示子宫内膜癌。子宫间质癌可能表现为异常子宫出血或疼痛。

诊断和分期

绝经后妇女如出现任何子宫出血迹象，甚至是点状出血，都应进行子宫内膜癌的筛查。检查包括子宫内膜取样以及评估子宫内膜外观的影像学检查（绝经后正常子宫内膜厚度 ≤ 4 mm）在内的全面妇科检查。子宫内膜活检可在诊室进行，且当子宫内膜厚度在 11 mm 或以下时，活检的灵敏度较高。如果整体内膜较厚，建议进行诊断性刮宫以进一步评估，以明确排除恶性肿瘤。在两次月经之间持续出血的绝经前妇女，尤其是那些已知具有子宫内膜癌风险因素的妇女，也应接受子宫内膜取样和影像学评估。

如果在子宫内膜采样中发现高级别癌症，则建议进行针对腹部和盆腔的 CT 检查，以评估是否存在转移性疾病。

子宫内膜癌的分期是通过手术完成的。FIGO Ⅰ 期定义为局限于子宫的肿瘤，Ⅱ 期为侵犯宫颈基质的肿瘤。Ⅲ 期肿瘤累及卵巢、输卵管及区域淋巴结。Ⅳ 期定义为肿瘤出现腹膜播散、肝转移或腹盆腔以外的其他部位转移。

治疗方法

如果术前影像学检查没有发现广泛转移，子宫内膜癌的标准治疗方法是子宫切除术（图 8.1）联合双侧卵巢输卵管切除术，并同时评估淋巴结转移情况。如果子宫较小，可采用腹腔镜或机器人辅助腹腔镜技术进行手术。如果子宫较大且无法经阴道取出，则可能

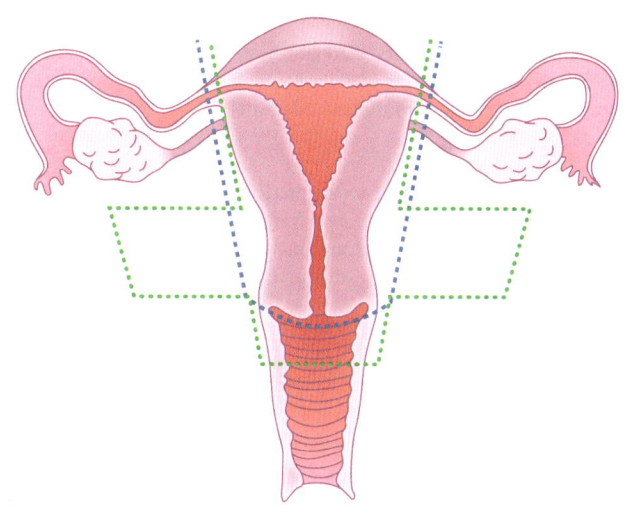

----- 单纯子宫切除术
仅切除子宫底和子宫颈

----- 根治性子宫切除术
包括宫颈周围的宫旁组织和阴道近端

图 8.1 单纯子宫切除术对子宫的切除包括子宫底和子宫颈。根治性子宫切除术扩大手术范围至周围宫旁组织和阴道近端

需要开腹手术。前哨淋巴结评估已在很大程度上取代了全盆腔和主动脉旁淋巴结切除术。操作流程是向宫颈注射染料，并清除那些积聚了染料的淋巴结。前哨淋巴结清扫的优点是手术范围局限，手术针对性更强，包括下肢淋巴水肿在内的手术并发症风险更低。

组织学分级较低且侵犯子宫肌层深度小于 50% 的早期子宫内膜癌，单纯手术的预后极佳，存在治愈可能。子宫内膜癌手术分期后的辅助治疗方案非常复杂。在制订治疗计划的过程中，多学科团队对病理风险因素进行仔细核查并兼顾合并症显得尤为重要。治疗推荐包括阴道袖带近距离放射治疗、盆腔放疗和（或）化疗。侵及子宫肌层深度 50% 以上的 1 期肿瘤通常采用阴道放射治疗，以防止局部复发。宫颈基质受累的肿瘤，则采用额外的全盆腔放射治疗。如发现淋巴结转移或子宫以外的其他转移病灶，则通常采用卡铂和紫杉醇的静脉化疗联合或不联合放疗。一些高级别肿瘤（如浆液性癌）患者，即使肿瘤仅局限于子宫，也可能从化疗中获益。

复发性子宫内膜癌的治疗根据复发部位而制定。阴道复发通常采用局部放射治疗。远处复发通常需要以铂类为基础的联合化疗；而低级别的转移性子宫内膜癌可能单用抗雌激素内分泌治疗就能有治疗反应。对于一线化疗进展的患者，应考虑进入临床试验。迄今为止，美国食品药物管理局还没有批准针对这些患者的二线或三线治疗药物。

一部分患有早期子宫内膜癌的女性可能会选择放弃标准的子宫切除术，包括希望保留生育能力的年轻女性，以及手术风险较高的老年或体弱女性。这些患者可以使用分泌孕酮的宫内节育器或口服片剂进行大剂量孕酮治疗。有报道称，对于在治疗前磁共振成像中没有子宫肌层受侵证据的低级别癌症患者，成功率超过 80%。

MRI imaging. Ongoing surveillance or hysterectomy when childbearing is complete is recommended for young patients. For frail patients, progesterone therapy is continued indefinitely.

Prognosis
Endometrial cancer isolated to the uterus is curable in 80% to 90% of cases. Rates of cure for more advanced disease are lower, while advanced stage IV disease remains incurable. Sadly, for women with endometrial cancer presenting with carcinomatosis, the 5-year survival rate is less than 25%.

CERVICAL CANCER

Epidemiology
Cervical cancer is the most preventable gynecologic cancer. Unfortunately, it remains the most common malignancy of the female reproductive tract worldwide and is a leading cause of cancer-related death in developing countries. In the United States, it is the third most common gynecologic cancer. The primary risk factor for developing cervical cancer is infection with a high-risk subtype of the human papillomavirus (HPV). As nearly all cancers of the cervix are the result of HPV-associated cytopathologic changes, infection with the virus is considered a necessary cause in disease development. The incidence and mortality of cervical cancer are influenced by access to screening programs. Thus, resource poor settings with limited access to Pap screening have higher rates of cervical cancer morbidity and mortality. Other risk factors for cervical cancer include smoking, immunosuppression, and diethylstilbestrol (DES) exposure.

HPV infects the female genital tract via sexual transmission. Subtypes are termed high-risk (HR) when they are associated with preinvasive and invasive cervical disease. There are 15 primary HRHPV subtypes associated with the development of cervical cancer; however, HPV-16 and -18 are responsible for 50% and 20% of cervical cancer cases, respectively. While many individuals will clear the HPV virus, persistence of HPV infection is associated with an increased risk for developing preinvasive neoplasia or invasive cervical cancer. Due to the causal relationship of HPV and cervical cancer, vaccines have been developed targeting HRHPV subtypes to prevent the development of HPV associated cervical pathology. In 2006, the FDA approved use of the Gardasil quadrivalent vaccine for the prevention of anogenital lesions, which covered six HRHPV subtypes for females aged 9 to 26 years old. Currently, the only FDA-approved vaccine in the US is Gardasil 9, covering HPV types 6, 11, 16, 18, 31, 33, 45, 52, and 58 for females and males ages 9 to 45 years old.

Pathology
The outer cellular layer of the cervix that lies within the vagina is comprised of squamous epithelium. The endocervical canal is comprised of columnar epithelium. The region where endocervical columnar epithelium is replaced by squamous epithelium—the transformation zone—serves as the primary site of HPV-related preinvasive and invasive lesions of the cervix. The majority of cervical cancers are squamous carcinomas (75%) and adenocarcinomas (25%). Other extremely rare types of cervical cancer include neuroendocrine, adenosquamous, clear cell, and undifferentiated carcinoma.

Clinical Presentation
In early stage disease, patients do not typically experience symptoms. If symptoms are present, they often include abnormal vaginal bleeding, bleeding with intercourse, discharge, or pelvic discomfort.

Cervical cancer spreads by local extension to surrounding tissues, followed by nodal metastasis and then hematologic dissemination. Patients with advanced stage disease may have symptoms related to involvement of surrounding structures. Local tumor infiltration may result in significant vaginal bleeding and pelvic pain or urinary or bowel complaints. These patients are often noted to have a large cervical mass on physical examination or imaging.

Diagnosis and Staging
The majority of cervical cancers are diagnosed through cervical biopsies performed as a result of a screening Pap that identifies abnormal cervical cytology or persistent HRHPV. In patients who have not undergone routine Pap screening, cervical cancer is diagnosed through biopsies of grossly abnormal appearing cervical tissue or masses. Regardless of PAP smear cytology, patients with persistent HRHPV subtypes should have a diagnostic biopsy for the presence of cervical pathology.

Cervical cancer is clinically and radiographically staged FIGO I through IV. Subcategories within each stage are based on the extent of disease. Cervical cancer is categorized into early stage disease (stages IA-IB1), locally advanced disease (stages IB2-IVA), and metastatic disease (stage IVB). Early stage cancers are small tumors limited to the cervix. Locally advanced disease refers to larger tumors and tumors that have invaded beyond the uterus and extend into nearby pelvic structures, including the bladder and rectum. Metastatic disease refers to cancer that has spread beyond the pelvic organs to distant sites. A complete physical examination and thorough pelvic examination is important in evaluating both localized and distant spread of disease.

Helpful imaging modalities in assessing the extent of disease in cervical cancer include CT of the chest, abdomen, and pelvis; positron emission tomography–computed tomography (PET/CT), which is often helpful in evaluation of nodal involvement or smaller metastasis; and MRI, which can aid in assessment of local spread to soft tissues and adjacent pelvic structures. If imaging identifies sites of metastatic disease, image-guided biopsy should be performed for confirmation of stage.

Treatment
Treatment for cervical cancer is dependent on whether the disease is early, locally advanced or has distant metastases. Both early stage tumors and locally advanced tumors are treated with curative intent. Early stage disease is managed surgically with simple hysterectomy or radical hysterectomy (see Fig. 61.1). Pelvic lymph node dissection is performed as part of the procedure, with the exception of smaller tumors (<3 mm depth of invasion) and no evidence for lymphovascular space invasion. In reproductive age patients with early stage disease who would like to maintain fertility, options include cone excisional procedures or trachelectomy (surgical removal of only the cervix), and the uterus is left intact for future childbearing.

For larger cervical tumors (>4 cm) and locally advanced disease, concurrent chemotherapy and radiation are the mainstays of treatment. The addition of chemotherapy (cisplatin or cisplatin and 5-fluorouracil) to radiation is utilized as a radiosensitizer to increase the effectiveness of radiation. Chemoradiation in locally advanced disease is associated with improved survival and reduction in recurrence rates. Surgical management is not favored for larger cervical tumors and locally advanced disease, because the goal of surgery is to obtain negative margins. With surgery, large tumors and locally advanced disease have higher rates of recurrence, decreased survival, and a high likelihood for requiring postoperative radiation, which is associated with increased complication rates when compared with radiation without prior surgery.

Unfortunately, widely metastatic cervical cancer is not considered curable and treatment is aimed at controlling the spread of disease and palliating bothersome symptoms. Treatment involves combination platinum-based chemotherapy with the addition of bevacizumab to improve survival outcomes. Pelvic radiation in these patients is

对于年轻患者，可采取持续监测或在生产结束时切除子宫。对于体弱的患者，可无限期地使用黄体酮治疗。

预后

如果病变局限于子宫，则有 80%～90% 的子宫内膜癌患者可以治愈。进展期疾病的治愈率较低，而Ⅳ期疾病仍然无法治愈。遗憾的是，对于患有子宫内膜癌并伴有癌播散的患者来说，5 年生存率不足 25%。

宫颈癌

流行病学

宫颈癌是最可有效预防的妇科癌症。不幸的是，它仍然是全球女性生殖系统最常见的恶性肿瘤，并且是发展中国家癌症相关死亡的主要原因。在美国，宫颈癌是第三常见的妇科癌症。发生宫颈癌的主要危险因素是感染人乳头瘤病毒（HPV）的高危亚型。由于几乎所有的宫颈癌都是 HPV 相关的细胞病理学改变的结果，所以病毒感染被认为是疾病发展的必要原因。宫颈癌的发病率和死亡率与筛查项目的可及性有关，因此在巴氏染色涂片筛查资源匮乏的环境中宫颈癌发病率和死亡率较高。宫颈癌的其他危险因素还包括吸烟、免疫抑制和己烯雌酚（DES）暴露。

HPV 通过性传播途径感染女性生殖道。与癌前病变和浸润性癌相关的 HPV 亚型定义为高危（high-risk，HR）亚型。有 15 种主要的 HRHPV 亚型与宫颈癌的发生相关；其中，HPV-16 和 HPV-18 分别占宫颈癌病例的 50% 和 20%。虽然许多感染者的 HPV 病毒可自然清除，但 HPV 感染的持续存在与发生癌前瘤变或浸润性宫颈癌的风险增加相关。因为 HPV 与宫颈癌有这样的因果关系，针对 HRHPV 亚型开发的疫苗可以预防 HPV 相关宫颈病变的发生。2006 年，Gardasil 四价疫苗首先获得 FDA 批准用于预防肛门生殖器病变，该疫苗针对 9～26 岁女性，覆盖了 6 种 HRHPV 亚型。目前，美国仅有 Gardasil 9 获得 FDA 批准，覆盖 HPV 6、11、16、18、31、33、45、52 和 58 型，用于 9～45 岁的女性和男性。

病理学

位于阴道内的宫颈表面被覆鳞状上皮，宫颈管内为柱状上皮。宫颈内柱状上皮被鳞状上皮所取代的区域——移行区——是 HPV 相关的宫颈浸润前和浸润性病变发生的主要部位。宫颈癌主要为鳞状细胞癌（75%）和腺癌（25%）。其他极为罕见的宫颈癌病理类型包括神经内分泌癌、腺鳞癌、透明细胞癌和未分化癌。

临床表现

在疾病早期，患者通常不会出现症状。如果出现症状，常包括异常阴道出血、性交出血、排液或盆腔不适。

宫颈癌通过局部进展侵犯周围组织，随后出现淋巴结转移，然后是血行播散。

晚期宫颈癌患者可以出现宫颈周围组织器官受累的相关症状。局部肿瘤浸润可能引起明显的阴道出血和盆腔疼痛，或泌尿系统或肠道不适。这些患者通常在体格检查或影像学检查时发现大的宫颈肿物。

诊断和分期

大多数宫颈癌是通过巴氏染色涂片筛查发现宫颈细胞学异常或持续 HRHPV 感染后进行的宫颈活检确诊的。未接受常规巴氏筛查的患者，则通过对明显异常的宫颈组织或肿物进行活检来诊断宫颈癌。无论巴氏染色涂片细胞学检查如何，HRHPV 亚型持续存在的患者均应进行诊断性活检，以确定是否存在宫颈病变。

宫颈癌的临床和影像学分期为 FIGO Ⅰ～Ⅳ期，各期别中的亚分期主要依据疾病侵犯程度。宫颈癌分为早期疾病（ⅠA～ⅠB1 期）、局部晚期疾病（ⅠB2～ⅣA 期）和转移性疾病（ⅣB 期）。早期宫颈癌是局限于宫颈的小肿瘤。局部晚期疾病是指体积较大的肿瘤，已侵犯子宫外并累及附近盆腔组织器官，包括膀胱和直肠。转移性疾病是指已扩散到盆腔器官以外的远处部位。完整的体格检查和全面的盆腔检查在评估疾病的局部和远处扩散方面至关重要。

有助于评估宫颈癌病变范围的影像检查方法包括胸部、腹部和盆腔 CT；正电子发射断层成像-计算机断层成像（PET/CT）通常有助于评估淋巴结转移或较小的转移灶；以及 MRI 有助于评估软组织和邻近盆腔结构的局部侵犯。如果影像学检查提示了转移部位，应进行影像引导下活检以确认分期。

治疗

宫颈癌的治疗取决于疾病是早期、局部晚期还是有远处转移。早期肿瘤和局部晚期肿瘤均采用根治性治疗。早期病变采用单纯子宫切除术或根治性子宫切除术（图 61.1）。除了肿瘤较小（浸润深度 < 3 mm），并且没有淋巴血管间隙浸润证据的患者，其他患者均应接受盆腔淋巴结清扫。对于希望保留生育功能的育龄期早期宫颈癌患者，可选择宫颈锥形切除术或宫颈切除术（仅手术切除宫颈），保持子宫完整以备未来生育。

对于较大的宫颈肿瘤（> 4 cm）和局部晚期疾病，同步放化疗是主要的治疗手段。放疗基础上加用化疗（顺铂或顺铂联合 5- 氟尿嘧啶）作为放疗增敏剂，以提高放疗的疗效。局部晚期疾病的放化疗与生存率改善和复发率降低相关。因为手术的目标是获得阴性切缘，所以较大的宫颈肿瘤和局部晚期疾病不推荐手术治疗，如果手术，较大肿瘤和局部晚期疾病的术后复发率较高，生存率降低，需要术后放疗的可能性更大，与既往未接受手术患者的放疗相比，术后放疗的并发症发生率明显增加。

不幸的是，广泛转移的宫颈癌通常无法治愈，治疗旨在控制疾病进展和缓解患者不适症状。治疗方案包括铂类为基础的化疗联合贝伐珠单抗，以改善生存结局。

reserved for palliative treatment intended to decrease symptomatic pelvic disease burden or to control vaginal bleeding. For those who experience recurrence despite first-line chemotherapy, testing for PD-L1 is recommended because the FDA has approved the immune checkpoint inhibitor pembrolizumab for use in these patients if their tumors are positive.

For patients with recurrent disease localized to the central pelvis and no evidence of distant metastatic spread, pelvic exenterative procedures that remove remaining pelvic structures with urinary and stool diversion may be curative but are associated with high rates of perioperative morbidity. For patients with recurrent disease who are not candidates for operative management or radiation therapy, chemotherapy such as cisplatin with paclitaxel or gemcitabine can help control disease.

New advances in the treatment of cervical cancer are now examining the role of HPV vaccination for active disease, as well as the utilization of immunotherapy as part of systemic treatment.

Prognosis

Outcomes in cervical cancer depend on stage at diagnosis. Patients with nodal disease have higher rates of relapse and poorer prognosis. Five-year survival rates are roughly 92%, 56%, and 17% for localized, regional, and distant disease, respectively.

VULVAR CANCER

Epidemiology

Vulvar cancer is the most frequently overlooked gynecologic cancer and is the fourth most common gynecologic cancer in the United States. A woman's lifetime risk of developing vulvar cancer is roughly 0.3%. Most vulvar cancers arise from either oncogenic HPV-associated preinvasive vulvar intraepithelial neoplasia (VIN) or through autoimmune or inflammatory related changes, such as lichen sclerosus, leading to differentiated VIN (dVIN). While vulvar cancer most commonly occurs in women over the age of 60, HPV-related vulvar cancer occurs more commonly in younger women. Atypical moles of vulva are associated with an increased risk for the development of vulvar melanomas. Other risk factors for developing vulvar cancer include advanced age, smoking, HIV, and a personal history of cervical cancer or preinvasive cervical lesions.

Pathology

The vulva includes the clitoris, mons, labia majora and minora, vestibule, and the perineal body. Squamous cell carcinoma (SCC) accounts for more than 80% of all vulvar cancers. Melanomas are the second most common type accounting for 10%, followed by basal cell carcinomas (2% to 4%), verrucous carcinomas—an indolent variant of SCC—and sarcomas (1% to 2%). Paget's disease of the vulva is a glandular-like intraepithelial neoplasm that can develop into or harbor underlying adenocarcinoma. Bartholin gland carcinomas account for 0.1% to 5% of vulvar cancers and are typically adenocarcinomas. Other rarer types of vulvar cancers include germ cell tumors, urothelial/transitional cell carcinoma, and neuroendocrine tumors.

Clinical Presentation

Vulvar cancers typically present as an irritated or pruritic solitary vulvar lesion that may be flat, raised, indurated, cauliform, ulcerated or discolored. Occasionally the lesions can be multifocal or may be associated with vulvar bleeding or dysuria. Vulvar cancers metastasize by local extension, lymphatic drainage to the inguinofemoral nodes, and hematogenous spread to distant sites. Patients with more advanced stage disease may present with evidence of a large ulcerated or verrucous (wartlike) mass extending to surrounding tissues or involving large areas of the vulva, vagina, or the anal verge. Often, enlarged groin lymph nodes can be palpated. Other signs related to local extension may include profound vulvar pain, urinary outlet obstruction or dysuria. As the development of vulvar cancer generally has an indolent growth rate, most patients presenting with locally advanced or advanced stage disease are elderly women who are disconnected from routine gynecologic care, or women with limited access to gynecologic care.

Diagnosis and Staging

Vulvar cancer is pathologically diagnosed and staged. Both patients and providers frequently ignore symptoms of perineal itching and discomfort that are typical for the cancer. Patients who present with a suspicious or bothersome lesion on the vulva should undergo a biopsy to evaluate for the presence of vulvar cancer. In addition to biopsy of the gross lesion for histologic confirmation, a complete pelvic examination should be performed including visual inspection of the entire vulva, vagina, cervix, and anus. The groin nodes are palpated to assess for inguinofemoral adenopathy. Enlarged lymph nodes should be biopsied to confirm the presence of disease versus reactive nodes.

After histologic confirmation, the next step is determining the extent of disease. Vulvar cancer is staged with a combination of clinical examination, pathologic confirmation, and radiographic findings. Helpful imaging modalities include CT of the chest, abdomen, and pelvis, or PET/CT. MRI can often be helpful in ambiguous cases to better characterize local extension of disease into surrounding soft tissues and can aid in operative decision making.

Vulvar cancers spread by local extension, and by lymphatic channels to inguinofemoral nodes then pelvic nodes. FIGO stage I disease defines tumor confined to the vulva. Stage II disease involves cancer extending to the adjacent perineal structures including the urethra, anus, and lower one third of the vagina. Stage III disease is comprised of tumor involving the inguinofemoral lymph nodes and stage IV tumor involves the upper two thirds of the urethra and vagina or any distant structures. Roughly 60% of vulvar cancers are localized to the primary site at diagnosis, approximately one third are diagnosed with regional spread, and roughly 6% present with distant metastasis.

Treatment

Treatment of vulvar cancer depends on the histologic subtype and stage of the disease. Treatment courses for vulvar cancer should be individualized because many affected patients are elderly or medically frail.

For patients with apparent early stage disease, treatment includes a radical wide local excision of the lesion with at least a 2-cm lateral margin. Because inguinofemoral node status is the most important prognostic factor, groin nodal evaluation should be assessed for tumors having more than 1 mm depth of invasion. Sentinel lymph node dissection to diagnose nodal involvement has largely replaced full groin nodal dissection because it is associated with less perioperative morbidity. Bilateral groin nodes are evaluated for midline tumors and tumors larger than 4 cm. Postoperative radiation therapy is typically recommended if two or more lymph nodes are involved or nodal extracapsular spread is present and is associated with improved survival outcomes.

For vulvar cancers that have spread beyond the vulva, treatment is highly individualized with careful consideration of goals of care and patient functional status. These tumors are typically not amenable to surgical management and treatment options include primary chemoradiation, radiation alone, palliative radiation to burdensome disease sites or

盆腔放疗可以作为姑息性治疗，用于减轻盆腔肿瘤引起的症状，或控制阴道出血。对于一线化疗后疾病进展的患者，建议检测 PD-L1 表达，FDA 已批准免疫检查点抑制剂帕博利珠单抗（Pembrolizumab）用于 PD-L1 阳性晚期宫颈癌患者。

对于复发疾病局限于骨盆中央且无远处转移的患者，通过尿路分流和消化道重建切除盆腔剩余结构的全盆腔脏器切除术可能治愈肿瘤，但围术期并发症发生率较高。不适合接受手术或放疗的复发患者，化疗（如顺铂联合紫杉醇或吉西他滨）有助于控制疾病进展。

目前，宫颈癌治疗的新进展包括研究 HPV 疫苗对活动性宫颈癌的作用，以及如何把免疫治疗纳入系统治疗的一部分。

预后

宫颈癌的预后取决于诊断时的分期。淋巴结转移患者的复发率较高，预后较差。局限于宫颈、局部区域侵犯和远处转移患者的 5 年生存率分别约为 92%、56% 和 17%。

外阴癌

流行病学

外阴癌是最常被忽视的妇科癌症，是美国第四大常见妇科癌症。女性一生中发生外阴癌的风险约为 0.3%。大多数外阴癌源于致癌性 HPV 相关癌前病变外阴上皮内瘤变（VIN）或自身免疫或炎症相关变化，如硬化性苔藓导致的分化型 VIN（dVIN）。虽然外阴癌最常见于 60 岁以上的女性，但 HPV 相关外阴癌更常见于年轻女性。外阴不典型痣与外阴黑色素瘤发生的风险增加有关。发生外阴癌的其他危险因素包括高龄、吸烟、HIV 感染和宫颈癌或宫颈癌前病变病史。

病理

外阴包括阴蒂、阴阜、大小阴唇、前庭和会阴体。鳞状细胞癌（SCC）占所有外阴癌的 80% 以上。黑色素瘤是第二常见类型，占 10%，其次是基底细胞癌（2%～4%）、疣状癌（SCC 的一种惰性变异型）和肉瘤（1%～2%）。外阴佩吉特病是一种腺样上皮内肿瘤，可发展成为或包含潜在的腺癌。前庭大腺癌占外阴癌的 0.1%～5%，通常为腺癌。外阴癌的其他罕见类型包括生殖细胞肿瘤、尿道/移行细胞癌和神经内分泌肿瘤。

临床表现

外阴癌通常表现为伴有刺激感或瘙痒的孤立性外阴病变，可呈扁平、隆起、硬结、菜花样、溃疡或色素脱失。偶尔病变可为多灶性，也可伴有外阴出血或排尿困难。外阴癌可局部侵犯，通过淋巴引流至腹股沟区淋巴结，和血行播散至远处。疾病分期更晚的患者可能出现大溃疡或疣状肿块，延伸至周围组织或累及外阴、阴道或肛缘的大片区域。查体常可扪及肿大的腹股沟区淋巴结。与肿瘤局部进展相关的其他症状可能包括严重外阴疼痛、尿道出口梗阻或排尿困难。由于外阴癌通常进展缓慢，因此大多数局部晚期或晚期患者是脱离了常规妇科诊疗的老年女性，或接受妇科诊疗机会有限的女性。

诊断和分期

外阴癌需病理诊断和分期。患者和医务人员经常忽略会阴瘙痒和不适的症状，这是外阴癌的典型症状。对于外阴出现可疑或引起不适症状的病变应进行活检，以评估是否存在外阴癌。除了对肉眼可见病变进行活检以进行组织学确认外，还应进行完整的盆腔检查，包括整个外阴、阴道、宫颈和肛门的视诊。触诊腹股沟淋巴结，以评估腹股沟区是否有淋巴结肿大。应对肿大的淋巴结进行活检，以确认淋巴结是癌症转移还是反应性的。

组织学诊断证实后，下一步需明确分期。要结合临床检查、病理诊断和影像学表现对外阴癌进行分期。有助于分期的影像学检查方法包括胸部、腹部和盆腔 CT 或 PET/CT。在分期困难的病例中，MRI 可以更好地显示疾病局部扩展至周围软组织的特征，协助制定手术决策。

外阴癌的进展包括肿瘤局部侵犯，并通过淋巴道转移至腹股沟股淋巴结，而后转移至盆腔淋巴结。FIGO Ⅰ 期定义为肿瘤局限于外阴。Ⅱ 期肿瘤侵犯至邻近会阴结构（包括尿道下 1/3、肛门和阴道下 1/3）。Ⅲ 期肿瘤有腹股沟股淋巴结转移，Ⅳ 期肿瘤累及尿道和阴道的上 2/3 或出现任何远处转移。确诊时，大约 60% 外阴癌局限在原发部位，约 1/3 为局部晚期，约 6% 出现远处转移。

治疗

外阴癌的治疗取决于疾病的组织学亚型和分期。由于许多患者为老年或身体虚弱者，所以外阴癌的治疗应个体化。

明显早期疾病的患者的治疗包括根治性局部广泛切除，侧切缘距肿瘤至少 2 cm。由于腹股沟区淋巴结状态是最重要的预后因素，因此对于原发肿瘤浸润深度超过 1 mm 的患者，腹股沟区淋巴结都应进行检查评估。因为前哨淋巴结切除的围术期并发症发生率较低，所以通过该方式来诊断淋巴结受累情况在很大程度上取代了全腹股沟区淋巴结清扫术。中线肿瘤和大于 4 cm 的肿瘤需检查双侧腹股沟区淋巴结。如果两个或多个淋巴结受累或存在淋巴结包膜外侵犯，建议患者术后接受放射治疗以改善生存。

扩散至外阴外的外阴癌应仔细斟酌治疗目标和患者功能状态，制定高度个体化的治疗方案。这些肿瘤通常不适合手术治疗，治疗选择包括初始放化疗、单纯放疗、高瘤负荷部位的姑息性放疗或系统性化疗。对于局

systemic chemotherapy. Chemoradiation with sensitizing cisplatin chemotherapy is considered superior to radiation alone for locally advanced disease. Radiation fields typically include the primary tumor site, inguinofemoral nodes, and pelvic lymph nodes. If there is residual primary tumor after radiation, resection, if technically feasible, may improve survival or alleviate symptoms. A palliative care approach to provide supportive care is important for patients with advanced stage disease because they often have a high symptom burden pre- and postradiation.

Patients who present with distant metastasis are treated with systemic chemotherapy such as carboplatin and paclitaxel, and radiation can be offered in palliative doses to highly symptomatic disease sites. Recurrent vulvar cancer is treated with surgical excision if localized to the vulva. Systemic carboplatin/paclitaxel is administered for recurrent vulvar cancer at distant sites.

Prognosis
The most important prognostic factor in vulvar cancer is inguinofemoral nodal involvement. Estimated 5-year survival rates for localized, regional, and distant disease are 86%, 53%, and 19%, respectively. Risk factors for recurrent disease include inguinofemoral nodal involvement, close postoperative surgical margins (<5 mm), and higher stage of disease at diagnosis. Patients with HPV-associated vulvar cancers have improved outcomes with radiation treatment relative to non-HPV-associated vulvar cancers.

VAGINAL CANCER
Epidemiology
Primary vaginal cancer is the rarest gynecologic cancer, accounting for only 1% to 2% of gynecologic malignancies. Extension of primary cancers of the uterus, cervix, and vulva, or metastasis from another primary site, should be ruled out to confirm vaginal origin. Vaginal cancer is typically diagnosed in patients older than 60 years. Risk factors include HRHPV, in utero DES exposure, HIV, history of pre-cancers or cancers of the cervix, and the presence of high-grade vaginal intraepithelial neoplasia.

Pathology
The main histopathologic subtype of vaginal cancer is squamous cell carcinoma (90%). Less common types include adenocarcinomas such as clear cells (8% to 14%), melanomas, sarcomas, lymphomas, neuroendocrine, and yolk sac tumors.

Clinical Presentation
Most patients with vaginal cancer present with vaginal bleeding or abnormal vaginal discharge. Alternatively, asymptomatic patients are diagnosed via biopsy of a grossly abnormal appearing lesion at time of routine annual pelvic examination or colposcopic directed biopsy after abnormal cervical or vaginal cytology is detected. Lesions have a variety of appearances and can be soft, friable, nodular, raised, papillary, flat, erythematous, hyper- or hypopigmented. Lesions are most commonly found in the upper one third of the vagina, but distal lesions can be seen as well. Primary vaginal cancers spread by direct extension, the lymphatics, and hematologically to distant sites. The lymphatic drainage of the upper vagina involves the internal iliac lymph nodes and the lower vagina drains to the inguinal lymph nodes. Patients with more advanced disease may present with symptoms related to local extension such as painful urination or defecation; pelvic, vulvar or vaginal pain; hematochezia or hematuria.

Diagnosis and Staging
The diagnosis of vaginal cancer is made by histologic confirmation via biopsy of visible tumor. Because most vaginal cancers are the result of metastasis from another primary site, it is important to rule out other primary gynecologic cancers of the cervix, uterus, ovaries, or vulva as well as nongynecologic cancers that may have vaginal extension such as colorectal or urethral/bladder cancers.

FIGO stage I vaginal cancer includes small tumors limited to the vagina. Stage II disease has extended through the vaginal walls. Stage III tumors invade into the pelvic wall or lower one third of the vagina and may obstruct urinary outflow or cause hydronephrosis. Stage IV tumors include nodal metastasis and spread to the rectum, bladder or distant sites.

Vaginal cancer is the only gynecologic cancer that remains clinically staged (physical examination, cystoscopy, proctoscopy, chest radiograph); however, more advanced imaging modalities such as pelvic MRI, PET/CT or CT chest, abdomen, and pelvis can be used to help assess the full extent of disease not detected by clinical examination alone. While these studies help to guide treatment, they are not currently used to assign the stage of disease.

Treatment
Treatment for vaginal cancer is based on location of tumor and stage of the disease. Aside from stage I disease confined to the mucosa, vaginal cancer is typically treated with a combination of primary chemotherapy and radiation.

An important consideration for surgical resection in vaginal cancer is location (upper vagina or lower vagina) and size of the lesion, as the goal is to achieve negative resection margins. Candidates for primary operative management of vaginal cancers include stage I disease limited to the upper or lower vagina. These lesions are best treated surgically when superficial and smaller than 2 cm. Surgery has become the mainstay of treatment for such lesions, with survival rates ranging from 75% to 100%. If the vaginal tumor includes the upper vagina, a radical hysterectomy with a radical upper vaginectomy and pelvic lymph node dissection may be performed. For stage I disease in the lower vagina, a radical vaginectomy and potentially a vulvovaginectomy may be performed with an inguinofemoral nodal dissection.

For stage II to IV tumors, primary chemoradiation is the mainstay of treatment because it is associated with improved disease control and reduction in locoregional recurrence rates. Due to the rarity of vaginal cancer, studies are few and treatment approaches are often derived from favorable outcomes demonstrated in cervical cancers utilizing a combination of chemotherapy and radiation. For a central pelvic recurrence of vaginal cancer after radiation treatment, total pelvic exenteration may be curative in approximately 50% of correctly selected cases.

Prognosis
Outcomes in vaginal cancer vary by stage at diagnosis, reflecting the size of the tumor and spread of disease. Stage I disease has the most favorable prognosis with survival rates ranging from 70% to 90%, and treatment at this early stage can be curative. Overall, 5-year relative survival rates in vaginal cancer are 67%, 52%, and 19% for localized, regional, and distant disease, respectively. Vaginal melanoma has an extremely poor prognosis with 5-year survival of 15%.

GESTATIONAL TROPHOBLASTIC DISEASE AND GESTATIONAL TROPHOBLASTIC NEOPLASIA
Epidemiology
Gestational trophoblastic disease (GTD) and gestational trophoblastic neoplasia (GTN) are unusual gynecologic conditions as they arise from fetal tissue. GTD is a benign growth of placental tissue arising from an

部晚期疾病，放疗联合顺铂增敏优于单纯放疗。放射野通常包括原发肿瘤部位、腹股沟区淋巴结和盆腔淋巴结。如果技术上可行，切除放疗后残留的原发肿瘤，可能改善患者生存或缓解症状。晚期疾病患者通常在放疗前后有明显的症状，对症支持治疗也非常重要。

出现远处转移的患者应采用系统性化疗，如卡铂和紫杉醇，症状明显的部位可以接受姑息放疗。外阴癌局部复发可以采用手术切除。远处复发性外阴癌应接受卡铂/紫杉醇方案的系统性化疗。

预后

外阴癌最重要的预后因素是腹股沟区淋巴结受累。局限于外阴、局部区域侵犯和远处转移患者的预期5年生存率分别为86%、53%和19%。疾病复发的风险因素包括腹股沟区淋巴结受累、手术切缘近（<5 mm）和诊断时疾病分期较晚。与非HPV相关外阴癌相比，HPV相关外阴癌患者接受放射治疗后可获得更好的生存。

阴道癌

流行病学

原发性阴道癌是最罕见的妇科癌症，仅占妇科恶性肿瘤的1%~2%。要确认阴道来源，需排除子宫、宫颈和外阴原发癌的局部进展，或其他原发部位肿瘤的转移。阴道癌通常见于60岁以上患者。风险因素包括HRHPV、宫内DES暴露、HIV、宫颈癌前病变或宫颈癌病史，以及存在阴道高级别上皮内瘤变。

病理

阴道癌的主要组织病理学亚型是鳞状细胞癌（90%）。较少见的类型包括腺癌［如透明细胞癌（8%~14%）］、黑色素瘤、肉瘤、淋巴瘤、神经内分泌肿瘤和卵黄囊瘤。

临床表现

大多数阴道癌患者表现为阴道出血或异常阴道分泌物，亦有无症状患者在每年例行盆腔检查时发现异常，或发现宫颈或阴道细胞学异常后接受阴道镜检查，进行活检后诊断。病变有多种表现，包括柔软、易碎、结节状、隆起、乳头状、扁平状、红斑状、色素沉着或色素脱失。病变最常见于阴道上1/3，但也可出现下段病变。原发性阴道癌可直接侵犯、淋巴转移和血行扩散至远处。阴道上段淋巴引流累及髂内淋巴结，阴道下段引流至腹股沟淋巴结。晚期患者可出现与局部进展有关的症状，如排尿或排便疼痛，盆腔、外阴或阴道疼痛，便血或血尿。

诊断和分期

阴道癌的诊断是通过对可见肿瘤进行活检，经组织病理学检查证实。因为大多数阴道恶性肿瘤来源于其他原发部位肿瘤的转移，因此诊断的关键是排除其他原发性妇科癌症如宫颈癌、子宫癌、卵巢癌或外阴癌以及可能有阴道侵犯的非妇科癌症，如结直肠癌或尿道/膀胱癌。

FIGO Ⅰ期阴道癌包括局限于阴道的小肿瘤。Ⅱ期病变穿透阴道壁。Ⅲ期肿瘤侵入盆壁或阴道下1/3处并可阻碍尿液流出或引起肾积水。Ⅳ期肿瘤包括淋巴结转移和侵犯直肠、膀胱或远处转移。

阴道癌是唯一临床分期（体格检查、膀胱镜检查、直肠镜检查、胸部X线检查）的妇科癌症。虽然更先进的影像学检查方法，如盆腔MRI、PET/CT或胸部、腹部和盆腔CT，可协助全面评估临床检查方法无法检测到的肿瘤，有助于指导治疗，但目前并不用于确定疾病分期。

治疗

阴道癌的治疗方法取决于肿瘤的部位和疾病的分期。除局限于黏膜的Ⅰ期疾病外，阴道癌的初始治疗通常采用化疗和放疗联合的方式。

阴道癌手术切除的目标是实现切缘阴性，因此病变的位置（阴道上段或阴道下段）和大小是重要的考量因素。初始手术治疗的方法适用于疾病局限在阴道上段或下段的Ⅰ期阴道癌，尤其是病变位置表浅且小于2 cm。手术是此类病变的主要治疗手段，生存率为75%~100%。如果阴道肿瘤位于阴道上段，可行根治性子宫切除术联合根治性阴道上段切除和盆腔淋巴结清扫术。位于阴道下段的Ⅰ期疾病，需要根治性阴道切除术，有可能需外阴阴道联合切除，并进行腹股沟股淋巴结清扫。

对于Ⅱ~Ⅳ期肿瘤，放化疗是主要的初始治疗手段，可以提高疾病控制和降低局部复发风险。由于阴道癌罕见，相关研究很少，治疗方法通常来自于放化疗联合治疗宫颈癌的利好研究结果。放射治疗后中央盆腔复发的阴道癌，经正确选择的患者接受全盆腔脏器切除术后约50%可能治愈。

预后

阴道癌的预后与诊断时的分期，即肿瘤的大小和疾病的范围相关。Ⅰ期预后最佳，治疗后可能获得治愈，生存率为70%~90%。总体而言，局限于阴道，局部区域侵犯和远处转移的5年相对生存率分别为67%、52%和19%。阴道黑色素瘤预后极差，5年生存率为15%。

妊娠滋养细胞疾病（GTD）和妊娠滋养细胞肿瘤（GTN）

流行病学

妊娠滋养细胞疾病（GTD）和妊娠滋养细胞肿瘤（GTN）是少见的起源于胎儿组织的妇科疾病。GTD是来自异常妊娠的胎盘组织的良性生长。在美国的发

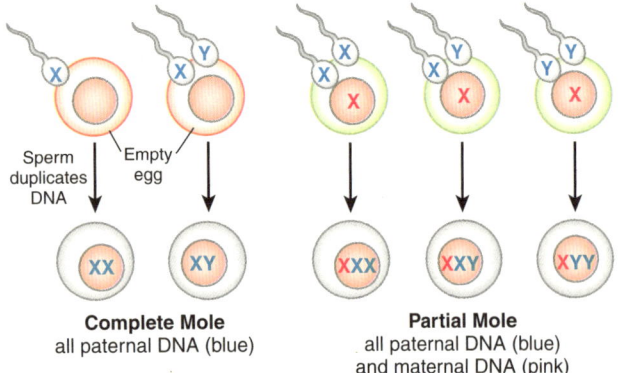

Fig. 8.2 Complete molar pregnancy versus partial molar pregnancy. (Adapted from Ning F, et al. F1000Research 2019;8:428.)

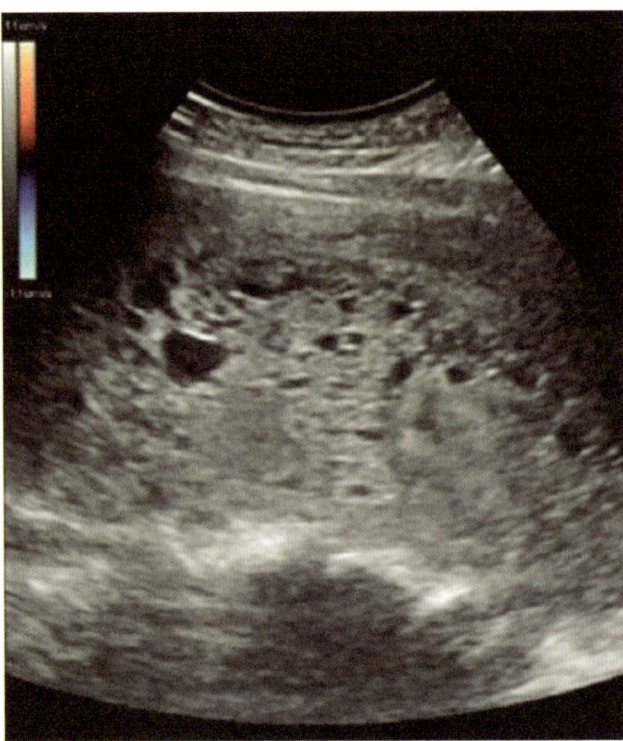

Fig. 8.3 Ultrasound showing classic snowstorm pattern of a complete mole at 24 weeks' gestation. (From J Ultrasound Med 2020;39:597-613.)

abnormal pregnancy. The frequency is 1:1000 to 1:1500 pregnancies in the United States and 1:125 pregnancies in Asia. Proposed reasons for the regional variation include heredity and dietary differences such as low vitamin A and low animal fat diet in the East. While GTD is considered benign, it may be a precursor to GTN, which is a neoplastic process associated with pregnancy. GTN includes invasive molar pregnancy, choriocarcinoma, placental site trophoblastic tumor (PSTT), and epithelioid trophoblastic tumors (ETT).

Pathology

The term "complete mole" refers to an abnormal pregnancy that contains only paternal DNA. For example, an egg devoid of maternal DNA may be fertilized by one sperm that duplicates or two sperm (most commonly XX or XY, with all paternal DNA). A "partial" mole refers to an egg with maternal DNA that has been fertilized by two sperm (69 XXX, 69 XXY or 69XYY) (Fig. 8.2). An invasive mole is a molar pregnancy that has grown into myometrial tissue. Choriocarcinoma is an aggressive form of cancer that can occur following a normal pregnancy, abortion, or complete molar pregnancy, and is comprised of cytotrophoblast and syncytiotrophoblast. It may be associated with local extension beyond the uterus and metastatic disease. PSTT arises in the placental bed of an antecedent pregnancy and has the pathologic appearance of sheets of intermediate trophoblast invading the myometrial wall of the uterus. ETT is composed of neoplastic chorionic-type intermediate trophoblast. Choriocarcinoma, PSTT, and ETT may occur after molar and non-molar pregnancies.

Clinical Presentation

The majority of molar pregnancies present with symptoms of bleeding, pain, hyperemesis, and uterine size too large for suspected dates. The pregnancy hormone, human chorionic gonadotropin (hCG), is abnormally elevated in cases of complete molar pregnancy. Pelvic ultrasound usually shows globular vesicles that are pathognomonic for the disease (Fig. 8.3). Other rarer symptoms may include ovarian theca lutein cysts and hyperthyroidism caused by the alpha subunit of hCG mimicking the effects of thyroid stimulating hormone.

Invasive moles typically present with bleeding due to uterine or vaginal disease. GTN may also present with symptoms of hemoptysis (lung disease), abdominal complaints (abdominal disease), or neurologic symptoms (brain disease). Choriocarcinoma often presents with high hCG levels and bleeding metastatic sites. PSTT and ETT can present years after a prior pregnancy and typically have low elevations in hCG levels and a uterine mass on imaging.

Diagnosis and Staging

When clinical presentation and imaging suggest a molar pregnancy, pathologic evaluation of products of conception obtained at time of D&C confirm the diagnosis. Although most patients with molar pregnancy are cured with D&C alone, 20% of patients will have a plateau, increase, or persistence of hCG over time not explained by other causes, which confirms the diagnosis of GTN. When this occurs, a metastatic work-up should be performed including physical exam for vaginal metastasis, chest radiograph, CT imaging of abdomen and pelvis or chest, and consideration of head CT or MRI. Biopsy of GTN is hazardous because these lesions are prone to excessive bleeding; therefore, tissue sampling is not required for diagnosis.

The most commonly used staging systems for GTN are the FIGO staging system, which reflects sites of metastases, and the WHO prognostic scoring system, which takes into account a number of prognostic factors including the patient's age, type and timing of antecedent pregnancy, pretreatment hCG level, tumor size, sites and number of metastases, and chemotherapy treatment. Low-risk metastases include disease in lungs and vagina, while high-risk metastases involve other organs including the brain and liver.

Treatment

The primary treatment of a molar pregnancy is a D&C, followed by weekly monitoring of hCG levels until undetectable. For an invasive mole isolated to the uterus, hysterectomy can be a curative treatment for women who do not wish to preserve fertility. Otherwise GTN is treated with chemotherapy, and regimens are determined by stratifying patients into low-risk and high-risk categories. If no evidence of metastatic disease is identified (low risk), then single agent chemotherapy is administered using methotrexate or dactinomycin. If high-risk metastatic disease is identified, or if disease persists despite single agent treatment, then patients are treated with an aggressive regimen such as

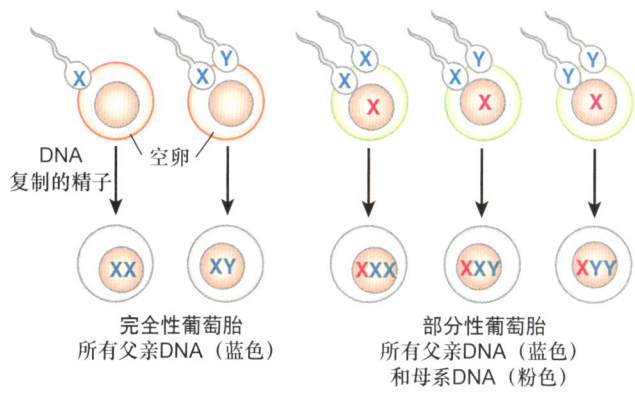

图 8.2 完全性葡萄胎妊娠和部分性葡萄胎妊娠（改编自 Ning F，et al. F1000Research 2019；8：428.）

生率为 1 : 1000 至 1 : 1500 例妊娠，在亚洲为 1 : 125 例妊娠。出现上述地区差异的原因包括遗传和饮食的不同，如东方人群饮食维生素 A 和动物脂肪含量低。GTD 是良性疾病，可能是 GTN 的前兆，GTN 是一种与妊娠相关的肿瘤。GTN 包括侵蚀性葡萄胎妊娠、绒毛膜癌、胎盘部位滋养细胞肿瘤（PSTT）和上皮样滋养细胞肿瘤（ETT）。

病理学

"完全性葡萄胎"一词是指仅含有父系 DNA 的异常妊娠。例如，一个缺乏母体 DNA 的卵子可能与一个复制成两倍体的精子受精，或与两个精子（最常见的是 XX 或 XY，携带所有父系 DNA）受精。"部分性"葡萄胎是指携带母体 DNA 的卵子已被两个精子受精（69 XXX、69 XXY 或 69XYY）（图 8.2）。侵蚀性葡萄胎是指葡萄胎妊娠已侵入子宫肌层组织。绒毛膜癌是一种侵袭性癌症，发生在正常妊娠、流产或完全性葡萄胎妊娠之后，由细胞滋养细胞和合体滋养细胞组成。它可以局部侵犯至子宫外和出现远处转移。PSTT 起源于妊娠早期的胎盘床，病理表现为成片的中间型滋养细胞浸润子宫肌壁。ETT 由肿瘤性绒毛膜型中间型滋养细胞组成。葡萄胎和非葡萄胎妊娠后可能发生绒毛膜癌、PSTT 和 ETT。

临床表现

大多数葡萄胎妊娠表现为出血、疼痛、剧吐和子宫大小超过孕龄相应的大小。孕激素、人绒毛膜促性腺激素（hCG）在完全性葡萄胎妊娠时异常升高。盆腔超声通常显示特有的球状囊泡（图 8.3）。其他较罕见的症状可能包括卵巢黄素化囊肿和与促甲状腺激素相似的 hCG 的 α 亚基引起的甲状腺功能亢进。

侵蚀性葡萄胎通常表现为子宫或阴道出血。GTN 还可以出现咯血（肺转移）、腹部不适（腹腔转移）或神经系统症状（脑转移）。绒毛膜癌常表现为 hCG 水平升高和转移部位出血。PSTT 和 ETT 可以在既往妊娠后数年出现，通常 hCG 水平升高幅度较低，影像检查发现子宫肿块。

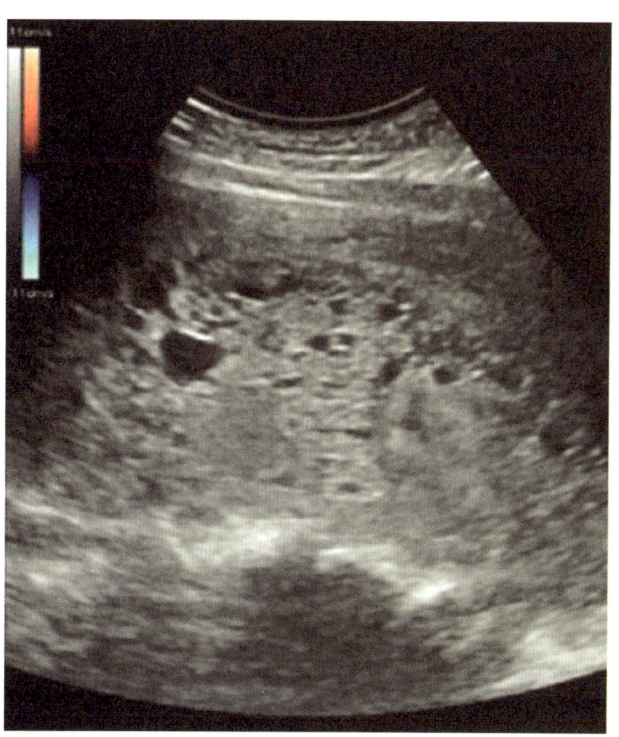

图 8.3 超声显示完全性葡萄胎 24 周妊娠时的经典型"暴风雪"征（引自 J Ultrasound Med 2020；39：597-613.）

诊断和分期

当临床表现和影像检查提示葡萄胎妊娠时，对刮宫术时清除的组织进行病理学检查可以明确诊断。虽然大多数葡萄胎妊娠患者单纯用刮宫术可以治愈，但 20% 的患者会出现其他原因不能解释的血 hCG 水平处于高平台、升高或持续，可证实 GTN 的诊断。当发生这种情况时，应进行转移病灶的检查，包括阴道转移的体格检查，胸片、腹部和盆腔或胸部 CT，并考虑头部 CT 或 MRI。因 GTN 病变容易出血过多，肿瘤活检有危险，因此无需组织活检即可诊断。

GTN 最常用的分期系统是可反映转移部位的 FIGO 分期系统和 WHO 预后评分系统，后者纳入了许多预后因素，包括患者的年龄、前期妊娠的类型和时间、治疗前 hCG 水平、肿瘤大小、转移部位和数量以及化疗治疗。低危转移包括肺和阴道转移，其他部位转移为高危转移，包括脑和肝转移。

治疗

葡萄胎妊娠的主要治疗是刮宫术，随后每周监测 hCG 水平，直至检测不到。如侵蚀性葡萄胎病变局限于子宫，无保留生育能力要求的妇女可以通过子宫切除术治愈疾病。否则，GTN 采用化疗治疗，并通过将患者分为低危组和高危组来确定治疗方案。如果无肿瘤转移证据（低风险），则使用甲氨蝶呤或放线菌素 D 单药化疗。如果确定为高危转移性疾病，或尽管接受了单药治疗疾病仍持续存在，推荐患者接受积极的治疗方案，如依托

the combination of etoposide, methotrexate, dactinomycin, calcium leucovorin, cyclophosphamide, and vincristine (EMA-CO). PSTT and ETT differ in that they are less chemoresponsive and thus are typically treated with hysterectomy and surgical removal of metastatic sites. The use of chemotherapy for PSTT and ETT is controversial.

Prognosis

For patients with low-risk GTN, the cure rate with single agent chemotherapy is nearly 100%. Cure rates with metastatic disease depend on the site of disease. Survival rates for lung, brain, and liver metastases are greater than 90%, 70% to 90%, and 40% to 50%, respectively. Prognosis is poor if metastatic PSTT or ETT is identified.

SUGGESTED READINGS

Brown J, Naumann RW, Seckl MJ, Schink J: 15 years of progress in gestational trophoblastic disease: scoring, standardization, and salvage, Gynecol Oncol 144(1):200–207, 2017.

Harkenrider MM, Markham MJ, Dizon DS, et al: Moving forward in cervical cancer—enhancing susceptibility to DNA repair inhibition and damage: NCI clinical trials planning meeting report, J Natl Cancer Inst djaa041, 2020. https://doi.org/10.1093/jnci/djaa041.

Konstantinopoulos PA, Lheureux S, Moore KNL: PARP inhibitors for ovarian cancer: current indications, future combinations, and novel assets in development to target DNA damage repair. American Society of Clinical Oncology Educational Book 40 (April 30, 2020):e116-e131. https://doi.org/10.1200/EDBK_288015.

Liontos M, Kyriazoglou A, Dimitriadis I, et al: Systemic therapy in cervical cancer: 30 years in review, Crit Rev Oncol Hematol 137:9–17, 2019.

McAlpine J, Leon-Castillo A, Bosse T: The rise of a novel classification system for endometrial carcinoma; integration of molecular subclasses, J Pathol 244(5):538–549, 2018.

Wright AA, Bohlke K, Armstrong DK, et al: Neoadjuvant chemotherapy for newly diagnosed, advanced ovarian cancer: society of gynecologic oncology and American society of clinical oncology clinical practice guideline, J Clin Oncol 34(28):3460–3473, 2016.

泊苷、甲氨蝶呤、放线菌素 D、亚叶酸钙、环磷酰胺和长春新碱联合治疗（EMA-CO）。PSTT 和 ETT 对化疗反应较差，因此通常采用子宫切除术和手术切除转移病灶治疗。化疗用于 PSTT 和 ETT 存在争议。

预后

对于低危 GTN 患者，单药化疗的治愈率接近 100%。转移性疾病的治愈率取决于转移部位。肺、脑和肝转移患者的生存率分别为超过 90%、70%～90% 和 40%～50%。转移性 PSTT 或 ETT 预后较差。

推荐阅读

Brown J, Naumann RW, Seckl MJ, Schink J: 15 years of progress in gestational trophoblastic disease: scoring, standardization, and salvage, Gynecol Oncol 144(1):200–207, 2017.

Harkenrider MM, Markham MJ, Dizon DS, et al: Moving forward in cervical cancer—enhancing susceptibility to DNA repair inhibition and damage: NCI clinical trials planning meeting report, J Natl Cancer Inst djaa041, 2020. https://doi.org/10.1093/jnci/djaa041.

Konstantinopoulos PA, Lheureux S, Moore KNL: PARP inhibitors for ovarian cancer: current indications, future combinations, and novel assets in development to target DNA damage repair. American Society of Clinical Oncology Educational Book 40 (April 30, 2020):e116-e131. https://doi.org/10.1200/EDBK_288015.

Liontos M, Kyriazoglou A, Dimitriadis I, et al: Systemic therapy in cervical cancer: 30 years in review, Crit Rev Oncol Hematol 137:9–17, 2019.

McAlpine J, Leon-Castillo A, Bosse T: The rise of a novel classification system for endometrial carcinoma; integration of molecular subclasses, J Pathol 244(5):538–549, 2018.

Wright AA, Bohlke K, Armstrong DK, et al: Neoadjuvant chemotherapy for newly diagnosed, advanced ovarian cancer: society of gynecologic oncology and American society of clinical oncology clinical practice guideline, J Clin Oncol 34(28):3460–3473, 2016.

Other Solid Tumors (Head and Neck, Sarcomas, Melanoma, Unknown Primary)

Christopher G. Azzoli, Ariel E. Birnbaum, Maria Constantinou, Thomas A. Ollila

INTRODUCTION

Head and neck cancer, melanoma, sarcoma, and carcinoma of unknown primary site (CUP) are distinct malignancies each with its own epidemiology, pathology, treatment, and prognosis. Head and neck cancers and melanoma are more common, and sarcomas and CUP are relatively rare. Recent advances in understanding of the molecular biology of cancer and immune therapies have refined diagnosis and improved treatment for each of these diseases.

HEAD AND NECK CANCER

Definition and Epidemiology

Head and neck cancers are squamous cell carcinomas that arise from the mucosal lining of the oral cavity, oropharynx, hypopharynx, and larynx. Other cancers arising from the head and neck include salivary gland cancers and thyroid cancers. These differ in regard to biology, presentation, natural history, pathology, and therapy.

Head and neck cancer accounts for 4% of new cancer diagnoses in the United States. In 2019, it was estimated that 53,000 patients would be diagnosed with, and 10,860 Americans would die of, head and neck cancer. Historically, tobacco and alcohol have been the strongest risk factors for developing this disease. Over the last 20 years, human papilloma virus (HPV) has been responsible for an increase in the incidence of oropharyngeal squamous cell carcinoma. Patients with HPV-associated oropharyngeal cancer are typically younger than patients with HPV-negative disease, and often have minimal tobacco or alcohol use. Nasopharyngeal squamous cell carcinoma is uncommon in the United States and is distinct from other head and neck cancers given its association with Epstein-Barr virus (EBV).

Pathology

Approximately 95% of all cancers arising from the squamous epithelium of the head and neck are squamous cell carcinomas. Other cancers include mucosal melanoma, adenocarcinomas, and neuroendocrine cancers. Poorly differentiated cancers have a worse prognosis.

The increasingly common HPV-associated oropharyngeal cancers differ in molecular profile from HPV-negative cancers. HPV-negative cancers are associated with mutations in the tumor suppressor gene TP53 and decreased expression of the cell cycle regulatory protein p16-INK4a. HPV-positive cancers display a wild-type TP53 with increased expression of p16-INK4a. P16 expression by immunohistochemistry staining of greater than 70% establishes the diagnosis of HPV-positive disease. Most but not all nasopharyngeal carcinomas are non-keratinizing and associated with EBV infection, which is detected by immunohistochemistry for Epstein-Barr–encoding RNAs (EBER).

Clinical Presentation

The presenting symptoms of head and neck cancer depend on the location of the primary cancer and extent of local disease. Tumors of the nasopharynx can present with a blocked eustachian tube or epistaxis. Oral cavity cancers present with a painful ulcerative lesion. HPV-associated oropharyngeal cancers present with enlarged cervical lymph nodes, often larger than the primary lesion. Laryngeal and hypopharyngeal cancers present with dysphagia and hoarseness.

Diagnosis and Staging

The diagnosis of a squamous cell carcinoma requires a biopsy. A direct laryngoscopy and biopsy is recommended to find the site of origin. Patients who have cervical lymphadenopathy and no apparent primary site require random biopsies of the tongue base and the surrounding tissues and often a tonsillectomy. CT scan, MRI, and positron emission tomography (PET) are used to detect nodal involvement and metastatic disease.

Treatment and Prognosis

Prognosis of head and neck cancer depends on tumor stage. The American Joint Committee of Cancer (AJCC) TNM, 8th edition, incorporates HPV status into its staging system, specifically for the base of tongue and tonsil. Patients with early-stage disease (no cervical lymphadenopathy) have an excellent prognosis. The majority of cancers are diagnosed at the locally advanced stage that has spread to the cervical lymph nodes. Average 5-year survival for all patients is approximately 50%.

Prognosis for HPV-associated disease is usually better. Both biology of disease and comorbidities impact prognosis. HPV-negative patients are at higher risk for developing second primary cancers of the lung and esophagus.

Surgery and radiation therapy are potentially curative treatments for head and neck cancer. Stage IV head and neck cancer may still be cured if all disease can be encompassed by treatment. Chemotherapy by itself is not curative. The combination of chemotherapy and radiation therapy improves rates of cure. The combination is also more toxic than radiation by itself. Choice of treatment is determined by location of the cancer and extent of disease. Locally advanced cancers usually require a combination of surgery, radiation therapy, and chemotherapy. Radiation treatment may be used instead of surgery to preserve organ function. In laryngeal cancer, chemoradiation therapy can be used without the need to remove the larynx. Chemoradiation therapy may permit organ preservation, but it has both acute and chronic toxicity.

Disease that has spread through the blood to distant sites is not curable. Chemotherapy may be used to control the disease and extend life.

其他实体瘤（头颈癌、肉瘤、黑色素瘤、原发部位不明的癌症）

公小蕾 译 葛郁平 赵林 审校 巴一 通审

引言

头颈癌、黑色素瘤、肉瘤及原发部位不明的癌症（CUP）是不同的恶性肿瘤，均有各自的流行病学、病理、治疗及预后。头颈癌及黑色素瘤更加常见，肉瘤和CUP相对少见。近年来，随着对肿瘤分子生物学和免疫疗法的认识逐渐加深，这些疾病的诊断和治疗在不断进步。

头颈癌

定义和流行病学

头颈癌是指发生于口腔、口咽、下咽和喉黏膜的鳞状细胞癌。其他来源于头颈部的肿瘤还包括涎腺癌和甲状腺癌等，其生物学、临床表现、自然病程、病理和治疗方面均有所不同。

头颈癌占美国新发肿瘤的4%。2019年全美约有53 000名患者被诊断为头颈癌，10 860名患者死于头颈癌。从历史上看，烟草和酒精一直是引发这种疾病最主要的危险因素。过去20年中，人乳头瘤病毒（HPV）被发现是导致口咽鳞状细胞癌发病率上升的原因。HPV相关性口咽癌患者通常比HPV阴性者年轻，且通常很少吸烟或饮酒。鼻咽鳞状细胞癌在美国并不常见，且不同于其他头颈癌，与EB病毒（EBV）相关。

病理

起源于头颈部鳞状上皮的所有肿瘤中，约95%为鳞状细胞癌。其他肿瘤包括黏膜黑色素瘤、腺癌和神经内分泌癌。低分化肿瘤预后较差。

日益常见的HPV相关性口咽癌与HPV阴性口咽癌在分子特征上有所不同。HPV阴性肿瘤与抑癌基因 *TP53* 的突变和细胞周期调节蛋白p16-INK4a的表达减少相关。HPV阳性肿瘤显示野生型 *TP53*，同时p16-INK4a表达增加。免疫组化染色显示当P16表达超过70%时，即可诊断HPV阳性肿瘤。大多数（并非所有）鼻咽癌为非角化性，与EBV感染相关，可以通过EB病毒编码RNA（EBER）的免疫组化染色来检测。

临床表现

头颈癌的症状取决于原发灶的部位和局部病变的侵犯程度。鼻咽癌可表现为咽鼓管堵塞或鼻出血。口腔癌表现为痛性溃疡。HPV相关性口咽癌表现为颈部淋巴结肿大，通常比原发灶更大。喉癌和下咽癌可表现为吞咽困难和声音嘶哑。

诊断和分期

鳞状细胞癌的诊断依赖于活检。为明确原发灶，建议进行直接喉镜检查，同时行活检。有颈部淋巴结肿大但无明确原发灶的患者，需要对舌根和周围组织进行随机活检，通常还需行扁桃体切除。CT扫描、MRI和正电子发射断层成像（PET）可用于检测淋巴结受累和转移病变。

治疗和预后

头颈癌的预后取决于肿瘤分期。美国癌症联合委员会（AJCC）的TNM第8版将HPV状态纳入分期系统，特别是对于舌根癌和扁桃体癌。早期（无颈部淋巴结受累）患者预后良好。大多数肿瘤诊断时为局部晚期，肿瘤已扩散至颈部淋巴结。所有患者5年生存率约为50%。

HPV相关性肿瘤的预后通常较好。肿瘤的生物学特性和合并症均会影响预后。HPV阴性患者罹患第二肿瘤肺癌和食管癌的风险较高。

手术和放射治疗是头颈癌的潜在治愈方法。即使Ⅳ期的头颈癌，如果所有的病灶都能通过治疗得到控制，肿瘤仍有可能治愈。化疗本身并不能治愈肿瘤。化疗和放疗联合可提高治愈率，但毒性也较单独放疗严重。治疗方法的选择取决于原发灶部位和病变范围。局部晚期肿瘤通常需要手术、放疗和化疗相结合的综合治疗。放疗可以代替手术来保存器官功能。在喉癌中，放化疗可以替代喉切除手术。放化疗可保留器官，但可引起急性和慢性毒性。

通过血液扩散到远处的肿瘤是无法治愈的。化疗可用于控制疾病和延长生存。转移性头颈癌药物治疗的重

A major advance in medical therapy for metastatic head and neck cancer are anti-PD1 immune checkpoint inhibitors (pembrolizumab and nivolumab) that can provide immune-mediated and durable control for a subset of patients. As with other metastatic cancers, enrollment in clinical trials and early integration of palliative care consultants is recommend for optimal patient care.

MELANOMA

Definition and Epidemiology

Melanoma is an aggressive form of skin cancer that originates from melanocytes, a pigment-producing cell found in the basal layer of the epidermis. Melanoma accounts for 1% of all skin cancers but it represents the fifth most common cancer in men and women.

The incidence of melanoma has been rising rapidly over the past five decades. An estimated 96,480 cases of melanoma were diagnosed in the United States in 2019 with approximately 7230 deaths. Melanoma is more common among people aged 65 to 74. Ultraviolet (UV) sun exposure is the main risk factor for development of melanoma.

Individuals with high recreational/intermittent sun exposure, history of blistering sunburns in childhood or adolescence, and exposure to artificial UV radiation from use of tanning beds have a higher risk for developing melanoma. In addition, family history of melanoma and certain phenotypic traits such as fair skin, red/blonde hair, light eyes, the presence of multiple nevi, and atypical or congenital nevi appear to also increase the risk.

Pathology

Melanoma can be classified based on four major histopathologic subtypes: superficial spreading melanoma (SSM), nodular melanoma (NM), lentigo maligna melanoma (LMM), and acral lentiginous melanoma (ALM).

SSM is the most common subtype, representing 70% of all melanomas. It typically affects individuals between the ages of 30 and 50 years. These melanomas spread in a radial growth pattern and develop in intermittently sun-exposed skin, often in a preexisting nevus. It commonly appears on the trunk in males and legs in females. It clinically presents as a flat lesion with irregular borders.

NM accounts for 10% to 15% of all melanomas. It has a vertical growth phase and is usually associated with dermal invasion at the time of diagnosis, hence a worse prognosis. It clinically presents as a deeply pigmented nodule, typically blue-black or polypoid, but 5% of nodular melanomas may be amelanotic (no pigment). It usually develops de novo on the trunk, head, and neck of middle-aged individuals.

LMM accounts for 5% of all melanomas. It affects older individuals with peak incidence in the seventh to eighth decade of life. It originates from a large brown patch on chronically sun-damaged skin (lentigo). Lentigo maligna is associated with slow progression and may evolve for decades before invading into the dermis.

ALM is uncommon and represents less than 5% of all melanomas. It is the most common type seen among Asians and African Americans. The median age of diagnosis is 65. ALM arises on palmar, plantar, and subungual surfaces, the nail matrix being the most common site, and it is not associated with sun exposure. Clinically, it appears as a dark brown to black patch on the palms, soles or under the nails.

Pathologic features that have prognostic relevance include the depth of invasion (Breslow thickness) and the presence of ulceration. Breslow thickness represents the depth of melanoma invasion from the upper epidermal layer. It is measured in mm and it defines the T stage. It is one of the most important prognostic and predictive factors for lymph node involvement. The risk of nodal spread increases with the depth of invasion. The presence of lymph node metastases in melanomas with Breslow thickness less than 0.8 mm is less than 5% and increases to 40% in patients with primary melanomas with Breslow thickness greater than 4 mm.

Another adverse predictor for the development of melanoma metastasis is the presence of microscopic ulceration within the primary site. Patients with ulcerated localized melanoma have a significant decrease in 5 year survival, from 80 to 55%.

Clinical Presentation

Most patients with cutaneous melanoma present with disease confined to the primary site.

Approximately 10% of patients have disease spread to regional lymph nodes, and 4% have distant metastasis at the time of diagnosis. A number of benign lesions share morphologic features with melanoma, making the diagnosis challenging. A lesion that is changing in shape, size, or color should be considered suspicious. Melanomas commonly arise within a preexisting nevus in sun-exposed areas such as the face, upper back, and extremities.

The ABCDE criteria encompass several features that increase the accuracy of skin examination for detection of melanoma: asymmetry (A), border irregularity (B), color change (C), diameter greater than 6 mm (D), and evolution or change (E).

Melanoma can metastasize to regional sites such as the nearby skin, subcutaneous tissue, and lymph nodes or distant sites such as skin, lung, liver, brain, and bone. Regional skin and nodal examination should be performed regularly. Symptoms of advanced disease are highly variable.

Diagnosis and Differential Diagnosis

Pathologic examination with an excisional biopsy is the "gold standard" for diagnosis of melanoma. Such approach allows sufficient depth assessment to ensure that the lesion is not transected at the base of the biopsy. The depth of invasion guides surgical decision making regarding the need for a sentinel lymph node biopsy (sampling the first lymph node that cancer cells are likely to spread to) and the optimal size of resection margin with subsequent excision. If an excisional biopsy cannot be performed, a full-thickness punch biopsy is recommended. Shave biopsies may lead to inadequate sampling and underestimation of the depth of the lesion. The histologic diagnosis is based on characteristic morphology and on immunohistochemical staining for markers such as S100, HMB45, and MART1/Melan A.

In general, imaging investigations for staging purposes are not required for patients with thin (<1 mm) or intermediate-thickness melanoma (1-4 mm). The likelihood of demonstrating metastatic disease is low. Patients with thick melanomas (>4 mm) or lymph node metastasis detected on clinical examination or by sentinel lymph node biopsy are at high risk for disease dissemination and need radiographic staging by CT of the chest, abdomen, and pelvis. Metastasis to the brain is observed in 10% to 40% of melanoma patients and imaging with a brain MRI is warranted for any patient with neurologic symptoms.

Treatment and Prognosis

The prognosis of melanoma can be accurately estimated using the AJCC TNM staging system. Overall survival depends on the thickness of the primary tumor and the presence and number of regional lymph node metastases. Tumor ulceration and high mitotic rate are associated with a poor prognosis. Metastatic disease is incurable, and the clinical course depends on the pattern and extent of dissemination. An elevated serum lactate dehydrogenase (LDH) level is an independent poor prognostic factor for patients with metastases.

Surgery with wide margins is the cornerstone of curative therapy for nonmetastatic disease. The optimal margin depends on the depth of

大进展是抗 PD1 免疫检查点抑制剂（帕博利珠单抗和纳武利尤单抗），能为部分患者提供免疫介导的持久控制。与其他转移性肿瘤一样，我们鼓励患者参加临床试验，并尽早与缓和医疗团队合作，以获得最佳的患者照护。

黑色素瘤

定义和流行病学

黑色素瘤是一种侵袭性皮肤肿瘤，起源于黑色素细胞——一种位于表皮基底层能产生色素的细胞。黑色素瘤虽然仅占所有皮肤肿瘤的 1%，但它是男性和女性第五大常见恶性肿瘤。

过去 50 年，黑色素瘤的发病率迅速上升。2019 年美国诊断 96 480 例黑色素瘤，约 7230 例死亡。黑色素瘤更常见于 65～74 岁人群。紫外线（UV）暴露是黑色素瘤发病的主要危险因素。

休闲性或间歇性高强度日光暴露、童年或青春期有严重晒伤史，以及因使用日光浴床而暴露于人工紫外线辐射的个体，罹患黑色素瘤的风险更高。此外，黑色素瘤家族史和某些表型特征如白皙皮肤、红色/金色头发、浅色眼睛、多发痣以及非典型或先天性痣，似乎也会增加患病风险。

病理

黑色素瘤可分为 4 种主要的组织病理学亚型：表面扩散性黑色素瘤（SSM）、结节性黑色素瘤（NM）、恶性雀斑样痣黑色素瘤（LMM）和肢端雀斑样痣黑色素瘤（ALM）。

SSM 是最常见的亚型，占所有黑色素瘤的 70%。发病年龄通常在 30～50 岁。这些黑色素瘤以放射状生长模式扩散，并在间歇暴露于阳光的皮肤上发展，通常在先前存在的痣上形成。男性好发于躯干，女性好发于腿部。临床表现为边界不规则的扁平皮损。

NM 占所有黑色素瘤的 10%～15%。它有一垂直生长阶段，诊断时通常伴有真皮侵犯，因此预后较差。临床表现为深色素结节，通常呈蓝黑色或息肉状，但 5% 的 NM 也可能是无黑色素的（无色素）。通常新发于中年人的躯干、头部和颈部。

LMM 占所有黑色素瘤的 5%。好发于老年人，发病高峰期在 70～80 岁。起源于长期晒伤皮肤上的大片褐色斑块（雀斑样痣）。恶性雀斑样痣进展缓慢，可能会发展数十年才侵入真皮。

ALM 不常见，占所有黑色素瘤的比例不到 5%。它是亚洲人和非裔美国人最常见的类型。确诊的中位年龄为 65 岁。ALM 多发于手掌、足底和指甲下表面，指甲基质是最常见的部位，与日晒无关。临床表现为手掌、足底或指甲下的深褐色至黑色斑块。

与预后相关的病理特征包括浸润深度（Breslow 厚度）和是否存在溃疡。Breslow 厚度代表黑色素瘤从上表皮层浸润的深度。以毫米为单位测量，用于确定 T 分期。它是淋巴结受累最重要的预后和预测因素之一。淋巴结扩散的风险随浸润深度的增加而增加。Breslow 厚度小于 0.8 mm 的黑色素瘤，淋巴结转移的发生率小于 5%，而 Breslow 厚度大于 4 mm 的原发性黑色素瘤，淋巴结转移的发生率则增加到 40%。

黑色素瘤发生转移的另一个预后不利因素是原发部位存在镜下溃疡。伴有溃疡的局部黑色素瘤患者的 5 年生存率明显下降，从 80% 降至 55%。

临床表现

大多数皮肤黑色素瘤患者的病变局限于原发部位。

约 10% 的患者在诊断时肿瘤已扩散到区域淋巴结，4% 的患者存在远处转移。许多良性病变与黑色素瘤具有相同的形态特征，给诊断带来挑战。病变出现形状、大小或颜色变化时应怀疑恶变。黑色素瘤通常在面部、上背部和四肢等暴露于阳光部位的原有痣内发生。

ABCDE 法则包含如下特征，以提高皮肤检查中发现黑色素瘤的准确性：不对称（asymmetry，A）、边缘不规则（border，B）、颜色变化（color，C）、直径大于 6 mm（diameter，D）以及病变进展或变化（evolution，E）。

黑色素瘤可转移至邻近皮肤、皮下组织和淋巴结等区域部位，或远隔皮肤、肺、肝、脑和骨等远处部位。应定期进行区域皮肤和淋巴结检查。晚期疾病的表现多样。

诊断和鉴别诊断

组织切除后行病理检查是黑色素瘤诊断的"金标准"。这种方法能达到充分的深度评估，确保在活检的底部病变没有被横切。浸润深度可指导手术决策，决定是否需行前哨淋巴结活检（在癌细胞可能扩散到的第一个淋巴结取样），以及后续手术切除的最佳切缘大小。如果无法进行切除活检，则建议进行全层打孔活检。刮片活检可能造成取样不足，导致对病变深度的低估。组织学诊断基于特征性形态和标志物的免疫组化如 S100、HMB45 和 MART1/Melan A 等确立。

一般来说，对于薄（＜1 mm）或中等厚度（1～4 mm）黑色素瘤的患者，不需要影像学检查分期，因为出现远处转移的可能性很低。厚（＞4 mm）黑色素瘤、临床检查或前哨淋巴结活检发现淋巴结转移的黑色素瘤患者，肿瘤扩散的风险较高，需要通过胸腹盆 CT 进行影像学分期。10%～40% 的黑色素瘤患者会出现脑转移，任何有神经系统症状的患者都应进行脑 MRI 检查。

治疗和预后

AJCC 的 TNM 分期系统可准确估计黑色素瘤患者预后。总生存期取决于原发肿瘤厚度、是否存在区域淋巴结转移及其数目。肿瘤溃疡和高有丝分裂率与预后不良有关。转移性肿瘤是无法治愈的，临床病程取决于扩散的模式和程度。血清乳酸脱氢酶（LDH）水平升高是转移患者预后不良的独立危险因素。

宽切缘手术是非转移性疾病治愈的关键。最佳切缘取

invasion and the location of the primary lesion but is typically between 1 and 2 cm. Biopsy of the sentinel lymph node (first lymph node to which cancer cells are likely to spread) is recommended for all patients with intermediate-thickness melanoma (1-4 mm) and should also be considered in patients with T1b melanomas 0.8 to 1.0 mm or less than 0.8 mm with ulceration. Despite adequate surgical resection of the primary melanoma, 15% to 36% of patients with early-stage melanoma with no lymph node involvement will develop disease recurrence or metastasis.

Patients who are found to have micrometastatic disease to the sentinel node may choose careful observation with routine nodal ultrasonography or immediate complete lymph node dissection. However, studies have shown that immediate completion of lymph node dissection has not shown to improve melanoma-specific survival in this group of patients. All patients with enlarged lymph nodes that test positive for melanoma, in the absence of distant metastasis, should undergo complete lymph node dissection.

Anti–programmed death (PD-1) agents nivolumab and pembrolizumab have recently gained regulatory approval for treating patients with a high risk of recurrence after complete resection—that is, those with lymph node involvement. These monoclonal antibodies are immune checkpoint inhibitors that block negative regulators of T cell immune function, leading to immune system activation. A year of therapy is associated with significantly longer relapse-free survival.

Approximately 50% of cutaneous melanomas have activating mutations of the proto-oncogene *BRAF*, a component of the mitogen-activated protein kinase (MAPK) signaling pathway. The MAPK pathway plays an important role in cell proliferation, differentiation, and apoptosis. BRAF-MEK inhibition with combination dabrafenib plus trametinib therapy is associated with improved clinical benefit and is an alternative adjuvant option for patients whose tumor contains a *BRAF* V600 mutation.

Immunotherapy and kinase inhibitors are the backbone of systemic therapy for patients with metastatic melanoma. Anti-PD1 antibodies and anti-CTLA4 antibodies (ipilimumab) have shown durable responses with improvement in survival. In *BRAF* V600–mutant melanoma, the use of BRAF inhibitors with MEK inhibitors has led to high response rates (70%) and a rapid response to induction and symptom control, with a progression-free survival of approximately 12 months.

Cytotoxic chemotherapy is generally not effective for treatment of metastatic melanoma. Radiation therapy is often used for management of brain metastases or central nervous system symptoms, pain associated with bone metastases, spinal cord compression, and superficial skin and subcutaneous metastases.

SARCOMA

Definition and Epidemiology

Sarcomas are heterogeneous solid tumors of mesenchymal origin, with over 70 different clinicopathologic subtypes. These tumors are broadly categorized as sarcomas of bone or sarcomas of soft tissue. There were expected to be 12,750 new diagnoses of soft tissue sarcoma and 3500 new diagnoses of bone sarcoma in the United States in 2019, causing nearly 7000 deaths. Overall, sarcomas account for fewer than 1% of all new cancer diagnoses in adults; however, they are relatively common in children and represent 15% of all pediatric malignancies.

Most sarcomas are sporadic, but risk factors include prior radiation exposure, chemical carcinogens, and genetic predisposition (familial adenomatous polyposis [FAP] and Li-Fraumeni syndrome). Human herpesvirus 8 (HHV-8) infection is associated with the development of Kaposi's sarcoma. Most genetic abnormalities that define sarcomas are sporadic and not inherited.

Soft tissue sarcomas can be classified by their anatomic site of origin: head and neck, visceral, retroperitoneal, intra-abdominal, and extremity. This categorization is useful for staging, assessing prognosis, and establishing a therapeutic approach. The most common soft tissue sarcomas are gastrointestinal stromal tumors (GISTs), pleomorphic sarcoma, liposarcoma, leiomyosarcoma, and synovial sarcoma. The most commonly encountered sarcomas of bone are the Ewing family of sarcomas, chondrosarcomas, and osteosarcomas.

Clinical Presentation

Given the heterogeneity of this group of diseases, including differences in tumor biology and in anatomic site of origin, the clinical presentation is highly variable. Soft tissue sarcomas of the extremities and of the head and neck usually manifest as a progressively enlarging, often painless, mass. Visceral and intra-abdominal sarcomas including GISTs are often found incidentally and are not symptomatic until they are locally advanced. Symptoms are often nonspecific but may include early satiety, abdominal fullness, bloating, or discomfort. Bone sarcomas, such as Ewing sarcoma and osteosarcoma, typically manifest with pain. The most frequently involved locations are the femur, tibia, and humerus. The physical examination may reveal a palpable mass, which is often tender to palpation. Symptoms may be present for several months before diagnosis. Most patients have locally confined disease at diagnosis. The lungs and bone are the most common sites of metastatic spread.

Diagnosis and Differential Diagnosis

The diagnosis of sarcoma can only be established by histologic confirmation, which requires a tissue biopsy. Large biopsy specimens are often necessary to accurately identify and subclassify sarcoma. Sarcoma must be distinguished from more common malignancies such as lymphoma, melanoma, and poorly differentiated carcinoma. The diagnosis of sarcoma is based on characteristic morphology but may be aided by the use of immunohistochemical and molecular studies.

For example, Ewing sarcoma is often associated with a characteristic reciprocal translocation between chromosomes 11 and 22, t(11:22), resulting in gene rearrangements between the EWS and ETS family of genes. Synovial sarcoma is characterized by a reciprocal t(X;18) translocation resulting in a chimeric SS18-SSX fusion protein. Dozens of other gene rearrangements have been identified such that routine molecular pathology testing is often required to establish a specific diagnosis.

For bone sarcomas, plain films often demonstrate a mixture of lytic and blastic components with associated soft tissue edema. For osteosarcoma, the periosteal reaction produces a "sunburst" appearance as new bone forms at right angles to the tumor, as opposed to the "onion peel" appearance caused by layering of reactive bone, which is more commonly associated with Ewing sarcoma.

Treatment and Prognosis

Surgery is the primary therapy for locally confined disease. Radiotherapy before or after surgery may decrease the likelihood of local recurrence. Chemotherapy may be used in resectable sarcoma for certain histologic subtypes (primarily Ewing sarcoma and osteosarcoma) to improve local control and decrease the risk of distant recurrences; however, whether drugs improve overall survival in resectable sarcoma remains uncertain.

Patients with metastatic sarcoma may occasionally benefit from surgical removal of their disease. However, once metastatic dissemination has been detected, the intent of therapy is primarily to control the disease and not to cure. Chemotherapy can reduce the overall tumor burden and minimize cancer-related symptoms.

决于浸润深度和原发病灶的部位，通常在 1～2 cm 之间。建议对所有中等厚度的黑色素瘤（1～4 mm）患者进行前哨淋巴结（癌细胞可能扩散到的第一个淋巴结）活检。厚度为 0.8～1.0 mm 或小于 0.8 mm 并伴有溃疡的 T1b 黑色素瘤患者，也应考虑进行前哨淋巴结活检。尽管对原发黑色素瘤进行了充分的手术切除，仍有 15%～36% 未累及淋巴结的早期黑色素瘤患者会出现疾病的复发或转移。

发现前哨淋巴结有微转移的患者，可选择常规淋巴结超声进行仔细观察，或立即进行彻底的淋巴结清扫。然而，研究表明，立即完成淋巴结清扫术并不能提高这组患者的黑色素瘤特异性生存率。所有伴淋巴结肿大的黑色素瘤患者，在没有远处转移的情况下，都应进行彻底的淋巴结清扫。

抗程序性死亡（PD-1）药物纳武利尤单抗和帕博利珠单抗近期获得了监管部门批准，用于治疗完全切除后复发风险高的患者即淋巴结受累者。这些单克隆抗体是免疫检查点抑制剂，阻断 T 细胞免疫功能的负调控因子，激活免疫系统。为期 1 年的治疗可显著延长无复发生存期。

大约 50% 的皮肤黑色素瘤具有原癌基因 *BRAF* 的激活突变，BRAF 是丝裂原活化蛋白激酶（MAPK）信号通路的一个组成部分。MAPK 通路在细胞增殖、分化和凋亡中发挥着重要作用。达拉非尼联合曲美替尼通过抑制 BRAF-MEK 可提高临床疗效，是 *BRAF* V600 突变患者的另一种辅助治疗选择。

免疫治疗和激酶抑制剂是转移性黑色素瘤患者全身治疗的主要手段。抗 PD1 抗体和抗 CTLA4 抗体（伊匹木单抗）显示出持久疗效，并延长了生存时间。在 *BRAF* V600 突变的黑色素瘤中，使用 BRAF 抑制剂联合 MEK 抑制剂可获得较高反应率（70%），对诱导治疗的快速应答和症状控制，无进展生存期约为 12 个月。

细胞毒性化疗通常对转移性黑色素瘤无效。放射治疗通常用于治疗脑转移或控制中枢神经系统症状、骨转移相关疼痛、脊髓压迫以及浅表皮肤和皮下转移。

肉瘤

定义和流行病学

肉瘤是起源于间叶组织的具有异质性的实体肿瘤，有 70 多种不同的临床病理亚型。大体分为骨原发肉瘤或软组织肉瘤。2019 年，美国新发 12 750 例软组织肉瘤和 3500 例骨原发肉瘤，并导致近 7000 例死亡。总体来说，肉瘤占所有成人新诊断恶性肿瘤的比例不到 1%；尽管如此，肉瘤在儿童中相对常见，占所有儿童恶性肿瘤的 15%。

大多数肉瘤呈散发性，危险因素包括既往辐射暴露史、化学致癌物和遗传易感性［家族性腺瘤性息肉病（FAP）和 Li-Fraumeni 综合征］。人类疱疹病毒 8（HHV-8）感染与卡波西肉瘤的发生有关。大多数肉瘤的基因变异是散发性，而非遗传性的。

根据起病解剖部位的不同，可将软组织肉瘤分为：头颈、内脏、腹膜后、腹腔内和四肢肉瘤。这种分类方法对于确定分期、评估预后和制订治疗方案非常有用。最常见的软组织肉瘤为胃肠道间质瘤（GIST）、多形性肉瘤、脂肪肉瘤、平滑肌肉瘤和滑膜肉瘤。最常见的骨原发肉瘤是尤因肉瘤家族肿瘤、软骨肉瘤和骨肉瘤。

临床表现

鉴于这组疾病的异质性（包括肿瘤生物学特性和原发解剖部位的不同），肉瘤的临床表现差异很大。四肢和头颈部软组织肉瘤通常表现为进行性增大的无痛性肿块。包括胃肠道间质瘤的内脏和腹腔内肉瘤通常是偶然发现的，直到局部进展才会出现症状。症状通常非特异，但可能包括早饱、腹部饱满、腹胀或腹部不适。骨原发肉瘤如尤因肉瘤和骨肉瘤的典型表现是疼痛，最常受累的部位是股骨、胫骨和肱骨。体格检查可能会触及肿块且触痛阳性。症状可能发生在诊断前数月。大多数患者诊断时疾病局限。最常见的转移部位是肺和骨。

诊断和鉴别诊断

肉瘤只能依靠组织活检的病理来明确诊断。通常需要大块活检标本以准确识别肉瘤并对其进行分类。肉瘤必须与常见恶性肿瘤如淋巴瘤、黑色素瘤和低分化癌鉴别。肉瘤的诊断以形态学特征为基础，但也可能需要免疫组化和分子分析来辅助诊断。

例如，尤因肉瘤通常与 11 号和 22 号染色体之间的特征性易位 t（11;22）相关，导致 EWS 和 ETS 家族基因之间的基因重排。滑膜肉瘤的特征是 t（X;18）相互易位，导致嵌合的 SS18-SSX 融合蛋白。已发现数十种其他的基因重排，因此通常需要常规的分子病理学检测来确定特异性诊断。

对于骨原发肉瘤，平片通常显示溶骨性和成骨性成分的混合，并伴有软组织水肿。对于骨肉瘤，骨膜反应产生"日光放射"样外观，这是由于新骨与肿瘤形成直角，而不是由反应性骨分层造成的"洋葱皮"样外观，后者更常见于尤因肉瘤。

治疗和预后

手术是局限期肉瘤的主要治疗方法。术前或术后放疗可降低局部复发的可能性。化疗可用于某些组织学亚型（主要是尤因肉瘤和骨肉瘤）的可切除肉瘤，以加强局部控制并降低远处复发的风险；然而，药物治疗是否能改善可切除肉瘤的总生存仍不明确。

转移性肉瘤患者可能偶尔会从手术中获益。然而，一旦发现转移性扩散，治疗目的主要是控制疾病，而不是治愈。化疗可以减少总体肿瘤负荷，并减轻肿瘤相关症状。

Historically, the most active drugs for sarcoma were cytotoxic drugs like doxorubicin, ifosfamide, and gemcitabine. These drugs damage or block production of DNA and inhibit cell division. Newer drugs also block cell division. Trabectedin is a DNA damaging agent used as salvage treatment of metastatic liposarcoma, or leiomyosarcoma. Eribulin is a nontaxane inhibitor of microtubules, which blocks cell division and is used for previously treated liposarcoma.

Other new drugs have diverse mechanisms of action and reflect the diverse biology of sarcoma. Imatinib is a small-molecule tyrosine kinase inhibitor (TKI) that blocks the activity of KIT and is highly active in patients with GISTs, which are commonly driven by KIT mutations. Imatinib is used to control metastatic GIST and also improves survival when combined with surgery in patients with resectable GIST. Pazopanib and regorafenib are multitargeted TKIs that have been tested in patients with soft tissue sarcomas (excluding GIST and liposarcoma). The activity of these drugs is limited, and they provide only a few more months of disease control compared to placebo. Other multitargeted TKIs have limited activity against chondrosarcoma, chordoma, osteosarcoma, and desmoid tumors. A small percentage of sarcomas (less than 1%) have a mutation in the neurotrophic receptor tyrosine kinase (NTRK) gene that responds to TRK inhibitors (larotrectinib, entrectinib).

Currently available immune therapies have only limited activity in the treatment of sarcoma. Single-agent anti-PD1 therapy is rarely effective, except in the 1% of sarcomas that are microsatellite instability-high (MSI-H) or mismatch repair deficient (dMMR). A combination of anti-PD1 and anti-CTLA4 drugs is being developed for unselected patients. There is activity of chimeric antigen receptor (CAR) T cells for the treatment of synovial sarcoma on research protocols, making it one of the first solid tumors to be targeted with cellular immune therapy.

CANCER OF UNKNOWN PRIMARY SITE

Definition and Epidemiology

CUPs occur when a malignancy is identified, but no primary site can be identified following pathology review, complete diagnostic imaging or invasive procedures. Once accounting for 5% to 10% of malignancies, improvements in histopathologic techniques have lessened the frequency of CUPs to 3% to 5% of all malignancies. Patients with CUP tend to be older, with median age 65 to 90 years. CUPs are heterogeneous, with adenocarcinoma, squamous cell carcinoma, neuroendocrine tumors, and poorly differentiated carcinoma all fulfilling criteria. Debate exists as to whether CUPs are simply malignancies where the primary is not found, or if they are truly a separate entity.

Treatment typically includes platinum-based chemotherapy unless a high clinical suspicion for a primary site provides a more specific guide. Molecular profiling suggests that CUP is frequently a result of occult lung, kidney, bladder, or pancreaticobiliary cancer.

Clinical Presentation

Many patients with CUP present with advanced disease. Symptoms can be based upon location of metastatic disease or general nonspecific complaints including fatigue, fevers, anorexia or weight loss. Examples of presenting signs and symptoms can include neurologic deficit from brain or spinal cord metastatic disease, ascites, or general malignancy-associated symptoms such as increased risk for thrombotic events, hypercalcemia, paraneoplastic syndrome or pain. Some patients with CUP present earlier with only mild symptoms, such as an enlarged lymph node or skin lesion. Also, some are found incidentally on imaging performed for another indication.

Diagnosis and Pathology

When considering the origin of a metastatic cancer, it is important to do a thorough history and physical exam, including breast, GU/pelvic, and rectal exam; review of prior malignancies; and available imaging (CT scan of the chest/abdomen/pelvis, which should include neck if there is disease in axillary or supraclavicular lymph nodes). Careful pathologic review of biopsy material is essential. The first step in pathologic evaluation is through immunohistochemistry. Adenocarcinoma constitutes around 70% of CUPs, followed by poorly differentiated carcinoma at 20%, squamous cell carcinoma around 5%, and neuroendocrine carcinoma and other rare subtypes at under 1%. Caution must be used in evaluation of the poorly differentiated carcinomas, because choice of treatment for a specific disease could be radically different. For example, melanoma is typically treated with targeted or immune-based therapy rather than chemotherapy as would be the case for a CUP.

Immunohistochemistry may disclose the site of origin. For example, in the case of poorly differentiated tumors, the presence of S100 and HMB45 supports a diagnosis of melanoma, whereas CD45 supports a diagnosis of lymphoma. Chromogranin and synaptophysin suggest neuroendocrine differentiation. Cytokeratin 5 (CK5) and CK6 are strongly expressed by squamous cell carcinomas, whereas the expression pattern of CK7 and CK20 can limit the differential diagnosis of adenocarcinomas.

Multiple groups have attempted to define genetic and molecular features of CUPs. The success of gene expression profiling to determine the origin of CUP varies widely in published reports, from 33% to nearly 100%, depending on the technique and patient population studied. Gene expression profiling points to biliary tract, urothelial, colorectal, and lung as common sites.

Treatment and Prognosis

Outcomes in CUP remain poor with a median survival of 8 to 12 months. Despite advances in many cancers, survival of CUP patients has not improved in greater than 30 years. Because CUP is typically widespread at time of presentation, treatment is usually palliative rather than curative in intent. There are situations where the histology suggests a favorable type, for example a germ cell tumor and lymphoma, and cure might still be possible. Occasionally CUPs are identified as localized disease, in which case an attempt should be made at definitive treatment.

For example, a woman presenting with adenocarcinoma isolated to unilateral axillary lymph nodes should be evaluated and treated as for a locally advanced breast cancer, even if imaging does not demonstrate a primary breast malignancy. Likewise, a patient with squamous cell carcinoma isolated to cervical lymph nodes at presentation should receive therapy for locally advanced head and neck cancer, again even if a primary lesion is not identified. In both of these circumstances, therapy may prove curative. Another clinical scenario for which specific therapy is beneficial is that of a young man with a poorly differentiated midline chest tumor, in which case a favorable response to a chemotherapy regimen for germ cell cancers may lead to long-term survival.

Whether or not gene expression profiling and next-generation sequencing can improve outcomes remains to be seen. A multicenter phase II trial of 130 patients with gene expression–guided treatment versus empiric carboplatin and paclitaxel in CUP found non–statistically significant inferior outcomes with 1-year survival at 44% in the guided group versus 55% for the empiric group. Despite these results,

从历史上看，治疗肉瘤最有效的药物是细胞毒性药物，如阿霉素、异环磷酰胺和吉西他滨。这些药物破坏或阻断 DNA 的产生并抑制细胞分裂。新药也能阻止细胞分裂。曲贝替定是一种 DNA 损伤剂，用于转移性脂肪肉瘤或平滑肌肉瘤的挽救治疗。艾立布林是一种非紫杉烷类微管抑制剂，可阻断细胞分裂，用于经治的脂肪肉瘤。

其他新药的作用机制各不相同，也反映出肉瘤在生物学上的多样性。伊马替尼是一种小分子酪氨酸激酶抑制剂（TKI），可阻断 KIT 基因的活性，在通常由 KIT 突变驱动的胃肠道间质瘤（GIST）患者中具有高度活性。伊马替尼用于治疗转移性 GIST，同时与手术结合能改善可切除 GIST 患者的生存。培唑帕尼和瑞戈非尼是多靶点 TKI，已在软组织肉瘤（除外 GIST 和脂肪肉瘤）患者中进行了试验。这些药物的活性有限，与安慰剂相比，它们只能多增加几个月的病情控制。其他多靶点 TKI 对软骨肉瘤、脊索瘤、骨肉瘤和硬纤维瘤的活性也有限。小部分肉瘤（＜1%）存在神经营养受体酪氨酸激酶（NTRK）基因突变，对 TRK 抑制剂（拉罗替尼、恩曲替尼）有效。

目前可用的免疫疗法在肉瘤上疗效有限。除了占肉瘤 1% 的微卫星高度不稳定（MSI-H）或错配修复缺陷（dMMR）的肉瘤以外，单药抗 PD1 单抗治疗很少有效。在未经选择的肉瘤患者中，抗 PD1 和抗 CTLA-4 药物的联合方案正在研究中。研究发现，嵌合抗原受体（CAR）T 细胞治疗滑膜肉瘤具有一定活性，使滑膜肉瘤成为首批细胞免疫治疗的实体瘤之一。

原发部位不明的癌症

定义和流行病学

明确为恶性肿瘤，但经过病理检查、全面的诊断性影像检查或侵入性操作后仍无法确定原发病灶，称为原发部位不明的癌症（CUP）。CUP 曾占所有恶性肿瘤的 5%～10%，随着组织病理学技术的进步，CUP 的发病率已下降至所有恶性肿瘤的 3%～5%。CUP 患者多为老年人，中位年龄为 65～90 岁。CUP 具有异质性，可包括腺癌、鳞状细胞癌、神经内分泌肿瘤和低分化癌。至于 CUP 只是没有发现原发灶的恶性肿瘤，还是真正独立的疾病，目前仍存争议。

除非临床高度怀疑的原发部位可提供更具体的指南，CUP 的治疗通常包含铂类为基础的化疗。分子分析提示，CUP 通常是隐匿性的肺癌、肾癌、膀胱癌或胰腺胆管癌。

临床表现

很多 CUP 患者都是晚期患者。症状取决于转移灶的部位，也可以表现为一般的非特异性主诉，包括疲劳、发热、厌食或体重减轻。出现体征和症状的例子包括脑或脊髓转移性疾病引起的神经功能缺损、腹腔积液或恶性肿瘤相关的普遍症状如血栓事件、高钙血症、副肿瘤综合征或疼痛。有些 CUP 患者早期仅有轻微症状，如淋巴结肿大或皮肤损害。此外，有些 CUP 是因其他原因做影像检查时被偶然发现的。

诊断和病理

在寻找转移性肿瘤的原发灶时，重要的是进行全面的病史采集和体格检查（包括乳房、泌尿生殖/盆腔和直肠检查）、既往肿瘤病史的回顾，以及合适的影像学检查（胸部/腹部/盆腔 CT 扫描；如果腋窝或锁骨上淋巴结有病变，还应包括颈部）。对活检组织进行仔细的病理检查至关重要。病理评估的第一步是免疫组化。CUP 中腺癌约占 70%，其次是低分化癌，约占 20%，鳞状细胞癌约占 5%，神经内分泌癌和其他罕见亚型占比不到 1%。评估低分化癌时必须谨慎，因为针对特定肿瘤的治疗选择可能截然不同。例如，黑色素瘤通常采用靶向或免疫治疗，而不是像 CUP 那样的化疗。

免疫组化有助于揭示原发部位。如在低分化肿瘤中，S100 和 HMB45 的表达支持黑色素瘤的诊断，而 CD45 阳性支持淋巴瘤的诊断。嗜铬粒蛋白和突触素提示神经内分泌分化。细胞角蛋白 5（CK5）和 CK6 在鳞状细胞癌中强表达，而 CK7 和 CK20 的表达模式可以用于腺癌的鉴别诊断。

多个研究小组试图确定 CUP 的遗传和分子特征。在已发表的文献中，因技术和研究的患者人群不同，利用基因表达谱确定 CUP 起源的成功率差异很大，从 33% 到近 100% 不等。基因表达谱显示胆道、尿路上皮、结直肠和肺是常见的原发部位。

治疗和预后

CUP 的预后仍然很差，中位生存期仅为 8～12 个月。尽管许多癌症取得进展，但 30 多年来，CUP 患者的生存并未得到提高。由于 CUP 在发病时通常已经扩散，因此治疗经常是姑息性的，而非治愈性的。在某些情况下，如果组织学提示是较好的类型，例如生殖细胞肿瘤和淋巴瘤，则仍有可能治愈。有时 CUP 被确定为局限性疾病，在这种情况下，应尝试进行根治性治疗。

例如，一位表现为孤立的单侧腋窝淋巴结腺癌的女性患者，即使影像学未发现原发乳腺恶性肿瘤，也应按局部晚期乳腺癌进行评估和治疗。同样，就诊时发现的孤立颈部淋巴结鳞癌患者，即使未发现原发灶，也应按照局部晚期头颈癌进行治疗。在这两种情况下，治疗可能是治愈性的。另一种从特定疗法中获益的临床情况是患有低分化胸部中线肿瘤的年轻男性，对生殖细胞瘤的化疗方案反应良好，可能会获得长期生存。

基因表达谱和二代测序能否改善预后还有待观察。一项纳入 130 例 CUP 患者的多中心 II 期试验发现，接受基因表达指导治疗的患者对比经验性卡铂联合紫杉醇治疗的患者，1 年生存率分别为 44% 和 55%，无统

hope exists that with further study gene expression profiling can offer guidance to improve outcomes.

SUGGESTED READINGS

D'Angelo SP, Melchiori L, Merchant MS, et al: Antitumor activity associated with prolonged persistence of adoptively transferred NY-ESO-1 c259T cells in synovial sarcoma, Cancer Discov 8(8):944–957, 2018.

Drilon A, Laetsch TW, Kummar S, et al: Efficacy of larotrectinib in TRK fusion-positive cancers in adults and children, N Engl J Med 378(8):731–739, 2018.

El Rassy E, Pavlidis N: The current evidence for a biomarker-based approach in cancer of unknown primary, Cancer Treat Rev 67:21–28, 2018.

Hainsworth JD, Rubin MS, Spigel DR, et al: Molecular gene expression profiling to predict the tissue of origin and direct site-specific therapy in patients with carcinoma of unknown primary site: a prospective trial of the Sarah Cannon Research Institute, J Clin Oncol 31(2):217–223, 2013.

Hayashi H, Kurata T, Takiguchi Y, et al: Randomized phase II trial comparing site-specific treatment based on gene expression profiling with carboplatin and paclitaxel for patients with cancer of unknown primary site, J Clin Oncol 37(7):570–579, 2019.

Pollack SM, Ingham M, Spraker MB, Schwartz GK: Emerging targeted and immune-based therapies in sarcoma, J Clin Oncol 36(2):125–135, 2018.

Siegel RL, Miller KD, Jemal A: Cancer statistics, 2019, CA Cancer J Clin 69(1):7–34, 2019.

Tawbi HA, Burgess M, Bolejack V, et al: Pembrolizumab in advanced soft-tissue sarcoma and bone sarcoma (SARC028): a multicentre, two-cohort, single-arm, open-label, phase 2 trial, Lancet Oncol 18(11):1493–1501, 2017.

Wisco OJ, Sober AJ: Prognostic factors for melanoma, Dermatol Clin 30:469–485, 2012.

Zandberg DP, Bhargava R, Badin S, et al: The role of human papillomavirus in nongenital cancers, CA Cancer J Clin 63:57–81, 2013.

计学差异。尽管如此，基因表达谱仍有望通过进一步研究为改善预后提供指导。

推荐阅读

D'Angelo SP, Melchiori L, Merchant MS, et al: Antitumor activity associated with prolonged persistence of adoptively transferred NY-ESO-1 c259T cells in synovial sarcoma, Cancer Discov 8(8):944–957, 2018.

Drilon A, Laetsch TW, Kummar S, et al: Efficacy of larotrectinib in TRK fusion-positive cancers in adults and children, N Engl J Med 378(8):731–739, 2018.

El Rassy E, Pavlidis N: The current evidence for a biomarker-based approach in cancer of unknown primary, Cancer Treat Rev 67:21–28, 2018.

Hainsworth JD, Rubin MS, Spigel DR, et al: Molecular gene expression profiling to predict the tissue of origin and direct site-specific therapy in patients with carcinoma of unknown primary site: a prospective trial of the Sarah Cannon Research Institute, J Clin Oncol 31(2):217–223, 2013.

Hayashi H, Kurata T, Takiguchi Y, et al: Randomized phase II trial comparing site-specific treatment based on gene expression profiling with carboplatin and paclitaxel for patients with cancer of unknown primary site, J Clin Oncol 37(7):570–579, 2019.

Pollack SM, Ingham M, Spraker MB, Schwartz GK: Emerging targeted and immune-based therapies in sarcoma, J Clin Oncol 36(2):125–135, 2018.

Siegel RL, Miller KD, Jemal A: Cancer statistics, 2019, CA Cancer J Clin 69(1):7–34, 2019.

Tawbi HA, Burgess M, Bolejack V, et al: Pembrolizumab in advanced soft-tissue sarcoma and bone sarcoma (SARC028): a multicentre, two-cohort, single-arm, open-label, phase 2 trial, Lancet Oncol 18(11):1493–1501, 2017.

Wisco OJ, Sober AJ: Prognostic factors for melanoma, Dermatol Clin 30:469–485, 2012.

Zandberg DP, Bhargava R, Badin S, et al: The role of human papillomavirus in nongenital cancers, CA Cancer J Clin 63:57–81, 2013.

10

Complications of Cancer and Cancer Treatment

Pamela Egan, Ari Pelcovits, John Reagan

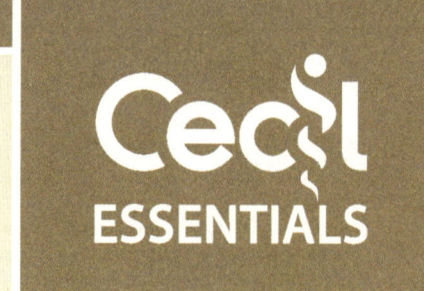

INTRODUCTION

The complications of cancer and its associated treatments are myriad. Although many of these complications require the expert management of hematologists and oncologists, all physicians who may encounter these patients should be prepared to recognize their manifestations and understand both their basic management and indications for specialist referral.

Cancer complications can be localized or systemic (Table 10.1). Cancer treatments, which can include radiation, chemotherapy, and hormonal therapy, have potentially significant side effects and complications. Most are temporary, but some, such as peripheral neuropathy, can become permanent (Table 10.2). Complications from cancer-directed therapy can affect not just quality of life for cancer patients, but can also result in treatment delays or discontinuation, hospitalization, and even death. The management of cancer- and treatment-related complications often requires a multidisciplinary approach. This chapter highlights some important complications of cancer and its treatment.

CANCER-ASSOCIATED THROMBOSIS

Epidemiology

Venous thromboembolism (VTE) is a common complication of cancer and is often its initial presenting event. Approximately 15% of patients with cancer develop VTEs during their illness, and it is a major cause of mortality among cancer patients.

Pathology

The primary drivers of the hypercoagulable state in cancer patients are the procoagulant factors associated with the tumor cells. Other contributing factors include immobilization due to illness, venous compression from tumor and resultant vascular stasis, chemotherapies such as platinum compounds and vascular endothelial growth factor (VEGF) inhibitors, hormonal therapies, and central venous catheters placed for treatment or in the setting of critical illness. Gastric, brain, and pancreas cancers pose the highest risk for development of VTE, but any tumor type can trigger a hypercoagulable state, including blood cancers.

Clinical Presentation

Symptoms and signs that should prompt a work-up for VTE include dyspnea, chest pain, tachycardia, unexplained low-grade fever, calf pain, and swelling of either the upper or lower extremities. Patients may present in either the inpatient or outpatient setting, and even those who are already anticoagulated may still thrombose. VTE may be discovered incidentally on staging scans; these should typically be treated even if asymptomatic.

The Khorana score is a widely used validated risk assessment tool that calculates the risk of developing VTE in cancer patients and may be used to guide consideration of prophylactic anticoagulation in these patients.

Treatment

Treatment of cancer-associated VTE with low-molecular-weight heparin (LMWH) has long been the "gold standard." In a pivotal trial, LMWH was shown to reduce VTE recurrence rate in cancer patients when compared with warfarin. More recently, the direct oral anticoagulants (DOACs) apixaban, edoxaban, and rivaroxaban have been studied in comparison with LMWH in cancer patients. Edoxaban was demonstrated to be noninferior to LMWH in reducing VTE recurrence risk, while apixaban and rivaroxaban were demonstrated to be superior with respect to this outcome. Some DOACs may have more bleeding complications in certain subsets of cancer patients, and the decision to use these agents should be made in consultation with a hematologist. Drug-drug interactions, including certain chemotherapeutic agents, may also preclude the use of DOACs. The duration of anticoagulation depends on the clinical scenario and requires a more nuanced approach than can be detailed here. In general, inferior vena cava (IVC) filters should only be placed if patients have a strong indication for anticoagulation that is contemporaneous with a strong contraindication.

SPINAL CORD COMPRESSION

Epidemiology

Approximately 3% of cancer patients will develop spinal cord compression as a result of their disease. Spinal cord compression is most prevalent in patients with lung and prostate cancers, as well as multiple myeloma.

Pathology

Most cases occur at the level of the thoracic spine, followed by the lumbar, then cervical spine. Spinal cord compression commonly develops when tumor extends from the bone into the epidural space, or as the result of a pathologic fracture. Compression of the spinal cord obstructs venous flow and results in vasogenic edema. When epidural disease occurs below the level of L1-L2 (where the conus medullaris terminates), cauda equina syndrome develops.

Clinical Presentation

The first symptom of spinal cord compression is typically pain. Patients will describe pain that is aggravated in the supine position or during a Valsalva maneuver, and may interfere with sleep. Motor weakness

肿瘤并发症及其治疗

朱以香 译 万蕊 段建春 审校 王洁 通审

引言

肿瘤的并发症及相关治疗是复杂的。尽管许多并发症需要由血液科和肿瘤科医生进行专业的治疗，但所有可能遇到这类患者的医生都应该对其临床表现、基本处理原则和转诊指征有所了解。

肿瘤的并发症既可表现于局部，也可以呈全身性（表10.1）。放疗、化疗和内分泌治疗等抗肿瘤治疗方案均具有潜在的副作用和并发症。这些大多数是一过性的，但也有可能是永久性的，比如周围神经毒性（表10.2）。抗肿瘤治疗带来的并发症不仅会影响患者的生活质量，还可能导致治疗延误或中断、需要住院甚至死亡。肿瘤及治疗导致的相关并发症管理通常需要多学科参与。本章重点介绍肿瘤的一些重要并发症及其治疗。

肿瘤相关性血栓

流行病学

静脉血栓栓塞（VTE）是肿瘤患者常见的并发症，亦常是其首发的临床表现。约15%的肿瘤患者在患病期间会发生VTE，是肿瘤患者死亡的主要原因之一。

病理学

肿瘤细胞相关促凝因子是促进肿瘤患者高凝状态的主要因素。此外，因病制动、肿瘤压迫所致血流凝滞、化疗药如铂类制剂、血管内皮生长因子抑制剂、内分泌治疗以及因治疗需要或危重情况下中心静脉置管等也会促进患者高凝状态。胃癌、中枢神经系统肿瘤和胰腺癌发生VTE的风险最高，但任何类型的肿瘤都可能引起高凝状态，包括血液系统肿瘤。

临床表现

VTE常见的症状和体征包括：呼吸困难、胸痛、心动过速、不明原因的低热、下肢疼痛和四肢肿胀。住院和门诊患者均可见，即使是那些已经使用了抗凝治疗的患者也可能发生血栓。部分VTE患者可能是在分期检查中偶然发现；即使无症状，也需要进行治疗。

Khorana评分是一种广泛用于评估肿瘤患者血栓栓塞风险的评分系统，可以评估肿瘤患者发生VTE的风险以及用来指导患者预防性抗凝治疗。

治疗

低分子量肝素（LMWH）是治疗肿瘤相关VTE的"金标准"。一项关键研究显示，LMWH对比华法林可降低肿瘤患者VTE的复发率。最新关于癌症患者口服抗凝剂（DOAC）阿哌沙班、依多沙班和利伐沙班与LMWH的比较显示：依多沙班在降低VTE的复发风险方面不劣于LMWH，而阿哌沙班和利伐沙班优于LMWH。部分DOAC对一些特定肿瘤患者可能增加出血的风险，是否使用口服抗凝剂治疗应咨询血液科医生。此外，药物间的相互作用，包括某些化疗药，也可能是使用DOAC的禁忌证。抗凝治疗时限取决于临床需要，在此不做详细阐述。通常情况下，下腔静脉（IVC）滤网置入仅适用于患者有强烈的抗凝指征，但又同时合并抗凝禁忌的患者。

脊髓压迫症

流行病学

约3%的肿瘤患者会因疾病本身发生脊髓压迫症。脊髓压迫症最常见于肺癌、前列腺癌以及多发性骨髓瘤的患者。

病理学

最常发生脊髓压迫症的部位是胸椎，其次是腰椎，然后是颈椎。脊髓压迫症常发生于肿瘤从骨扩散到硬膜外腔，或发生病理性骨折时。脊髓受压会阻碍静脉回流，导致血管源性水肿。当硬膜外病变发生在L1～L2水平以下（脊髓圆锥终止处）时，会发生马尾综合征。

临床表现

疼痛往往是脊髓压迫的首发症状。患者描述仰卧位或做Valsalva动作时疼痛加重，可能会影响睡眠。下肢无力和感觉减退，特别是鞍区麻木可作为诊断依据。

TABLE 10.1	Complications of Cancer
Localized	Systemic
Brain metastases	Anorexia/cachexia
Cancer-related pain	Cancer-associated thrombosis
Cord compression/cauda equina syndrome	Cancer-related anemia
Malignant effusions	Cancer-related fatigue
Pathologic fractures	Hypercalcemia
Superior vena cava syndrome	Paraneoplastic syndromes
Visceral obstruction	Tumor lysis syndrome

TABLE 10.2 Complications of Cancer Treatment
Alopecia
Central line thrombosis/infections
Cytopenias
Febrile neutropenia
Hot flashes
Hypertension
Nausea and vomiting
Peripheral neuropathy
Secondary malignancies
Skin toxicity
Stomatitis
Tumor lysis syndrome

and sensory deficits, specifically saddle anesthesia, can be present at diagnosis. These symptoms, however, typically herald advanced cord compression and are associated with a lower likelihood of functional recovery. Patients may also present with urinary retention (early) or bowel and bladder incontinence (later).

Diagnosis

A high clinical suspicion for spinal cord compression should develop when patients with known cancer present with any new back pain, and rapidly investigated with spinal imaging. Though plain radiographs of the vertebrae can certainly reveal abnormalities such as lytic lesions or vertebral fractures, time should not be wasted obtaining these studies because negative results in the setting of high clinical suspicion will not rule out spinal cord compression. Magnetic resonance imaging (MRI) is the preferred diagnostic imaging modality and should be obtained unless there is a contraindication to MRI, in which case computed tomography myelography should be performed. Imaging of the full spine is recommended even with localized symptoms because frequently multiple vertebral levels are affected.

Treatment

Dexamethasone and narcotic analgesia are the cornerstones of immediate treatment for cord compression. The optimal dose of corticosteroid is controversial. The most widely accepted dosing of dexamethasone is 10 mg IV followed by 4 to 6 mg IV every 6 hours, although some providers advocate an initial dose as high as 96 mg. This large dose, however, has been demonstrated to result in significant toxicity with questionable benefit.

Surgery and radiation therapy (RT) are the cornerstones of definitive therapy for spinal cord compression. Large randomized studies have demonstrated conflicting evidence about the benefits of surgery followed by RT versus RT alone. Though the presence of neurologic deficits is typically considered to be a clear indication for surgical intervention, goals of care, patient and tumor characteristics, and other comorbidities factor in to decision making regarding the most appropriate course of therapy.

SUPERIOR VENA CAVA SYNDROME

Definition

Superior vena cava (SVC) syndrome in malignancy is the result of flow obstruction by either external compression or intravascular thrombosis. The superior vena cava is thin walled and therefore easily compressed. The most common malignant causes are lung cancer and lymphoma.

Clinical Presentation

The presenting symptoms and signs of SVC syndrome depend on the rate of vessel obstruction. Slow compression allows for the development of collaterals from the azygos, internal mammary, paraspinous, lateral thoracic, and esophageal venous systems. Of these collateral tributaries the azygos vein is the most important because obstruction below its level is not well tolerated. Symptoms can be sudden or insidious. Most patients experience dyspnea (60% to 70%) and facial or neck swelling (50%). Cough, pain, arm swelling, and dysphagia are less common. Symptoms are frequently positional and exacerbated by leaning forward or lying down. Physical findings may include venous distention of neck and chest wall, facial edema, plethora, cyanosis, and upper extremity edema.

Diagnosis

Plain chest radiographs are usually abnormal; mediastinal widening (64%) and pleural effusion (26%) are the most common findings. The diagnosis is best established with contrast-enhanced computed tomographic scanning of the chest. It demonstrates the location and size of masses, the presence of intravascular thrombosis, and collateral venous drainage. When SVC syndrome is the initial manifestation of malignancy, pathologic diagnosis is the first step in establishing the proper initial treatment modality.

Treatment

The goals of treatment are to alleviate symptoms urgently and to treat the underlying malignancy. General supportive measures include head elevation and administration of glucocorticoids and diuretics. It is essential not to start radiation or glucocorticoids before obtaining a biopsy because these therapies can cloud the pathologic diagnosis. Specific management depends on the underlying pathology. Chemotherapy is the preferred first line of therapy for chemosensitive malignancies such as lymphoma, small cell lung cancer, or germ cell tumors. For non–small cell lung cancers and other less chemosensitive tumors, initial radiation therapy may be preferred.

Symptomatic relief can occur within 2 weeks but is often temporary; therefore, systemic management should be initiated as soon as possible with either chemotherapy, chemoradiation, or surgical resection. Persistent symptoms not relieved by chemotherapy or irradiation and those severe enough to warrant intervention before diagnosis can be successfully managed with endovascular stent placement with or without balloon angioplasty. The treatment of catheter-related SVC syndrome from thrombosis is anticoagulation. The decision regarding catheter removal is case dependent. Typically, catheters may remain in place provided they continue to function without evidence for clot propagation.

HYPERCALCEMIA

Epidemiology

Hypercalcemia complicates cancer in up to 10% of cases, occurring in both hematologic and solid malignancies. The most common etiologies are multiple myeloma, breast cancer, and squamous cell carcinoma.

表 10.1 肿瘤并发症	
局部	全身
脑转移	厌食／恶病质
癌症相关性疼痛	癌症相关性血栓
脊髓压迫／马尾综合征	癌症相关性贫血
恶性积液	癌症相关性乏力
病理性骨折	高钙血症
上腔静脉综合征	副肿瘤综合征
肠梗阻	肿瘤溶解综合征

表 10.2 癌症治疗性并发症
脱发
中央型血栓形成／感染
血细胞减少
发热性中性粒细胞减少
潮热
高血压
恶心呕吐
周围神经毒性
继发第二肿瘤
皮肤毒性
口腔炎
肿瘤溶解综合征

一旦出现上述症状往往预示为脊髓压迫症晚期，功能恢复的可能性较低。患者还可能会出现尿潴留（早期）或大小便失禁（晚期）。

诊断

当已确诊肿瘤的患者出现新发背部疼痛时，应高度怀疑脊髓压迫症，尽快完善脊椎影像学检查。尽管脊椎平片某些情况下会显示异常，如溶骨性病变或椎体骨折，但不应浪费时间在这些检查上，因为在临床高度怀疑脊髓压迫症的情况下，即使脊椎平片阴性也不能排除脊髓压迫症的可能性。磁共振成像（MRI）是首选的影像学检查，除非有禁忌证，优先推荐 MRI 检查明确诊断，如存在 MRI 禁忌证，应行计算机断层成像。即使为局部症状，也建议对整个脊椎进行检查，因为通常为多个椎体受累。

治疗

地塞米松和麻醉镇痛是脊髓压迫症紧急治疗的基石。皮质类固醇激素的最佳剂量尚存在争议。常用剂量为地塞米松 10 mg 静脉注射，之后 4～6 mg 每 6 h 一次静脉注射，也有部分单位推荐地塞米松的初始剂量达 96 mg。但这种大剂量给药方式已被证实会导致明显的不良反应且获益不明确。

手术和放射治疗（RT）是脊髓压迫症决定性治疗的基石。多项大型随机研究显示，手术后序贯 RT 与单纯 RT 的疗效比较结论不一。虽然神经功能障碍是手术治疗的明确适应证，但选择最佳治疗方案还需结合治疗目的、患者与肿瘤情况，以及其他合并症等因素。

上腔静脉综合征

定义

恶性肿瘤引起的上腔静脉（SVC）综合征是由于肿瘤压迫或血管内血栓形成造成血流阻塞所致。由于管壁较薄，上腔静脉很容易受到压迫。最常发生 SVC 综合征的恶性肿瘤是肺癌和淋巴瘤。

临床表现

上腔静脉综合征的症状和体征取决于血管阻塞发生的速度。缓慢的压迫可引起奇静脉、乳内静脉、胸骨旁静脉、胸外侧静脉和食管静脉系统的侧支扩张。其中，奇静脉最为关键，如果阻塞范围超过奇静脉，患者会出现明显的症状。这些症状可以突然发作，也可以为隐匿性。大部分患者会表现为呼吸困难（60%～70%）和面部或颈部肿胀（50%）。咳嗽、疼痛、手臂肿胀和吞咽困难较为少见。患者的症状与体位相关，前倾或平卧时会加重。体格检查会发现颈部和胸壁静脉扩张、面部水肿、淤血、发绀和上肢水肿。

诊断

胸部平片检查通常会提示异常；最常见的是纵隔增宽（64%）和胸腔积液（26%）。首选的诊断性检查是胸部增强计算机断层成像。不仅可以显示肿瘤的位置和大小、血管内的血栓情况，还可以观察侧支静脉回流。当 SVC 综合征是恶性肿瘤的初始症状时，首要任务是完善病理诊断以选择最佳的初始治疗方案。

治疗

治疗目的是快速缓解症状及治疗基础存在的恶性肿瘤。对症支持治疗包括抬高患者头部、使用糖皮质激素和利尿剂。在进行组织活检之前，切勿开始进行放射治疗或使用糖皮质激素，因为可能会干扰病理诊断。针对性治疗方案取决于病理类型。对于化疗敏感的恶性肿瘤（如淋巴瘤、小细胞肺癌或生殖细胞肿瘤）首选化疗。对于非小细胞肺癌及其他化疗敏感性较低的肿瘤，可首选放射治疗。

对症治疗 2 周内症状可以缓解，但通常是暂时的；应尽快开始系统性治疗，包括化疗、同步放化疗或手术切除。若症状经化疗或放疗无法缓解，或者病情严重、需要在诊断前进行治疗的患者，可以通过血管内支架置入伴／不伴球囊血管成形术治疗。由导管相关血栓导致的 SVC 综合征的治疗方法则是抗凝。是否拔出导管取决于病情需要。通常情况下，只要导管能继续使用且没有血栓扩散的迹象，可以保留导管。

高钙血症

流行病学

高达 10% 的肿瘤（包括血液系统肿瘤和实体瘤）患者会并发高钙血症。高钙血症最常见于多发性骨髓瘤、乳腺癌和鳞状细胞癌。

Pathology

Mechanisms leading to hypercalcemia include osteolysis due to bony involvement or tumor production of parathyroid hormone–related protein (PTHrP), calcitriol, or cytokines. Primary hyperparathyroidism should always be ruled out even in cancer patients. Because most cancer patients also have hypoalbuminemia, calcium levels should either be corrected or ionized calcium levels should be obtained.

Clinical Presentation

Early symptoms of hypercalcemia include altered mental status, constipation, polydipsia, polyuria, nausea, vomiting, and bradycardia. Many patients also have hypovolemia because of the polyuria. The severity of symptoms depends on the time course over which hypercalcemia has developed rather than the absolute calcium level.

Treatment

First and foremost, all calcium supplements, vitamin D, and diuretics should be stopped. Initial aggressive fluid resuscitation with normal saline at 200 to 300 mL/hour should be started to maintain a high urine output. This should be done carefully in patients with compromised cardiac or renal function while loop diuretics can be considered to maintain urine output in all patients who show signs of volume overload.

More definitive treatment for almost all cases of hypercalcemia in cancer patients is centered on bisphosphonates, which inhibit osteoclast activity and bone resorption. Intravenous pamidronate and zoledronic acid are the two most commonly used bisphosphonates. In a pooled analysis, zoledronic acid was associated with a higher rate of calcium normalization and longer control. Calcium response to bisphosphonates can take a few days, so if a rapid reduction in calcium is required then subcutaneous calcitonin (4 units/kg) can be given two to four times daily. Tachyphylaxis occurs with calcitonin so its use should be limited to 48 hours. Calcitonin works by increasing calcium renal excretion and reducing bone resorption. Ultimately, management should eventually include control of the underlying disease, which in the case of myeloma and lymphoma, includes glucocorticoids. Frequently new or recurring hypercalcemia indicates disease progression or treatment resistance and should be addressed with systemic therapy.

FEBRILE NEUTROPENIA

Definition

Febrile neutropenia is another common complication of chemotherapy and is defined as a temperature of 100.4° F sustained over 1 hour, or a one-time reading of 101.0° F in the setting of a neutrophil count lower than 1000/μL. The risk of febrile neutropenia increases with the intensity of the chemotherapy regimen and the severity and duration of neutropenia. It can lead to treatment delays or interruptions, prolonged hospitalizations, decreased quality of life, and increased morbidity and mortality. Febrile neutropenia is a medical emergency and delays in assessment and treatment should be avoided.

Treatment

Although most cases are managed in the hospital, low-risk patients may occasionally be successfully managed as outpatients. The American Society of Clinical Oncology (ASCO) has published guidelines for outpatient management that are based on a risk-stratified scoring system, including the Multinational Association for Supportive Care in Cancer (MASCC) and Clinical Index of Stable Febrile Neutropenia (CISNE) scores. All patients should have a history and physical examination to identify possible focal sources of infection. Attention should be given to the presence of mucositis and to swelling or induration and erythema around indwelling catheters as possible sources of infection. The initial work-up should include a full chemistry profile, complete blood count with differential, two sets of blood cultures, urinalysis, and chest radiography. ASCO guidelines allow for institutional variation in whether one set of blood cultures should be drawn from central venous access devices.

Prompt initiation of broad-spectrum antibiotics as soon as febrile neutropenia is identified is critical. Empirical antimicrobial therapy should consist of an antipseudomonal β-lactam such as cefepime or piperacillin-tazobactam for patients who require inpatient treatment and a fluoroquinolone for those whose risk profile allows for outpatient therapy. Patients with risk factors for antimicrobial resistance should have their regimens tailored accordingly; for example, vancomycin should be added if the clinical picture is consistent with pneumonia or there is hemodynamic instability. Often, no source is identified; in this case, antibiotics are continued until the neutrophil count exceeds 500 (provided that the fever resolves). When a source has been identified, antibiotic duration is dictated by the standard course for that particular type of infection. Certain high-risk chemotherapeutic regimens include the use of prophylactic myeloid growth factors such as filgrastim or pegfilgrastim to shorten the duration of neutropenia, and with that, the risk of developing febrile neutropenia. Routine use of growth factor support is not recommended in the management of febrile neutropenia in the absence of critical illness because there is little evidence to support its use in this clinical scenario.

CHEMOTHERAPY-INDUCED NAUSEA AND VOMITING

Definition

Nausea and vomiting are common adverse effects of chemotherapy, but prevention and management of this toxicity has evolved significantly in the last 2 decades. Nausea and emesis are typically categorized as acute, delayed, or anticipatory. Acute nausea and vomiting occur during the first 24 hours of treatment, whereas delayed nausea occurs 2 to 5 days after treatment initiation. Patients with high levels of anxiety or prior poor control of nausea may also suffer symptoms in anticipation of starting treatment. The risk of chemotherapy-induced nausea and vomiting is greater in younger patients, women, and those with a history of motion sickness.

Pathology

The mechanism by which chemotherapy induces nausea is complex. Proposed mechanisms involve the transmission of signals from neurotransmitter receptors in the gut to the nucleus tract solitarius, the area postrema, and the central pattern generator (in the brainstem) and involve the neurotransmitters dopamine, serotonin, and substance P.

Treatment

The best approach for treatment is prevention. The prophylactic antiemetic protocol depends on the chemotherapy regimen and emetic risk (Table 10.3). Randomized clinical trials have established that the combination of a neurokinin 1 (NK1) receptor antagonist (aprepitant or fosaprepitant), a 5HT3 serotonin receptor antagonist (ondansetron), olanzapine, and dexamethasone is the regimen of choice for highly emetogenic chemotherapy. For moderately emetogenic chemotherapy, a three-drug regimen of an NK1 receptor antagonist, 5HT3 antagonist with dexamethasone is recommended, although for some regimens just a 5HT3 receptor antagonist and dexamethasone alone may be adequate. All patients should be given a dopamine receptor antagonist such as prochlorperazine or a 5HT3 receptor antagonist

病理学

高钙血症的病理机制包括：由于骨转移或肿瘤释放的甲状旁腺激素相关蛋白（PTHrP）、骨化三醇或细胞因子引起骨溶解。即使是肿瘤患者，诊断肿瘤相关性高钙血症依然需要先排除原发性甲状旁腺功能亢进。由于大多数肿瘤患者会同时合并低白蛋白血症，因此，诊断时需要对钙离子浓度进行校正或检测游离钙浓度。

临床表现

高钙血症的早期症状包括神志改变、便秘、多饮、多尿、恶心、呕吐和心动过缓。由于多尿，患者可能会出现血容量不足。症状的严重程度取决于发生高钙血症的时间快慢，而非钙离子浓度的绝对水平。

治疗

首先，应停用所有钙补充剂、维生素 D 和利尿剂。采用生理盐水 200～300 ml/h 的速度开始积极补液，确保尿量。对心功能或肾功能受损的患者应谨慎补液，当患者出现容量超负荷时，可使用袢利尿剂利尿，保证尿量。

对高钙血症的癌症患者最有效的治疗方案是使用双膦酸盐，该药可以抑制破骨细胞活性，减少骨吸收。两种最常用的双膦酸盐是静脉用帕米膦酸和唑来膦酸。汇总分析显示，唑来膦酸具有更高的降血钙功效，且效果更持久。由于双膦酸盐的起效时间需要数天，如果需要快速降低血钙浓度，可采用皮下注射降钙素（4 单位/千克）每天 2～4 次进行治疗。由于降钙素存在快速耐药，治疗时间不应超过 48 h。降钙素可以增加肾对钙的排泄，减少骨的重吸收。最后，还需要尽可能控制基础疾病，如骨髓瘤和淋巴瘤，包括使用糖皮质激素等。如果反复出现新发或复发性高钙血症通常提示疾病进展或治疗抵抗，应考虑全身治疗。

发热性中性粒细胞减少

定义

发热性中粒细胞减少是化疗常见的并发症之一，是指中性粒细胞计数低于 1000/μl，且体温高于 38℃（100.4°F）超过 1 h，或 1 次最高体温达 38.3℃（101.0°F）。发热性中性粒细胞减少的发生风险会随着化疗方案的强度和中性粒细胞减少的严重程度及持续时间而增加。这会导致治疗延迟或中断、住院时间延长、生活质量下降以及发病率和死亡率增加。发热性中性粒细胞减少属于临床急症，应避免诊治延误。

治疗

虽然大多数患者需要住院治疗，但低风险的患者有时在门诊可以成功救治。美国临床肿瘤学会（ASCO）发布了基于风险分级评分系统的门诊治疗指南，包括癌症支持疗法多国学会（MASCC）和稳定状态发热性中性粒细胞减少临床指数（CISNE）评分系统。所有患者都应完善病史采集和体格检查，以识别可能的局部感染。需要注意是否存在黏膜炎以及留置导管周围肿胀、硬结或红斑等潜在的感染源。初步检查应包括全血生化、全血细胞计数和分类、两份血培养、尿液分析和胸部影像学检查。ASCO 指南允许各机构自行决定其中一份血培养是否从留置的中心静脉通道抽取。

一旦诊断发热性中性粒细胞减少，应立即使用广谱抗生素。对需要住院治疗的患者，经验性抗菌治疗应包括抗 β-内酰胺类药物，如头孢吡肟、哌拉西林-他唑巴坦；对经风险预测评估可以进行门诊治疗的患者，经验性抗菌治疗包括氟喹诺酮类药物。有抗菌药耐药风险的患者需相应个体化调整治疗方案；例如，临床症状支持肺炎诊断或存在血流动力学不稳定的情况，应加用万古霉素。通常情况下，在不能明确感染源时，应继续抗生素治疗直到中性粒细胞计数超过 500/μl（前提是体温正常）。当已经明确感染源后，抗生素的治疗时间取决于特殊感染的标准治疗疗程。对高风险化疗方案应预防性使用粒细胞生长因子，如非格司亭或长效非格司亭，以缩短中性粒细胞减少的持续时间，降低发生发热性中性粒细胞减少的风险。尚无证据支持在无危重症的情况下，常规使用粒细胞生长因子预防发热性中性粒细胞减少。

化疗诱发的恶心、呕吐

定义

恶心、呕吐是化疗常见的不良反应，在过去 20 年，针对它们的预防和处理取得了显著进步。化疗诱发的恶心、呕吐分为急性、延迟性和预期性。急性恶心、呕吐是指发生在治疗开始之后的 24 h 内，延迟性恶心、呕吐是指发生在治疗开始之后的 2～5 天。预期性恶心、呕吐是指高度焦虑或既往症状控制不佳的患者在开始治疗前出现恶心、呕吐。化疗诱发恶心、呕吐的高危风险因素包括：年轻、女性和有晕车史。

病理

关于化疗诱发恶心的发生机制十分复杂。可能涉及肠道中的神经递质受体向孤束核、延髓后区和中枢模式发生器（位于脑干）传递信号，涉及神经递质多巴胺、血清素和 P 物质。

治疗

针对化疗诱发的恶心呕吐的最佳治疗是预防。预防性止吐方案取决于化疗方案的致吐风险（表 10.3）。多项临床试验证实，对高致吐性化疗方案首选神经激肽 1（NK1）受体拮抗剂（阿瑞匹坦或福沙匹坦）、5HT3 受体拮抗剂（昂丹司琼）、奥氮平和地塞米松四药联合。对中度致吐性化疗方案，推荐使用 NK1 受体拮抗剂、5HT3 受体拮抗剂和地塞米松三药联合。然而，一些化疗方案仅使用 5HT3 受体拮抗剂和地塞米松双药联

TABLE 10.3 Nausea and Vomiting Risk With Cancer Therapy

Emetic Risk	Percentage of Patients Affected	Representative Agents	Recommended Preventive Antiemetic
High	>90	Cisplatin, high-dose cyclophosphamide	NK1 antagonist + 5HT3 antagonist + olanzapine + dexamethasone
Moderate	30–90	Oxaliplatin, doxorubicin, irinotecan	NK1 antagonist + 5HT3 antagonist + dexamethasone
Low	10–30	Paclitaxel, etoposide, gemcitabine	5HT3 antagonist OR dexamethasone
Minimal	<10	Vincristine, bleomycin	No routine prophylaxis

5HT3, Serotonin receptor; *NK1*, neurokinin 1.

such as ondansetron as rescue therapy for intermittent nausea, and the addition of olanzapine for breakthrough nausea and vomiting is appropriate in some circumstances.

Dexamethasone is the preferred treatment for delayed nausea and vomiting in highly and moderately emetogenic chemotherapy. Anticipatory nausea or vomiting is best treated with proper control of symptoms in the initial cycles. When it occurs, it is best treated with behavioral therapy, and benzodiazepines can be useful as adjunctive therapy.

DERMATOLOGIC TOXICITY

Many chemotherapeutic and targeted agents are associated with dermatologic toxicity, which can lead to patient morbidity, alter quality of life, and affect therapeutic dosing.

Clinical Presentation

Acneiform eruptions are observed with agents targeted against epidermal growth factor receptor (EGFR) in 70% to 80% of patients. The rash is usually erythematous with pustulopapular eruptions over the face, scalp, and upper trunk.

Palmar-plantar erythema, or so-called hand-foot syndrome, is seen with chemotherapeutic agents such as 5-fluorouracil and capecitabine or with tyrosine kinase inhibitors such as sorafenib, sunitinib, and regorafenib. Manifestations can differ slightly between classes of drugs, but they usually involve symmetrical redness of the palms or soles. Tingling and pain may accompany erythema. With progression, painful blistering or skin peeling may occur. Symptoms are frequently observed at pressure areas, such as on the soles of the feet after prolonged standing or running.

Treatment

Treatment of skin rash associated with anti-EGFR therapies is tailored to the severity of the rash and may include topical steroids, oral antibiotics (minocycline or doxycycline), and dose modification or cessation. Sunscreens, reduced sun exposure, and lotions for dry skin should be used for prevention. For hand-foot syndrome, preventive measures such as sunscreens and routine application of lotion to hands and feet are helpful. The most effective treatment is a brief treatment break (typically for several days, until complete resolution occurs), followed by resumption but with a reduced dose of the inciting agent.

TUMOR LYSIS SYNDROME

Definition

Tumor lysis syndrome (TLS) occurs when tumor cells break up and release toxic contents into the blood stream. It most commonly occurs in hematologic malignancies such as acute leukemias and non-Hodgkin's lymphoma, but can occur in almost any malignancy. It is typically triggered by the initiation of therapy in aggressive malignancies but can occur spontaneously, especially when there is a high tumor burden.

Pathology

Lysis of tumor cells causes the release of intracellular contents, including nucleic acids, potassium, and phosphate, into the bloodstream. The breakdown of nucleic acids results in high levels of uric acid, which can precipitate in the renal tubules and cause acute kidney injury (AKI). High levels of phosphate result in precipitation of calcium phosphate, which can cause symptomatic hypocalcemia, renal tubular injury and cardiac arrhythmias. High levels of potassium can also result in life-threatening cardiac arrhythmias.

Diagnosis

The recognition of patients who are at high risk for TLS should begin before therapy, and most patients in this category are given prophylactic allopurinol before initiation of treatment. The formal diagnosis of TLS is guided by the Cairo-Bishop criteria, which involves identifying both laboratory abnormalities suggestive of TLS (hyperkalemia, hypocalcemia, hyperphosphatemia, and hyperuricemia) and clinical criteria (AKI, cardiac arrhythmia, and seizure). The prompt diagnosis of TLS is critical to treatment and prevention of life-threatening electrolyte disturbances.

Treatment

Treatment involves aggressive hydration and meticulous management of electrolyte abnormalities. Patients are given 2 to 3 L of normal saline over 24 hours, which is sometimes augmented with loop diuretics to increase urine output. Allopurinol, if not given as a preventative measure, is given at a dose of 300 mg daily. If uric acid rises above 8, or is rapidly rising, rasburicase is given for a reduction in serum uric acid levels, although the magnitude of benefit with respect to preservation of renal function has not been solidly established. Most patients with a diagnosis of TLS require close monitoring, with laboratory checks three to four times a day and telemetry monitoring for cardiac arrhythmias, and sometimes require ICU level of care.

IMMUNE CHECKPOINT INHIBITOR TOXICITY

Definition

The use of recently discovered checkpoint inhibitors (e.g., pembrolizumab, nivolumab) is radically changing prognosis and treatment for several malignancies. With these new drugs, however, has also come new immunotherapy-induced toxicity. These are almost all related to an autoimmune-like response induced by these medications, resulting in inflammation of various organ systems. These include colitis, hepatitis, pneumonitis, dermatitis, encephalitis, and hypophysitis (panhypopituitarism).

表 10.3 癌症治疗诱发的恶心呕吐风险

致吐风险	发生患者百分比	代表药物	推荐的预防性止吐药
高	>90	顺铂，大剂量环磷酰胺	NK1 受体拮抗剂＋5HT3 受体拮抗剂＋奥氮平＋地塞米松
中等	30～90	奥沙利铂、多柔比星、伊立替康	NK1 受体拮抗剂＋5HT3 受体拮抗剂＋地塞米松
低	10～30	紫杉醇、依托泊苷、吉西他滨	5HT3 受体拮抗剂或地塞米松
轻微	<10	长春新碱、博来霉素	无需常规预防

5HT3，5-羟色胺受体；NK1，神经激肽 1。

合效果亦佳。口服多巴胺受体拮抗剂（如丙氯哌嗪）或 5HT3 受体拮抗剂（如昂丹司琼）可以作为所有患者间歇性恶心的补救措施。某些情况下，出现爆发性恶心、呕吐可以联用奥氮平治疗。

针对高度和中度致吐性化疗方案诱导的延迟性恶心呕吐的治疗首选地塞米松。对预期性恶心、呕吐的最佳治疗方法是在初始治疗时采用最佳的止吐方案。如果依然出现恶心、呕吐，优先采用行为疗法，可以辅助苯二氮䓬类药物。

皮肤毒性

许多化疗药物和靶向药物都会产生皮肤毒性，可能会导致患者患病、生活质量下降，以及影响药物剂量。

临床表现

70%～80% 的患者在使用表皮生长因子受体（EGFR）抑制剂时会出现痤疮样皮疹。皮疹通常表现为头面部和躯干上部脓疱疹样红斑。

掌跖红斑也称作手足综合征，常见于化疗药，如 5-氟尿嘧啶和卡培他滨，或酪氨酸激酶抑制剂，如索拉非尼、舒尼替尼和瑞戈非尼。不同类型的药物表现略有不同，但通常为手掌或足底的对称性红斑。局部可伴有刺痛和疼痛。随着病情发展，可能会出现疼痛性水疱或皮肤剥脱。常发生于受压部位，如长时间站立或跑步的足底区。

治疗

针对表皮生长因子受体抑制剂引起皮疹的治疗取决于皮疹的严重程度，包括局部使用类固醇激素、口服抗生素（米诺环素或多西环素）、药物减量或停药。另外，可预防性使用防晒霜，减少太阳照射，以及对干燥皮肤涂抹润肤乳。对于手足综合征，防晒霜和日常手足涂抹润肤露等预防措施具有一定帮助。针对手足综合征最有效的治疗方法是暂停治疗（通常为数天，至症状完全缓解），待症状完全缓解后降低剂量重新开始。

肿瘤溶解综合征

定义

肿瘤溶解综合征（TLS）是指肿瘤细胞破裂释放有毒细胞内物质到血液。最常见于血液系统肿瘤，如急性白血病和非霍奇金淋巴瘤，但可发生于任何恶性肿瘤。对侵袭性强的恶性肿瘤，肿瘤溶解综合征常发生于开始治疗之后，但也会自发出现，特别是在肿瘤负荷较高的情况下。

病理

肿瘤细胞的溶解会导致细胞内物质，如核酸、钾和磷酸盐释放到血液中。核酸分解会导致尿酸升高，尿酸在肾小管中沉积引起急性肾损伤（AKI）。高磷酸盐水平会导致磷酸钙沉积，从而引起有症状的低钙血症、肾小管损伤和心律失常。高血钾也可能引发危及生命的心律失常。

诊断

治疗前应识别 TLS 的高危患者，对于这类患者在开始治疗之前需预防性使用别嘌呤醇。TLS 的诊断参照 Cairo-Bishop 标准，包括提示 TLS 的实验室检查结果异常（高钾血症、低钙血症、高磷血症和高尿酸血症）和临床症状（AKI、心律失常和癫痫发作）。早期诊断 TLS 对治疗和预防危及生命的电解质紊乱至关重要。

治疗

治疗包括积极补液和纠正电解质紊乱。24 h 内需补 2～3 L 生理盐水，必要时使用袢利尿剂以保证尿量。如未进行过预防性处理，则需每天口服别嘌呤醇 300 mg 治疗。如果尿酸达 8 mg/dl 以上或快速升高，可口服拉布立酶降尿酸水平，尽管目前尚无证据支持拉布立酶对肾功能具有保护作用。大多数患者确诊 TLS 后都需要密切监测，每天进行 3～4 次实验室检查，对心律失常的患者进行心电监测，必要时需要重症监护病房级别的支持。

免疫检查点抑制剂毒性

定义

免疫检查点抑制剂（如帕博利珠单抗、纳武利尤单抗）的出现改变了多种癌症患者的预后和治疗格局。然而，随着这些新药的出现，免疫治疗导致的毒性也随之而来。这些毒性反应几乎都与药物诱导的自身免疫反应有关，表现为各脏器系统的炎症反应，包括结肠炎、肝炎、肺炎、皮炎、脑炎和垂体功能减退（全垂体功能减退）。

Pathophysiology

Immune checkpoint inhibitors work by "releasing the brakes" on the immune system imposed by cancer cells. Co-stimulatory cell surface antigens such as PD-1/PDL-1 and CTLA-4, needed for activation of the immune system, are often downregulated by tumor cell surface markers. Immunotherapy reactivates the immune system, removing the tumor blockades and allowing the body's own immune system to attack the tumor cells. In doing so, the immune system may be mobilized indiscriminately, resulting in its activation not only against the cancer but also against the patient's own healthy tissue.

Diagnosis

Immune-mediated toxicity should be considered in all patients on immunotherapy presenting with symptoms consistent with immune-mediated phenomena. These include diarrhea (colitis), shortness of breath or cough (pneumonitis), rash (dermatitis), or altered mentation (encephalitis). In addition, patients are also monitored for laboratory evidence of hepatitis and hypophysitis (most specifically hypothyroidism). These signs and symptoms can be mild and treated symptomatically, but on rare occasions can be life-threatening.

Treatment

Patients with mild signs and symptoms can often be treated symptomatically while remaining on the medication, or with a brief interruption in treatment, which can be restarted once signs and symptoms have resolved. Patients with findings of hypothyroidism can be started on thyroid hormone replacement without need for immune checkpoint discontinuation. In more severe cases, such as with new oxygen requirement, severe diarrhea, or significant elevations in liver function tests (LFTs), the immunotherapy needs to be discontinued and patients should be started on corticosteroids to try to decrease the inflammatory response, typically at doses of 1 to 2 mg/kg of methylprednisolone (or its equivalent) per day. In rare cases of severe toxicity, immunomodulatory medication such as mycophenolate mofetil or infliximab is utilized in addition to corticosteroids. In most cases, expert consultation should be obtained to guide the management of these toxicities.

For a deeper discussion on this topic, please see Chapter 73, "Thrombotic Disorders: Hypercoagulable States," Chapter 232, "The Parathyroid Glands, Hypercalcemia, and Hypocalcemia," and Chapter 372, "Mechanical and Other Lesions of the Spine, Nerve Roots, and Spinal Cord," in *Goldman-Cecil Medicine*, 26th Edition.

SUGGESTED READINGS

Hesketh P, Kris MG, Basch E, et al: Antiemetics: american society of clinical oncology clinical practice guideline update, J Clin Oncol 35(28):3240–3261, 2017.

Howard SC, Jones DP, Pui CH: The tumor lysis syndrome, N Engl J Med 364:1844–1854, 2011.

Kraaijpoel N, Carrier M: How I treat cancer-associated venous thromboembolism, Blood 133:291–298, 2019.

Lawton AJ, Lee KA, Cheville AL, et al: Assessment and management of patients with metastatic spinal cord compression: a multidisciplinary review, J Clin Oncol 37(1):61–71, 2019.

Postow MA, Sidlow R, Hellmann MD: Immune-related adverse events associated with immune checkpoint blockade, N Eng J Med 378:158, 2018.

Taplitz R, Kennedy EB, Bow EJ, et al: Outpatient management of fever and neutropenia in adults treated for malignancy: American Society of Clinical Oncology and Infectious Diseases Society of America Clinical Practice Guideline Update, J Clin Oncol 36(14):1443–1453, 2018.

病理生理

免疫检查点抑制剂的作用机制是"松开"癌细胞对免疫系统的"刹车"。肿瘤细胞的表面标记通常会下调免疫系统激活所需的共刺激细胞表面抗原，如 PD-1/PDL-1 和 CTLA-4 等。免疫治疗可以重新激活患者的免疫系统，消除肿瘤阻滞，从而使人体自身的免疫系统恢复对肿瘤细胞的攻击。在此过程中，免疫系统可能会无差异地激活，导致激活的免疫系统不仅靶向肿瘤，同时也针对患者本身的正常组织。

诊断

所有接受免疫治疗并出现相应症状的患者都应该考虑免疫相关毒副作用，包括腹泻（结肠炎）、呼吸困难或咳嗽（肺炎）、皮疹（皮炎）或神志改变（脑炎）。另外，需要完善实验室检查评估患者是否合并肝炎和垂体炎（尤其是甲状腺功能减退）等情况。通常而言，这些症状和体征较轻，只需对症治疗，但极少数情况也可能会危及生命。

治疗

症状和体征较轻微的患者在对症治疗的基础上可以继续用药，或短暂中断治疗，一旦症状和体征缓解，即可恢复治疗。合并甲状腺功能减退症的患者可以联用甲状腺激素替代药物，无需停用免疫检查点抑制剂。若出现新发缺氧、严重腹泻或肝功能指标（LFT）异常升高，则需要停用免疫检查点抑制剂，并使用皮质类固醇激素减轻炎症反应，推荐甲泼尼龙（或同等剂量其他类型药物）1～2 mg/kg 每天给药。在极少数毒副作用严重的患者中，除皮质类固醇激素外，还可以使用免疫调节剂，如霉酚酸酯或英夫利西单抗。建议在专科医生的指导下处理这些毒副作用。

有关此专题的深入讨论，请参阅 *Goldman-Cecil Medicine* 第 26 版第 73 章"血栓性疾病：高凝状态"、第 232 章"甲状旁腺、高钙血症和低钙血症"，以及第 372 章"脊柱、神经根和脊髓的机械性损伤和其他损伤"。

推荐阅读

Hesketh P, Kris MG, Basch E, et al: Antiemetics: american society of clinical oncology clinical practice guideline update, J Clin Oncol 35(28):3240–3261, 2017.

Howard SC, Jones DP, Pui CH: The tumor lysis syndrome, N Engl J Med 364:1844–1854, 2011.

Kraaijpoel N, Carrier M: How I treat cancer-associated venous thromboembolism, Blood 133:291–298, 2019.

Lawton AJ, Lee KA, Cheville AL, et al: Assessment and management of patients with metastatic spinal cord compression: a multidisciplinary review, J Clin Oncol 37(1):61–71, 2019.

Postow MA, Sidlow R, Hellmann MD: Immune-related adverse events associated with immune checkpoint blockade, N Eng J Med 378:158, 2018.

Taplitz R, Kennedy EB, Bow EJ, et al: Outpatient management of fever and neutropenia in adults treated for malignancy: American Society of Clinical Oncology and Infectious Diseases Society of America Clinical Practice Guideline Update, J Clin Oncol 36(14):1443–1453, 2018.

索引 Index

A

Acrallentiginous melanoma (ALM), 110
Adenocarcinomas, of lung, 44
Adenosquamous carcinomas, of lung, 46
Adjuvant chemotherapy, 36-38
Alcohol
    cancer risk and, 22
Alemtuzumab, 40t
ALK 2p23, lung cancer and, 46
All-*trans*-retinoic acid (ATRA), for acute promyelocytic leukemia, 40t
Anal cancer, 64-66
Androgen deprivation therapy, in prostate cancer, 76
Angiogenesis, 4, 16-18
Anticoagulation
    in cancer patient, hospitalized, 118, 120t
Antiemetic drugs, with cancer chemotherapy, 42
Apoptosis, 8, 8f-12f
    chemotherapy-induced, 38
Aromatase inhibitors, for breast cancer, 40
Asbestos
    lung cancer and, 44
Axitinib, 40t
Azacitidine, 40t

B

Barrett esophagus (BE), 56
Bevacizumab, 40t
Biomarkers, of cancer, 32
Bisphosphonates
    for hypercalcemia, 122
Bladder cancer, 72-74, 72f
Bone metastasis, breast cancer and, 88
Bone sarcomas, 112
Borderline ovarian neoplasms, 92
Bortezomib, 40t
Breast cancer, 80-90
    clinical presentation of, 80-84
    diagnosis of, 80-84
    dose-dense approach in, 36
    early-stage, 86-88
    endocrine therapy for, 40
    epidemiology of, 80, 82t
    gene expression in, 32
    genetics, 80
    histology of, 82-84
    hypercalcemia in, 120
    invasive, 82-84
    male, 90
    metastatic, 88
    in older women, 90
    risk factors of, 80, 82t
    screening, 30, 90
    staging, 84
    therapy for HR+, 88
    treatment of, 84-90
    triple-negative, 88
Bronchioloalveolar carcinomas, 44

C

Calcitonin

Page numbers followed by "f" indicate figures, "t" indicate tables, and "b" indicate boxes.

A

肢端雀斑样痣黑色素瘤（ALM），111
肺腺癌，45
肺腺鳞癌，47
辅助化疗，37-39
酒精
    癌症风险，23
阿仑单抗，41t
ALK 2p23，肺癌，47
全反式维甲酸（ATRA），治疗急性早幼粒细胞白血病，41t
肛门癌，65-67
雄激素剥夺治疗，见于前列腺癌，77
血管生成，5，17-19
抗凝治疗
    癌症患者，住院用药，119，121t
止吐药，癌症化疗，43
凋亡，9，9f-13f
    化疗诱导，39
芳香化酶抑制剂，治疗乳腺癌，41
石棉
    肺癌，45
阿昔替尼，41t
阿扎胞苷，41t

B

巴雷特食管（BE），57
贝伐珠单抗，41t
生物标志物，癌症，33
双膦酸盐
    高钙血症，123
膀胱癌，73-75，73f
骨转移，乳腺癌，89
骨肉瘤，113
交界性卵巢肿瘤，93
硼替佐米，41t
乳腺癌，81-91
    临床表现，81-85
    诊断，81-85
    "剂量密集"法，37
    早期，87-89
    内分泌治疗，41
    流行病学，81，83t
    基因表达，33
    遗传学，81
    组织学，83-85
    高钙血症，121
    浸润性，83-85
    男性，91
    转移性，89
    老年女性，91
    危险因素，81，83t
    筛查，31，91
    分期，85
    HR 阳性患者的治疗，89
    治疗，85-91
    三阴性，89
细支气管肺泡癌，45

C

降钙素

页码数字中，"f"代表"图"，"t"代表"表格"，"b"代表"框"。

索引 Index

for hypercalcemia, 122
Cancer
  apoptosis, 8, 8f-12f
  biology, 4-18
  complications of, 118-126
    febrile neutropenia, 122
    immune checkpoint inhibitor toxicity, 124-126
    spinal cord compression, 118-120
    superior vena cava syndrome, 120
    thrombosis, 118
  diagnosis of, 32
  epidemiology methods of, 20
  estimated cases and deaths from, 22t
  genetics of, 4, 6f
  hallmarks of, 4-18
  hereditary syndromes of, 26t
  metastatic, staging of, 32
  microenvironment of, 4, 6f
  mortality rates of, 24f
  prevention of, 28
    chemoprevention in, 28
    genetic testing and, 20-22, 26t
    lifestyle changes in, 28
    risk factors and, 20-28
  screening for, 28-30
  signaling, 14f-16f
  staging of, 32
  suppression, 4-8, 8f-12f
  treatment of, 32
    complications, 120t
    endocrine therapy in, 38-40
    evaluation of response in, 42
    immunotherapy in, 40-42
    palliative, 32-34
    personalized medicine in, 40
    supportive care in, 42
    surgery in, 32-34
    targeted therapy in, 38, 40t
Cancer of unknown primary site (CUP), 114-116
Castrate-resistant prostate cancer (CRPC), 76
Cervical cancer, 98-100
  human papillomaviruses and, 24
  screening for, 30
Cetuximab, 38, 40t
Chemicals, cancer risk and, 28
Chemopreventive agents, cancer, 28
Chemotherapy, 36t
  definition of, 36
  indications for, 36-38, 38t
  limitations of, 38
  in non-small cell lung cancer, 54
  side effects of, drugs for, 42
  in testicular cancer, 78
Chimeric antigen receptor-T (CAR-T) cell therapy, 42
Cholangiocarcinoma, 60
Cirrhosis
  hepatocellular carcinoma and, 60
Cisplatin, 36t
  in bladder cancer, 72
Clear cell carcinoma, renal, 68-72
Colon cancer, screening for, 30
Colonoscopy
  in colorectal cancer, 64
Colorectal cancer, 62-64
  clinical presentation of, 64
  diagnosis of, 64
  epidemiology of, 62
  pathology of, 62-64, 62f
  prognosis of, 64

高钙血症，123
癌症
  凋亡，9，9f-13f
  生物学，5-19
  并发症，119-127
    发热性中性粒细胞减少，123
    免疫检查点抑制剂毒性，125-127
    脊髓压迫症，119-121
    上腔静脉综合征，121
    血栓，119
  诊断，33
  流行病学研究方法，21
  预计病例和死亡人数，23t
  遗传学，5，7f
  特征，5-19
  遗传性综合征，27t
  转移，分期，33
  微环境，5，7f
  死亡率，25f
  预防，29
    化学预防，29
    基因检测，21-23，27t
    生活方式改变，29
    危险因素，21-29
  筛查，29-31
  信号，15f-17f
  分期，33
  抑制，5-9，9f-13f
  治疗，33
    并发症，121t
    内分泌治疗，39-41
    疗效评估，43
    免疫治疗，41-43
    姑息性，33-35
    个性化医疗，41
    支持性治疗，43
    手术，33-35
    靶向治疗，39，41t
原发部位不明的癌症（CUP），115-117
去势抵抗性前列腺癌（CRPC），77
宫颈癌，99-101
  人乳头瘤病毒，25
  筛查，31
西妥昔单抗，39，41t
化学物质，癌症风险，29
化学预防剂，癌症，29
化疗，37t
  定义，37
  适应证，37-39，39t
  局限性，39
  非小细胞肺癌，55
  副作用，药物，43
  睾丸癌，79
嵌合抗原受体-T（CAR-T）细胞治疗，43
胆管癌，61
肝硬化
  肝细胞癌，61
顺铂，37t
  膀胱癌，73
透明细胞癌，肾，69-73
结肠癌，筛查，31
结肠镜
  结直肠癌，65
结直肠癌，63-65
  临床表现，65
  诊断，65
  流行病学，63
  病理学，63-65，63f
  预后，65

screening for, 64
surveillance for, 64
treatment of, 64
    monoclonal antibodies in, 40t
Computed tomography (CT)
    of ovarian cancer, 92
    of renal cell carcinoma, 68
Condyloma acuminata, anal cancer and, 64
Crizotinib, 40t
Cyclophosphamide, 36t
Cytoreductive nephrectomy, for metastatic renal cell carcinoma, 70
Cytotoxic chemotherapy, for melanoma, 112

D

Dabrafenib, for melanoma, 112
Dasatinib, 40t
Dermatologic toxicity, 124
Desmoplastic reaction, in pancreatic cancer, 58
Doxorubicin, 36t
Ductal carcinoma in situ (DCIS), 82
Dysphagia
    in esophageal cancer, 56

E

Early-stage breast cancer, 86-88
EML4-ALK fusion, lung cancer and, 44
Endocrine therapy
    for cancer, 38-40
        compliance, breast cancer and, 90
Endometrial cancer, 94
Endoscopic ultrasound (EUS)
    for esophageal cancer, 56
Endoscopy
    gastrointestinal
        in esophageal cancer, 56
Epidermal growth factor receptor (EGFR), 32, 34f, 40t
    lung cancer and, 46, 54
Erlotinib, 40t
    for lung cancer, 54
ER-positive HER2-negative metastatic breast cancer, 88
Esophageal cancer, 56
Everolimus, 40t
Ewing sarcoma, 112

F

False-negative results, 30
False-positive results, 30
Familial adenomatous polyposis (FAP), 62-64
Febrile neutropenia, 122
Fertility preservation, breast cancer and, 90
α-fetoprotein, hepatocellular carcinoma, 32
Filgrastim, 42
Fluid resuscitation
    in hypercalcemia, 122
18-Fluorodeoxyglucose (FDG), in lung cancer, 50
5-Fluorouracil, 36t

G

Gallbladder cancer, 60
Gastric cancer, 58
Gastrointestinal cancers, 56-66
Gastrointestinal stromal tumors (GIST), 38, 40t
Gemcitabine, 36t
Genetic testing
    for hereditary cancer syndromes, 20-22, 26t
Genitourinary cancers, 68-78
Genome, lung cancer, 48

筛查，65
监测，65
治疗，65
    单克隆抗体，41t
计算机断层成像（CT）
    卵巢癌，93
    肾细胞癌，69
尖锐湿疣，肛门癌，65
克唑替尼，41t
环磷酰胺，37t
减瘤性或细胞减灭性肾切除术，治疗转移性肾细胞癌，71
细胞毒性化疗，治疗黑色素瘤，113

D

达拉非尼，治疗黑色素瘤，113
达沙替尼，41t
皮肤毒性，125
结缔组织增生反应，见于胰腺癌，59
多柔比星，37t
导管原位癌（DCIS），83
吞咽困难
    食管癌，57

E

早期乳腺癌，87-89
EML4-ALK（融合基因），肺癌，45
内分泌治疗
    癌症，39-41
        依从性，乳腺癌，91
子宫内膜癌，95
内镜超声（EUS）
    食管癌，57
内镜
    胃肠道
        食管癌，57
表皮生长因子受体（EGFR），33，35f，41t
    肺癌，47，55
厄洛替尼，41t
    肺癌，55
ER阳性HER2阴性转移性乳腺癌，89
食管癌，57
依维莫司，41t
尤因肉瘤，113

F

假阴性结果，31
假阳性结果，31
家族性腺瘤性息肉病（FAP），63-65
发热性中性粒细胞减少，123
保留生育能力，乳腺癌，91
甲胎蛋白，肝细胞癌，33
非格司亭，43
补液
    高钙血症，123
18-氟脱氧葡萄糖（FDG），肺癌，51
5-氟尿嘧啶，37t

G

胆囊癌，61
胃癌，59
胃肠道癌症，57-67
胃肠道间质瘤（GIST），39，41t
吉西他滨，37t
基因检测
    遗传性癌症综合征，21-23，27t
泌尿生殖系统肿瘤，69-79
基因组，肺癌，49

Genomic instability, 8-10
Germ cell tumors, 76
Gestational trophoblastic disease, 102-106, 104f
    clinical presentation of, 104
    diagnosis of, 104
    epidemiology of, 102-104
    pathology of, 104
    prognosis of, 106
    staging of, 104
    treatment of, 104-106
Gestational trophoblastic neoplasia, 102-106, 104f
    clinical presentation of, 104
    diagnosis of, 104
    epidemiology of, 102-104
    pathology of, 104
    prognosis of, 106
    staging of, 104
    treatment of, 104-106
Giant cell carcinoma, of lung, 46
Gleason scoring system, in prostate cancer, 74-76
Glucocorticoids
    for hypercalcemia, cancer-associated, 122
    for superior vena cava syndrome, 120
Goserelin, for prostate cancer, 40
Graft-*versus*-host disease (GVHD)
    in stem cell transplantation, 42
Graft-*versus*-tumor effect, in stem cell transplantation, 42
Granulocyte colony-stimulating factor (G-CSF)
    with chemotherapy, 42
Granulocyte-macrophage colony-stimulating factor (GM-CSF)
    with chemotherapy, 42
Gynecological cancer, 92-106
    cervical, 98-100
    gestational trophoblastic disease/neoplasia, 102-106, 104f
    ovarian, 92-94, 94t
    uterine, 94-98, 96f
    vaginal, 102
    vulvar, 100-102

H

Hamartomas, lung, 50
Hand-foot syndrome, 124
Head cancer, 108-110
Helicobacter pylori
    gastric cancer and, 58
Hematochezia
    colorectal cancer and, 64
Heparin
    in cancer patient, hospitalized, 118
Hepatocellular carcinoma, 60-62
Hereditary nonpolyposis colorectal cancer, 64
HLA-A gene, lung cancer and, 48
Horner syndrome
    lung cancer and, 48-50
HR+ breast cancer, therapy for, 88
Human epidermal growth factor receptor 2 (HER2), 56
Human papillomavirus (HPV), 98
    cervical cancer and, 22-24
Hypercalcemia
    cancer-associated, 120-122

I

Ibrutinib, 40t
Imatinib, 38, 40t
Immune checkpoint inhibitor toxicity, 124-126
Immune escape, 18, 18f
Infections
    cancer risk and, 22-24

基因组不稳定性，9-11
生殖细胞肿瘤，77
妊娠滋养细胞疾病，103-107，105f
    临床表现，105
    诊断，105
    流行病学，103-105
    病理学，105
    预后，107
    分期，105
    治疗，105-107
妊娠滋养细胞肿瘤，103-107，105f
    临床表现，105
    诊断，105
    流行病学，103-105
    病理学，105
    预后，107
    分期，105
    治疗，105-107
肺巨细胞癌，47
Gleason 评分系统，前列腺癌，75-77
糖皮质激素
    高钙血症，癌症相关，123
    上腔静脉综合征，121
戈舍瑞林，治疗前列腺癌，41
移植物抗宿主病（GVHD）
    干细胞移植，43
移植物抗肿瘤效应，见于干细胞移植，43
粒细胞集落刺激因子（G-CSF）
    化疗，43
粒细胞-巨噬细胞集落刺激因子（GM-CSF）
    化疗，43
妇科癌症，93-107
    宫颈癌，99-101
    妊娠滋养细胞疾病/肿瘤，103-107，105f
    卵巢癌，93-95，95t
    子宫癌，95-99，97f
    阴道癌，103
    外阴癌，101-103

H

错构瘤，肺，51
手足综合征，125
头部癌症，109-111
幽门螺杆菌
    胃癌，59
便血
    结直肠癌，65
肝素
    住院癌症患者，119
肝细胞癌，61-63
遗传性非息肉病性结直肠癌，65
HLA-A 基因，肺癌，49
霍纳综合征
    肺癌，49-51
HR 阳性乳腺癌的治疗，89
人表皮生长因子受体 2（HER2），57
人乳头瘤病毒（HPV），99
    宫颈癌，23-25
高钙血症
    癌症相关，121-123

I

伊布替尼，41t
伊马替尼，39，41t
免疫检查点抑制剂毒性，125-127
免疫逃逸，19，19f
感染
    癌症风险，23-25

Infiltrating ductal carcinoma (IDC), 82-84, 84f
Inflammatory breast cancer, 84, 86f
Invasion, 16-18
Invasive breast cancer, 82-84
Invasive lobular carcinoma (ILC), 82-84
Ionizing radiation, cancer risk and, 28
Ipilimumab, 40t
    for melanoma, 112
Irinotecan, 36t

J
Jaundice
    in pancreatic cancer, 58

K
KRAS oncogene, lung cancer and, 44-46

L
Lapatinib, 40t
Lead-time bias, 30
Length-time bias, 30
Lentigo maligna melanoma (LMM), 110
Leuprolide, for prostate cancer, 40
Lifestyle
    cancer risk and, 22-28, 26t
Liver transplantation
    for hepatocellular carcinoma, 62
Lobectomy, in non-small cell lung cancer, 54
Lobular carcinoma in situ (LCIS), 82
Lung cancer, 44-52
    clinical presentation of, 48-50
    definition of, 44
    diagnosis and differential diagnosis of, 50-52
    epidemiology of, 44
    genome, 48
    histologic subgroups of, 44-46
    molecular-genomic subtypes of, 46, 48t
    non-small cell, 44-46
    paraneoplastic syndromes associated with, 46t
    pathology of, 44-48
    prognosis of, 54
    screening for, 50
    small cell, 44-46
    staging of, 50, 52t
    treatment for, 52-54
Luteinizing hormone-releasing hormone (LHRH) agonists, for prostate cancer, 40, 76
Lymph nodes
    enlargement of, lung cancer and, 50
Lymphedema, breast cancer and, 90
Lynch syndrome, 64

M
Magnetic resonance imaging (MRI)
    of ovarian cancer, 92
Male breast cancer, 90
Mammography, screening, breast cancer and, 90
Masses
    renal, 68-70
Medullary carcinoma, 82-84
Melanocytes, 110
Melanoma, 110-112
Metastases, 16-18
Metastatic breast cancer, 88
Metastatic disease, bladder cancer and, 72-74
Methotrexate, 36t
Microsatellite instability (MSI), 8-10
Mitogen-activated protein kinase (MAPK) signaling pathway, 112

J
浸润性导管癌（IDC），83-85，85f
炎性乳腺癌，85，87f
侵袭，17-19
浸润性乳腺癌，83-85
浸润性小叶癌（ILC），83-85
电离辐射，癌症风险，29
伊匹木单抗，41t
    黑色素瘤，113
伊立替康，37t

J
黄疸
    胰腺癌黄疸，59

K
KRAS 癌基因，肺癌，45-47

L
拉帕替尼，41t
前导时间偏倚，31
长度时间偏倚，31
恶性雀斑样痣黑色素瘤（LMM），111
亮丙瑞林，治疗前列腺癌，41
生活方式
    癌症风险，23-29，27t
肝移植
    肝细胞癌，63
肺叶切除术，非小细胞肺癌，55
小叶原位癌（LCIS），83
肺癌，45-53
    临床表现，49-51
    定义，45
    诊断和鉴别诊断，51-53
    流行病学，45
    基因组，49
    病理亚型，45-47
    分子基因亚型，47，49t
    非小细胞，45-47
    相关的副肿瘤综合征，47t
    病理学，45-49
    预后，55
    筛查，51
    小细胞，45-47
    分期，51，53t
    治疗，53-55
促黄体素释放激素（LHRH）激动剂，治疗前列腺癌，41，77
淋巴结
    肿大，肺癌，51
淋巴水肿，乳腺癌，91
林奇综合征，65

M
磁共振成像（MRI）
    卵巢癌，93
男性乳腺癌，91
乳腺X线筛查，乳腺癌，91
肿物
    肾，69-71
髓样癌，83-85
黑色素细胞，111
黑色素瘤，111-113
转移，17-19
转移性乳腺癌，89
转移性疾病，膀胱癌，73-75
甲氨蝶呤，37t
微卫星不稳定性（MSI），9-11
丝裂原活化蛋白激酶（MAPK）信号通路，113

Monoclonal antibodies, as anticancer agents, 38, 40t
Mucinous breast cancer, 82-84
Mucosal melanoma, 108

N

National Comprehensive Cancer Network (NCCN) Guidelines, in breast cancer, 80, 82t
Nausea
    chemotherapy-induced, 122-124, 124t
Neck cancer, 108-110
Neoadjuvant chemotherapy, 38
    for breast cancer, 86
Nephrectomy, for metastatic renal cell carcinoma, 68
Neutropenia
    chemotherapy-induced, 42
    febrile, 122
Nodular melanoma (NM), 110
Nonepithelial ovarian cancers, 92
Non-ionizing radiation, cancer risk and, 28
Nonseminomas, 76
Non-small cell lung carcinomas, 44-46
    treatment for, 54
Nutrition
    cancer risk and, 22

O

Obesity
    risks associated with cancer, 22
Ofatumumab, 40t
Older adults
    breast cancer in, 90
Oncogenes, 10-14, 14f-16f
    lung cancer and, 44
Orchiopexy, in testis cancer, 76
Organ-confined disease, bladder cancer and, 72
Oropharyngeal cancer, HPV-associated, 108
Osteoporosis
    prostate cancer and, 76
Osteosarcoma, 112
Ovarian cancer, 92-94, 94t

P

Paclitaxel, 36t
Palliative cancer treatment, 32-34
Palmar-plantarerythema, 124
Pancoast tumors, 48-50
Pancreatic cancer, 58-60
Pancreatic neuroendocrine tumors, 58
Panitumumab, 40t
PD-L1 (programmed-death ligand 1), 18
Performance status, 32
Pertuzumab, 40t
P-glycoprotein, 38
Philadelphia chromosome, 38
Physical activity, cancer risk and, 22
Pleural effusion
    lung cancer and, 48-50
Polyps, colon cancers from, 62
Positron emission tomography (PET)
    in lung cancer, 50
Positron emission tomography-computed tomography (PET/CT), of cervical cancer, 98
Postobstructive pneumonia, lung cancer and, 50
Prostate cancer, 74-76, 76t
Prostatectomy, in prostate cancer, 76
Prostate-specific antigen (PSA)
    in prostate cancer, 74

单克隆抗体，抗癌药物，39，41t
黏液性乳腺癌，83-85
黏膜黑色素瘤，109

N

美国国家综合癌症网络（NCCN）乳腺癌指南，81，83t
恶心
    化疗诱发，123-125，125t
颈部癌，109-111
新辅助化疗，39
    乳腺癌，87
肾切除术，治疗转移性肾癌，69
中性粒细胞减少症
    化疗诱发，43
    发热性，123
结节性黑色素瘤（NM），111
非上皮性卵巢癌，93
非电离辐射，癌症风险，29
非精原细胞瘤，77
非小细胞肺癌，45-47
    治疗，55
营养
    癌症危险因素，23

O

肥胖
    癌症相关风险，23
奥法木单抗，41t
老年人
    乳腺癌，91
癌基因，11-15，15f-17f
    肺癌，45
睾丸固定术，治疗睾丸癌，77
局限于膀胱的疾病，膀胱癌，73
口咽癌，HPV相关性，109
骨质疏松症
    前列腺癌，77
骨肉瘤，113
卵巢癌，93-95，95t

P

紫杉醇，37t
癌症姑息性治疗，33-35
掌跖红斑，125
肺上沟瘤，49-51
胰腺癌，59-61
胰腺神经内分泌肿瘤，59
帕尼单抗，41t
PD-L1（程序性死亡配体-1），19
体力状态，33
培妥珠单抗，41t
P-糖蛋白，39
费城染色体，39
体育活动，癌症风险，23
胸腔积液
    肺癌，49-51
息肉，结肠癌，63
正电子发射断层成像（PET）
    肺癌，51
正电子发射断层成像-计算机断层成像（PET/CT），宫颈癌，99

阻塞性肺炎，肺癌，51
前列腺癌，75-77，77t
前列腺切除术，见于前列腺癌，77
前列腺特异性抗原（PSA）
    前列腺癌，75

R

Radiation, cancer risk and, 28
Radiation therapy, 34-36
    acute effects of, 36
    late effects of, 36
    in prostate cancer, 76
    for spinal cord compression, 120
Radon, lung cancer and, 44
Regorafenib, 40t
Renal cell carcinoma, 68-72
    therapeutic approaches in metastatic, 70t
Rituximab, 40t
ROS-1, lung cancer and, 46

S

Sarcoma, 112-114
Sargramostim, 42
Seminomas, 76
Sensitivity, of test, 28-30
Severe acute respiratory syndrome coronavirus 2 (SARS-CoV-2)
    cancer risk and, 26-28
Sexual dysfunction
    breast cancer and, 90
Signal transduction inhibitors, 38, 40t
Small cell lung carcinoma (SCLC), 44f-46f, 46
    treatment for, 52-54
Smoking
    bladder cancer and, 72
    lung cancer and, 44
Soft tissue sarcomas, 112
Solid tumors, 108-116
    cancer of unknown primary site, 114-116
    head and neck cancer, 108-110
    melanoma, 110-112
    sarcoma, 112-114
Solitary pulmonary nodule (SPN), 50-52
Sorafenib, 38, 40t
    for hepatocellular carcinoma, 62
Specificity, of test, 28-30
Squamous cell carcinomas
    of esophagus, 56
    of head and neck, 108
    of lung, 44-46, 44f-46f
Stem cell transplantation, 42
Sunitinib, 38
Superficial spreading melanoma (SSM), 110
Superior sulcus tumors, of lung, 48-50
Superior vena cava syndrome, cancer-associated, 120
Surgery
    for cancer, 32-34
    in metastatic renal cell carcinoma, 70
Survivorship, breast cancer and, 88-90
Systemic therapy, in metastatic renal cell carcinoma, 70, 70t

T

Tamoxifen
    for breast cancer, 40
Targeted therapy
    in cancer, 38, 40t
    in lung cancer, 54
Telomerase
    activation of, 4-8, 8f-12f
Testicular cancer, 76-78
Thrombosis
    cancer-associated, 118
Tobacco
    cancer risk and, 22, 26t
Topotecan, for small cell lung cancer, 52-54

R

辐射，癌症风险，29
放射治疗，35-37
    急性损伤，37
    迟发性损伤，37
    前列腺癌，77
    脊髓压迫症，121
氡，肺癌，45
瑞戈非尼，41t
肾细胞癌，69-73
    转移性肾细胞癌的治疗方法，71t
利妥昔单抗，41t
ROS-1，肺癌，47

S

肉瘤，113-115
沙格司亭，43
精原细胞瘤，77
敏感度，检查的敏感度，29-31
严重急性呼吸综合征冠状病毒2（SARS-CoV-2）
    癌症风险，27-29
性功能障碍
    乳腺癌，91
信号转导抑制剂，39，41t
小细胞肺癌（SCLC），45f-47f，47
    治疗，53-55
吸烟
    膀胱癌，73
    肺癌，45
软组织肉瘤，113
实体瘤，109-117
    原发部位不明的癌症，115-117
    头颈癌，109-111
    黑色素瘤，111-113
    肉瘤，113-115
孤立性肺结节（SPN），51-53
索拉非尼，39，41t
    肝细胞癌，63
特异性，检查的特异性，29-31
鳞状细胞癌
    食管，57
    头颈，109
    肺，45-47，45f-47f
干细胞移植，43
舒尼替尼，39
表面扩散性黑色素瘤（SSM），111
肺上沟瘤，49-51
上腔静脉综合征，癌症相关，121
手术
    癌症，33-35
    转移性肾细胞癌，71
幸存者，乳腺癌，89-91
系统治疗，转移性肾细胞癌，71，71t

T

他莫昔芬
    乳腺癌，41
靶向治疗
    癌症，39，41t
    肺癌，55
端粒酶
    激活，5-9，9f-13f
睾丸癌，77-79
血栓
    肿瘤相关，119
烟草
    癌症风险，23，27t
托泊替康，治疗小细胞肺癌，53-55

TP53 protein, 38
Transscrotal orchiectomy, in testicular cancer, 76-78
Transscrotal ultrasound, in testicular cancer, 76-78
Transurethral resection of bladder tumor (TURBT), 72
Trastuzumab, 32, 40t
    for esophageal cancer, 56
Triple-negative breast cancer, 88
Tubular breast cancer, 82-84
Tumor biomarker carbohydrate antigen 125 (CA 125), of ovarian cancer, 92
Tumor lysis syndrome, 124
Tumor suppressor genes, 14-16
Type 1 endometrial cancers, 96
Type 2 endometrial cancers, 96
Tyrosine kinase inhibitors, 38

U

Ultrasonography
    of ovarian cancer, 92
Urothelial carcinoma, of bladder (UCB), 72
Uterine cancer, 94-98, 96f

V

Vaginal cancer, 102
Vandetanib, 40t
Vascular endothelial growth factor (VEGF), 38, 40t
Vemurafenib, 40t
Venous thromboembolism
    cancer-associated, 118
    in pancreatic cancer, 58
Vincristine, 36t
Vomiting
    chemotherapy-induced, 42, 122-124, 124t
Vulvar cancer, 100-102

W

Warburg effect, 16-18
Wedge resections, in non-small cell lung cancer, 54
Weight loss, esophageal cancer and, 56

TP53蛋白，39
经阴囊睾丸切除术，治疗睾丸癌，77-79
阴囊超声，用于睾丸癌，77-79
经尿道膀胱肿瘤切除术（TURBT），73
曲妥珠单抗，33，41t
    食管癌，57
三阴性乳腺癌，89
管状乳腺癌，83-85
糖类抗原125（CA125），卵巢癌，93

肿瘤溶解综合征，125
抑癌基因，15-17
1型子宫内膜癌，97
2型子宫内膜癌，97
酪氨酸激酶抑制剂，39

U

超声
    卵巢癌，93
膀胱尿路上皮细胞癌（UCB），73
子宫癌，95-99，97f

V

阴道癌，103
凡德他尼，41t
血管内皮生长因子（VEGF），39，41t
维莫非尼，41t
静脉血栓栓塞
    肿瘤相关，119
    胰腺癌，59
长春新碱，37t
呕吐
    化疗诱发，43，123-125，125t
外阴癌，101-103

W

Warburg效应，17-19
楔形切除，见于非小细胞肺癌，55
体重减轻，食管癌，57